THE DOCTORS BOOK
OF

HOME REMEDIES®

for Seniors

An A-to-Z Guide to Staying Physically
Active, Mentally Sharp, and Disease-Free

By Doug Dollemore
and the Editors of

PREVENTION
HEALTH BOOKS *for* **SENIORS**™

Medical Advisor: W. Steven Pray, Ph.D., R.Ph.,
professor of nonprescription drug products
at Southwestern Oklahoma State University in Weatherford

Rodale Press, Inc.
Emmaus, Pennsylvania

"Waking Up Your Flex Life" text on page 376 is reprinted by permission from Clark, J., 1992, *Full Life Fitness* (Champaign, Ill.: Human Kinetics), 67, 76, 96, 97–98, 101–2, 103, 105.

Library of Congress Cataloging-in-Publication Data

Dollemore, Doug.
    The doctors book of home remedies for seniors : an A-to-Z guide to staying physically active, mentally sharp, and disease-free / by Doug Dollemore and the Editors of Prevention Health Books for Seniors.
        p.   cm.
    Includes index.
    ISBN 1–57954–011–2   hardcover
    1. Aged—Health and hygiene.   2. Self-care, Health.   3. Medicine, Popular.
I. Prevention Health Books for Seniors.   II. Title.   III. Title: Home remedies for seniors.
RA77.6.D653   1999
613'.0438—dc21   99–11451

Distributed to the book trade by St. Martin's Press

2 4 6 8 10 9 7 5 3 1   hardcover

Visit us on the Web at www.rodaleremedies.com or call us toll-free at (800) 848-4735

OUR PURPOSE

*"We inspire and enable people to improve
their lives and the world around them."*

About *Prevention* Health Books

The editors of *Prevention* Health Books are dedicated to providing you with authoritative, trustworthy, and innovative advice for a healthy active lifestyle. In all of our books, our goal is to keep you thoroughly informed about the latest breakthroughs in natural healing, medical research, alternative health, herbs, nutrition, fitness, and weight loss. We cut through the confusion of today's conflicting health reports to deliver clear, concise, and definitive health information that you can trust. And we explain in practical terms what each new breakthrough means to you, so you can take immediate, practical steps to improve your health and well-being.

Every recommendation in *Prevention* Health Books is based upon interviews with highly qualified health authorities, including medical doctors and practitioners of alternative medicine. In addition, we consult with the *Prevention* Health Books Board of Advisors to ensure that all of the health information is safe, practical, and up-to-date. *Prevention* Health Books are thoroughly factchecked for accuracy, and we make every effort to verify recommendations, dosages, and cautions.

The advice in this book will help keep you well-informed about your personal choices in health care—to help you lead a happier, healthier, and longer life.

Notice

This book is intended as a reference volume only, not as a medical manual. The information given here is designed to help you make informed decisions about your health. It is not intended as a substitute for any treatment that may have been prescribed by your doctor. If you are under treatment for any health problem, you should check with your doctor before trying any home remedies. If you are taking any medication, do not take any vitamin, mineral, herb, or other supplement without consulting with your doctor. If you suspect that you have a medical problem, we urge you to seek competent medical help.

The Doctors Book of Home Remedies for Seniors Staff

Editor: Stephen C. George
Contributing Editor: Edward Claflin
Author: Doug Dollemore
Contributing Writers: Alisa Bauman, Bill Doherty,
Bridget Doherty, Patricia Dooley,
Diane Gardiner Kozak, Jorden Matus,
Terry McManus, Tom Monte,
Bebe Raupe, Christine Seliga,
Nora Villagran
Art Director: Darlene Schneck
Cover and Interior Designer: Richard Kershner
Illustrators: Melanie Powell, Gwendolyn Wong
Assistant Research Manager: Anita C. Small
Lead Researcher: Jennifer L. Kaas
Editorial Researchers: Jennifer Abel, Adrien S. Drozdowski,
Carol J. Gilmore, Grete Haentjens,
Toby Hanlon, Bella Hebrew,
Patricia Iannelli, Terry Sutton Kravitz,
Paris Mihely-Muchanic, Elizabeth B. Price,
Jennifer P. Reimert, Jesse L. Reish,
Staci Ann Sander, Teresa A. Yeykal,
Nancy Zelko, Shea Zukowski
Copy Editors: Kathryn A. Cressman, Marilyn Hauptly
Layout Designer: Keith Biery
Assistant Studio Manager: Thomas P. Aczel
Manufacturing Coordinators: Brenda Miller, Jodi Schaffer,
Patrick T. Smith

PUBLISHER: Brian Carnahan
VICE PRESIDENT AND EDITORIAL DIRECTOR: Debora T. Yost
EDITORIAL DIRECTOR: Michael Ward
MARKETING DIRECTOR: Karen Arbegast
PRODUCT MARKETING MANAGER: Denyse Corelli
BOOK MANUFACTURING DIRECTOR: Helen Clogston
MANUFACTURING MANAGERS: Eileen Bauder, Mark Krahforst
RESEARCH MANAGER: Ann Gossy Yermish
COPY MANAGER: Lisa D. Andruscavage
PRODUCTION MANAGER: Robert V. Anderson Jr.
OFFICE MANAGER: Roberta Mulliner
OFFICE STAFF: Julie Kehs, Suzanne Lynch, Mary Lou Stephen

Foundation, in Valhalla, New York, and an expert on nutrition and cancer for the National Cancer Institute and the American Cancer Society

Maria A. Fiatarone Singh, M.D. Scientist I in the nutrition, exercise physiology, and sarcopenia laboratory at the Jean Mayer USDA Human Nutrition Research Center on Aging at Tufts University in Boston, associate professor at Tufts University School of Nutrition Science and Policy in Medford, Massachusetts, and professor of exercise and sports science and medicine at the School of Health Sciences at the University of Sydney in Australia

Yvonne S. Thornton, M.D. Associate clinical professor of obstetrics and gynecology at Columbia University College of Physicians and Surgeons in New York City and director of the perinatal diagnostic testing center at Morristown Memorial Hospital in New Jersey

Lila Amdurska Wallis, M.D., M.A.C.P. Clinical professor of medicine at Cornell University Medical College in New York City, past president of the American Medical Women's Association, founding president of the National Council on Women's Health, director of continuing medical education programs for physicians, and Master and Laureate of the American College of Physicians

Andrew T. Weil, M.D. Director of the program of integrative medicine and clinical professor of internal medicine at the University of Arizona College of Medicine in Tucson

E. Douglas Whitehead, M.D. Associate clinical professor of urology at Albert Einstein College of Medicine in the Bronx, associate attending physician in urology at Beth Israel Medical Center and co-founder and director of the Association for Male Sexual Dysfunction, both in New York City

Richard J. Wood, Ph.D. Laboratory chief of the mineral bioavailability laboratory at the Jean Mayer USDA Human Nutrition Research Center on Aging at Tufts University in Boston and associate professor at the Tufts University School of Nutrition Science and Policy in Medford, Massachusetts

Susan Zelitch Yanovski, M.D. Director of the obesity and eating disorders program in the division of digestive diseases and nutrition at the National Institute of Diabetes and Digestive and Kidney Diseases in Bethesda, Maryland

CONTENTS

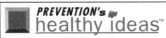

PREVENTION's
healthy ideas™

For the best interactive guide to healthy active
living, visit our Web site at **www.healthyideas.com**

INTRODUCTION

Beating the Little Big Things

Older Americans are bombarded with news about heart disease, stroke, cancer, and other catastrophic ailments. Yet these probably aren't the problems that you and your friends talk about when someone mentions aging.

You're concerned about the things you're facing now—the hundreds of little big things that make getting older so difficult. Things like arthritis, bunions, corns, calluses, memory loss, morning aches, shingles, dry mouth, hearing loss, and cold feet and hands. You're concerned about the things that nip away at self-reliance, independence, and self-confidence and threaten to make you feel older than your years.

For years, we've been listening to your concerns, through your letters to *Prevention* magazine and our research with our readership. And now we're here to help you with *The Doctors Book of Home Remedies for Seniors*. In the pages that follow, more than 350 doctors and other health care practitioners who specialize in the treatment of older Americans share tips and techniques that can help you care for yourself and remain robust for years to come.

Part one, "Help Yourself to Healthier Living," offers a five-step action plan to help you stay healthy and independent for life. You'll find tips to help you stay mentally sharp, eat well, get enough exercise, prevent accidents, and get the best possible care from your doctors.

Part two, "Home Remedies for Seniors," includes more than 1,500 doctor-recommended remedies that can help you prevent, relieve, and even self-treat more than 120 ailments that commonly affect older Americans. From aches and pains to varicose veins, you'll find the solutions to many of your most vexing health problems. For your convenience, each chapter has a special section called

"Try This First" that highlights the remedy doctors deem the simplest, safest, and most effective way to relieve a particular condition. Additional safe and effective remedies are listed under "Other Wise Ways." Many chapters in part two also offer advice about managing your medications.

From the first page to the last, *The Doctors Book of Home Remedies for Seniors* truly is a comprehensive guide to beating the little big things that make you feel older. But much more than that, we sincerely hope reading it will allow you to live well and bask in that time of life that famed choreographer Martha Graham called "the glory of years."

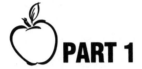**PART 1**

HELP YOURSELF TO HEALTHIER LIVING

CARE FOR YOUR HEALTH

Older Americans are healthier than ever before. Studies have found that as many as 89 percent of Americans ages 65 to 74 report having no serious disabilities. And nearly 40 percent of people over age 65 and 31 percent of those over age 85 rate their health as very good or excellent.

Certainly, medical breakthroughs have played a role in this encouraging trend. But the real driving force behind all of this is simple: Seniors are taking better care of themselves, says Harrison Bloom, M.D., vice chairman of clinical affairs in the department of geriatrics and adult development at Mount Sinai Medical Center in New York City. Older Americans smoke less, get more exercise, eat less fat, and are more apt to seek preventive care than seniors did 40 years ago.

As a result, the prevalence of emphysema, arthritis, arteriosclerosis (hardening of the arteries), stroke, and high blood pressure has dipped, and the average number of diseases afflicting a typical older person has plunged.

But even if you've smoked, drunk, and eaten too much and exercised far too little in the past few decades, there is still time to help yourself achieve healthy living in later life, Dr. Bloom points out. "It's nonsense to think that you're too old to begin living in more healthy ways," he declares. "It just makes sense to do everything you can to prevent as many ailments as possible as you get older."

In fact, preventive care, including getting regular screening tests and knowing how to manage your medications, is essential if you want to remain independent and self-reliant as you age, according to Dr. Bloom. Here are some basic preventive strategies that should help you achieve and maintain a healthy senior lifestyle.

Check Your Checkups

Certainly, what you can do for yourself at home is the core of good preventive care. But there also is much that you and your doctor can do in partnership to ensure that you will stay healthy for many years to come.

Get regular health examinations. In most instances, the annual head-to-toe physical is as arcane as the Studebaker, Dr. Bloom says. It's better to get regular health exams that are tailored to your age, lifestyle, and physical condition.

Cholesterol screening, for instance, isn't as accurate a gauge of heart attack risk in seniors as it is among younger people. So your doctor may forgo cholesterol screening after you are in your seventies unless you have a family history of heart disease. Other important optional tests for seniors, depending on health and medical history, include pap smears for women and digital rectal exams and prostate-specific antigen (PSA) blood screenings for men.

Get immunized. Everyone over 65 should have a flu shot each fall, Dr. Bloom says. At age 65, you should have a one-time immunization to prevent pneumonia. Every 10 years—at 55, 65, and 75, for instance—you should get a tetanus-diphtheria shot.

Get your blood pressure checked. Your blood pressure should be checked by a doctor or nurse at least once a year. High blood pressure (readings consistently above 140/90) is an important risk factor for stroke and heart disease.

Get screened for colon cancer. Each year, nearly 18,000 deaths from colon and rectal cancer could be prevented if all men and women over age 50 were screened for these diseases. Typically, this means having an annual stool test, an examination of the rectum and lower colon every 5 years, and a thorough examination of the entire colon every 10 years. If you have a family history of colorectal cancer, your doctor will likely want to screen you more often, Dr. Bloom suggests.

Get a complete skin inspection. Examine your skin at least once a month for suspicious-looking moles or sores that might be signs of skin cancer. Ask your doctor to do a thorough examination of your skin at least once a year.

Get out of the habit. About 23 percent of people over age 65 still smoke. If you're one of them, ask your doctor about new drug treatments that can help you quit. In addition, there are self-help smoking cessation programs that are tailored specifically for people over age 50.

Women, get regular breast exams. Women over 50 should have mammograms every one or two years to detect breast cancer, Dr. Bloom says.

Manage Your Medications

Americans over age 65 purchase 30 percent of all prescription drugs and 40 percent of all over-the-counter (OTC) drugs, according to the U.S. Food and Drug Administration. But arthritis, poor eyesight, and memory lapses can make it difficult for some seniors to take their medications properly, Dr. Bloom says. In fact, some studies suggest that between 40 and 75 percent of older adults don't take their medications at the right times or in the right amounts. Here are a few ways you can sidestep these problems.

Explore the alternatives. Ask your doctor if, instead of taking a medicine, you first can try a nondrug treatment such as diet, stress management, and exercise, Dr. Bloom suggests.

Learn all you can about the drug. Before you leave your doctor's office or pharmacy with a new prescription, make sure you fully understand how to take the drug properly, Dr. Bloom says. Ask the following questions.

- What is the name of the drug and what will it do?
- How often should I take it?
- How long should I take it?
- When should I take it? As needed? Before, with, after, or between meals? At bedtime?
- If I forget to take it, what should I do?
- What side effects might I expect? Should I report them?
- Will I need periodic blood or urine tests to monitor adverse effects?
- Is there any information about this drug that I can take home with me?

Follow directions. Always take the medicine in the exact amount and on the same schedule prescribed by your doctor. Make sure you're taking the right drug, says Dr. Bloom. To prevent mistakes, read the label every time you take the medication.

Tweak your memory. Set an alarm clock, carry a pillbox, or mark a calendar. Do whatever is necessary to remind yourself to take your medication.

Ask your pharmacist for a hand. Request an oversized, easy-to-open bottle, says W. Steven Pray, Ph.D., R.Ph., professor of non-prescription drug products at Southwestern Oklahoma State University in Weatherford. If the label is hard to read, ask the pharmacist to use large type.

Pitch the ancient wonders. Check expiration dates on your medicine bottles. Throw out any drugs that have expired.

Keep it to yourself. Never take drugs prescribed for another person or give your medication to someone else, Dr. Pray says.

Keep a daily record of all of the drugs you take. Include prescription and OTC drugs. Jot down the name of each drug, the doctor who prescribed it, the amount you take, and the times of day you take it, Dr. Pray suggests. Keep a copy in your medicine cabinet and one in your wallet or pocketbook so it can easily be found in an emergency.

Finish what you start. Even if you are feeling better, never stop taking a prescription medication without a doctor's consent, Dr. Bloom says. If you think the medication is causing a problem, consult your physician.

Recognize Side Effects

Drugs can do wondrous things. They can relieve pain, eliminate the need for surgery, and even keep you alive. But as you get older, your metabolism slows, so drugs stay in your system longer and are more apt to cause side effects, according to Dr. Bloom. In addition, taking two or more medications—as two-thirds of older Americans do each day—puts you at even greater risk of an adverse reaction.

Here's how Dr. Bloom and Dr. Pray say you can minimize the risks.

• Always tell your doctor about past problems that you've had with drugs, including rashes, drowsiness, insomnia, allergies, dehydration, faintness, diarrhea, or indigestion.

• Take a list of all your medicines—including OTC drugs—with you each time you visit your doctor. Ask your doctor if you can reduce any dosages or if you can safely stop taking any medication. If you have several physicians, make sure they all know what the others are prescribing, and ask your primary-care physician to coordinate your use of these medications.

• Keep alcohol out of the mix. Don't use alcohol when you are taking any medication unless your doctor says it's okay. Some drugs simply don't work as well or may make you ill or drowsy if taken with alcohol.

GET YOUR EXERCISE

G rab an unopened jar out of the cupboard and try to open it. It's a task that 92 percent of people ages 40 to 60 can do in an instant. But after age 60, unless you regularly engage in strength-building exercise, odds are that you won't be able to open it without some help.

Now sit in a living room chair, get up, and walk briskly into the kitchen as if something on the stove were burning. Then rush back into the living room and sit down again. Repeat this three times in rapid succession. If you're like three out of four people over 60 who don't get regular aerobic exercise, you're likely to feel out of breath after this effort.

Regular exercise makes the little chores of life possible after age 60. With it, even the little everyday tasks that normally wear you out can be easier to deal with—and can leave you with energy to spare. In fact, keeping active may be the most important thing an older person can do to stay healthy and self-reliant, says Walter M. Bortz II, M.D., former president of the American Geriatrics Society and clinical associate professor at the Stanford University School of Medicine.

And you don't have to run a marathon, take up windsurfing, or climb mountains to make your everyday life easier. Just a little bit of exercise can go a long way. Moderate exercise like bowling, golf, gardening, and walking can enhance your physical condition.

"It's never ever too late to start. The more exercise you can do in later life, the better off you will be," Dr. Bortz says.

Don't Take It Easy, Exercise

Regular exercise can slow or reverse many of the natural physical consequences we traditionally associate with aging, according to Dr. Bortz. Older people who are inactive, for instance, have less efficient hearts, weaker muscles, and diminished lung capacity compared to seniors who are constantly on the go. But what you may not know is that inactivity also makes it harder for your aging body to process sugars in the bloodstream. And as blood sugars rise, the chances of developing diabetes increase. Lack of regular exercise also accelerates bone loss in people over 60, he says.

"Humans were extremely active 4.5 million years ago," says Dr. Bortz, who studied with famed anthropologist Louis Leakey. "If you take a bone from a Neanderthal and pound it with a hammer, the hammer will break before the bone will. But if you take a modern human bone, you can break it with your hands. Why? Because we are less active."

But just 20 minutes of regular exercise every day can do wonders for your bones, heart, and lungs. It can help you feel more energetic and confident. Here's just a sampling of what exercise can do for you after age 60.

• Swimming, walking, and other aerobic activities raise your heart rate and can reduce stiffening of the arteries. Stiff arteries are a major cause of high blood pressure among seniors, which can lead to heart disease and stroke.

• Older Americans who are physically active are less likely to develop adult-onset diabetes and can control it better if they do have it. Exercise increases the body's ability to control blood sugar levels.

• Strength training can reduce arthritis pain. It doesn't cure arthritis, but stronger muscles lessen the strain on joints and, therefore, the pain.

• Walking and other modest exercise may be good for your mental health, according to the National Institute on Aging.

Stretch, Strengthen, and Build Stamina

Even if you have a few chronic illnesses like heart disease, arthritis, or diabetes, you can do almost any activity, including walking, bicycling, dancing, hiking, swimming, tennis, and working with weights, Dr. Bortz says. Ideally, any exercise program should include a mix of stretching, strength training, and aerobic activity. Begin with stretching and strength training, then add aerobics later. Aerobics are safer once you can maintain your balance and your muscles are stronger. Here are a few advantages of each of these basic activities.

Stretching increases blood flow and gets your body ready to exercise. It improves flexibility, relieves stress, and cuts the risk of injury and muscle strain. A regular stretching routine can help loosen up muscles in the neck, shoulders, back, chest, stomach, arms, thighs, and calves. Stretching should be done slowly and carefully before all types of exercise. Allow 5 to 10 minutes to stretch before and after you work out.

For a simple warmup, Dr. Bortz recommends these stretches. Do each stretch five times.

• Take a deep breath through your nose and exhale slowly through your mouth. Raise your shoulders when you breathe in. Exhale as you return your shoulders to the starting position.

• Extend your arms out to your sides so that they are parallel with the floor. Move your arms slowly in small one-foot circles, first clockwise and then counterclockwise.

• Turn your head slowly to the left side, come back to the center, and turn to the right side.

• Sitting in a chair, clasp your hands behind your left knee and raise it toward your chest. Repeat on the other side.

• Lift your left shoulder toward your left ear. Allow both arms to hang by your sides. Then release your left shoulder, using your muscles to lower it as far as you comfortably can. Repeat on the right side. Then, lift both shoulders at the same time, leaving both arms hanging at your sides. Stretch up and push down in the same way.

• While standing, raise your body up on the balls of your feet, then lower yourself.

• Stand or sit with your hands clasped behind your head. Turn your trunk slowly from side to side.

• Start with your arms at your sides. Lift both arms out to the sides and up over your head, then slowly lower them.

Strength training maintains bones, improves balance, and increases muscle strength. This can prevent or slow bone-weakening osteoporosis and lower the risk of hip fractures and other injuries caused by falls, says Maria A. Fiatarone Singh, M.D., associate professor of nutrition at Tufts University and a scientist at the Jean Mayer USDA Human Nutrition Research Center on Aging at Tufts in Boston.

Strengthening exercises can be done by lifting weights, using elastic resistance bands, or working out on machines. Good instructional materials are a must. Without information on the proper technique, you can get hurt. With proper advice, you can work your way up to many of the same weight-lifting routines that younger men and women use. Once you know what to do, you can do your routine at home using free weights or in a gym using machines.

MANAGING YOUR MEDS

If you have diabetes and use insulin, avoid injecting the insulin into an area that is going to be exercised, says W. Steven Pray, Ph.D., R.Ph., professor of nonprescription drug products at Southwestern Oklahoma State University in Weatherford.

Exercise will increase blood flow into the muscles around the tissues, causing the insulin to be absorbed faster than normal, and that could possibly trigger dangerous fluctuations in blood sugar. For instance, don't inject insulin into your leg before you go out jogging, says Dr. Pray.

In addition, avoid taking over-the-counter (OTC) cold medications containing decongestants like phenylpropanolamine or pseudoephedrine. These products could cause arrhythmias—irregular heartbeats—during exercise. They can cause fluctuations in blood sugar even when you do not exercise, so they should be avoided by all people with diabetes, says Dr. Pray. Phenylpropanolamine and pseudoephedrine are found in OTC products such as Sudafed, Dimetapp, and Contac.

If you are interested in lifting weights, it is important to start with a weight that you can lift all the way up using proper form with only a moderate amount of effort.

One- or five-pound dumbbells work well if you are a beginner, says Dr. Singh. If you have chosen a weight that is too heavy, you will be unable to lift it in proper form all the way up, so back off to a slightly lower weight until you find the correct one. Once you have selected the proper weights for your workout, here's how you can make strength training work for you, she says.

• Using no weight at all, practice the exercise you want to perform. Make sure you can perform it correctly without pain. Pay attention to the positioning of your arms, legs, and trunk because injuries usually occur from improper positioning or movements. You should not feel any pain during the exercise unless you have preexisting joint problems. If you do have joint problems, you initially may need to limit your range of motion to the pain-free zone of movement. This pain-free range will very likely improve during the course of strength training.

• Lift the weight eight times, rest for a minute, then do it again. This is two sets. You may either lift both arms or legs together, or alternate right and left arms and legs, depending upon the exercise and amount of time you have.

• Every couple of sessions, try to increase the weight you are lifting, until the effort feels like an 8 on a scale of 1 to 10. This should feel hard to very hard to lift, but you should be able to do it in proper form. As soon as you can complete a set of eight and it no longer feels hard, you should increase the weight you are using for that exercise.

• Allow one day of rest between the same exercises.

• Exercise each muscle group three days per week. If all you can manage is two days, that will work almost as well as long as you are progressing with the weight.

• Always breathe out during the lifting portion of any movement and breath in during the lowering phase. Never hold your breath during weight-lifting exercises. You may take a breath in and out during a rest between repetitions, if you need to.

• Perform repetitions slowly. Take about three seconds to lift the weight, hold for one or two seconds at the fully extended position, then take another three to five seconds to lower the weight. It is much better to do eight slow repetitions than 16 rapid ones.

Aerobic exercise, also known as endurance exercise, strengthens the heart and improves overall fitness by increasing the body's ability to use oxygen, Dr. Bortz says. Some high-impact aerobic workouts like jogging and jumping rope may not be your best choice after age 60, because they can be hard on muscles and joints. Here's a look at a few of the more common aerobic activities and why they are good for seniors.

• Walking is the simplest endurance activity that a person over 60 can do, according to Dr. Singh. It doesn't require any athletic prowess or special equipment except for comfortable shoes. It builds up muscle endurance, improves blood circulation, and can reduce spasms and stiffness in the back and leg muscles. Walking works out more muscles than many other aerobic activities, including bicycling. To increase the intensity of walking, you can avoid high-impact activity such as jogging by advancing to stair-

---

IS THIS WORKOUT RIGHT FOR YOU?

There are literally dozens of fun, energizing workouts any older person can do. Here are a few things to consider before you take up a new activity, says Walter M. Bortz II, M.D., former president of the American Geriatrics Society and clinical associate professor at the Stanford University School of Medicine.

• Is it enjoyable? The activity should be fun. If you just do it for the workout it gives you, you probably won't stick with it.
• Is it an activity you can easily fit into your daily schedule? Are facilities nearby? Is it something you can do alone or do you need a partner (tennis) or a group (line dancing)?
• Will the activity offer you a feeling of success and a feeling of increased vigor and strength? If it is a group activity, are the instructor and your fellow classmates compatible and friendly?

climbing (on real stairs, not on a machine), hiking, or power walking, or a combination of these activities.

• Bicycling is less stressful on the joints than walking, making it ideal for many older people, including those with diabetes who may have difficulty hiking or strolling. It can also be done indoors on a stationary bicycle, which is a good choice if you have balance problems, Dr. Singh says.

• Swimming is the ultimate gentle, low-impact endurance exercise, says Dr. Singh. If you have arthritis, swimming in warm water

PLAY IT SAFE

As Americans over 65 have become more active, the number of sports-related injuries in this age group has mushroomed, according to the U.S. Consumer Product Safety Commission in Washington, D.C. Approximately 53,000 are injured in sporting accidents each year—greater than 50 percent more than a decade ago. Bicycling, calisthenics and weight lifting, golfing, snow skiing, and fishing were the five most common injury-causing activities.

Here are seven ways you can prevent injuries when you are participating in activities, according to Maria A. Fiatarone Singh, M.D., associate professor of nutrition at Tufts University and a scientist at the Jean Mayer USDA Human Nutrition Research Center on Aging at Tufts in Boston.

• Always wear appropriate safety gear. If you bike, always wear a helmet. Wear the appropriate shoes for each sport. A podiatrist or a trained clerk at a local sports specialty shop may be able to give you footwear recommendations. If you have diabetes, hardening of the arteries, or any loss of sensation in your foot, you are at higher risk for foot injuries and ulcerations during repetitive impact activities such as walking.

• Warm up before you exercise. Slowly walk, stretch, swing your arms, or do the same exercise movement that you are about to do (such as pedaling on a bike without resistance) for a couple of minutes before you increase your pace or add resistance. What you are trying to do is increase the temperature of the muscle you are about to use, so the muscle is less likely to be torn or injured during the workout. Warming up also gradually increases your heart rate so that it does not suddenly jump to very high levels.

is a great way to relieve pain and maintain range of motion. To get aerobic benefit from swimming, you have to swim at a pace that raises your heart rate or add aerobic water exercises and equipment made to add resistance to the arm and leg movements in the water.

• Dancing, whether it is line dancing, square dancing, or ballroom dancing, is so much fun that it may be hard to think of it as exercise, Dr. Singh says. But dancing actually is a good aerobic workout that also can improve your sense of balance, coordination, and muscle endurance. Because it is a weight-bearing exercise that places some impact on bones and joints, it is a positive stimulus for

---

• Follow the 10 percent rule. Never increase your routine more than 10 percent a week. So if you walk a mile a day this week, for instance, walk no more than 1.1 miles a day next week.

• Try not to do the same routine two days in a row. You'll be less likely to injure overtaxed muscles and joints. If you lift weights today, take a walk or swim tomorrow.

• If you work out on exercise equipment like a rowing machine, be sure to read the instructions carefully before you start. If necessary, ask a qualified fitness instructor for help.

• Check treadmills and other exercise equipment before using them, to ensure that they are in good working order.

• Avoid exercising in extreme heat or humidity. When you do work out, make sure you drink enough fluids before and during exercise to prevent dehydration. Unless you are biking or running a marathon, one to two glasses of water or juice should be sufficient for most exercise sessions. Increase this amount if it is extremely hot or humid.

Be careful if you take diuretics or have just had a fever, vomiting, or diarrhea, as you may be starting from a dehydrated state and be more susceptible to heatstroke. Don't use caffeine-containing beverages or alcohol to replace fluids, as these drinks cause you to urinate. There is no need for special sports drinks. Although they are absorbed a little faster, their benefit is lost to all but high-level athletic performers.

bone formation, although it may not be tolerable for those with severe arthritis.

• The slow, mindful movements of tai chi, an ancient Chinese exercise technique performed while standing, enhance balance and body awareness, can increase your mobility, and can reduce your risk of falling, says Steven L. Wolf, Ph.D., professor of rehabilitation medicine at Emory University School of Medicine in Atlanta.

Get Off on the Right Foot

It may take a little effort to make exercise a part of your life. But once you start, your endurance, strength, and mood will probably skyrocket, and those are three of the most powerful motivations you can have for staying active, Dr. Bortz says. Here are a few pointers from him to get you started.

• A class can be good way to plunge into an activity, particularly if it's been a long time since you've exercised. A qualified teacher can help you learn to work out the right way.

• Go slow. It will take time for you to overcome years of inactivity. Set realistic goals such as "I'm going to take the stairs instead of the elevator this morning" or "I'm going to work out for 5 minutes today." Gradually, work your way up to 20 minutes of activity a day.

• If you feel like taking a 20-minute walk every day, great. But you don't have to get your 20 minutes of daily exercise all at once. Short bursts of activity like two 10-minute walks or four 5-minute swings around the dance floor also can contribute to your overall well-being.

• Wear loose-fitting clothing that breathes. Use layers of clothing to both keep you warm and help protect you from overheating by dispelling perspiration and heat.

• Wear athletic socks designed to absorb perspiration away from your feet. Be certain that your shoes fit and support your feet.

• Avoid working out so vigorously that you can't talk and exercise at the same time. Stop working out if you feel pain, become light-headed, or become short of breath.

BALANCE YOUR DIET

In mythology, ambrosia was the food of the Greek gods that conferred everlasting beauty and youth.

These days, there aren't a lot of Greek gods around. But a modern version of ambrosia—the promise of a robust and healthy lifestyle in your later years—isn't just a fable. It exists in the very foods you eat—that is, if you choose your foods wisely.

"It's very clear that a diet low in fat and cholesterol and high in fiber, fruits, and vegetables will reduce the incidence of heart disease and cancer and help an older person remain healthy," says Nancy Betts, R.D., Ph.D., associate professor of nutritional science and dietetics at the University of Nebraska in Lincoln. Here are a few ways you can become a savvy senior connoisseur.

Meet Your Basic Nutritional Needs

Variety is not only the spice of life, it is probably the best way to meet your nutritional needs as you age, according to Chris Rosenbloom, R.D., Ph.D., professor of nutrition at Georgia State University in Atlanta. Since no single food provides everything you need, the best meal-planning tactic is to include a mix of dairy products, whole grains, vegetables, and protein. Following is what dietary experts suggest that people over 50 try to include in their daily menus.

- Milk or cheese: 2 servings (1 serving is 1 cup of milk or yogurt or 2 ounces of processed cheese)
- Cereals and breads: 6 to 11 servings (1 serving equals 1 ounce of dry cereal, a slice of bread, or ½ cup of cooked brown rice)
- Fruits: 2 to 4 servings (1 serving is a medium-size apple, orange, or banana)

- Vegetables: 3 to 5 servings (1 serving equals 1 cup of raw leafy vegetables, ½ cup of cooked vegetables, or ½ cup of raw chopped vegetables)
- Protein: 2 to 3 servings of lean meat or poultry, eggs, nuts, or dried beans
- Water: 8 to 10 eight-ounce glasses. Water is an important part of the diet that is often overlooked by seniors, Dr. Rosenbloom says. People over 50 frequently have a diminished sense of thirst and don't realize they need water. Dehydration can develop gradually and is a serious problem. Drink a glass of water every couple of hours, especially after exertion.

Take Stock of Supplements

Getting enough of the more than 40 nutrients needed for good health can be more difficult as you age. Poor teeth or dentures can make chewing torturous. Shopping and cooking can be a challenge because of arthritis, walking problems, or a lack of transportation. Loneliness and depression can sharply diminish your appetite. But no matter what the cause, you still need adequate nutrients to lead an active lifestyle. For that reason, many seniors rely on vitamin and mineral supplements to make up for deficiencies in their diets.

But some seniors take too many supplements, says Mark E. Williams, M.D., director of the program on aging at the University of North Carolina at Chapel Hill School of Medicine and author of *The American Geriatrics Society's Complete Guide to Aging and Health*.

In one study, researchers found that 1 in 10 older men was consuming 10 times the recommended amounts of vitamins B-complex, C, D, and E. These researchers also found that 10 percent of women were getting 10 times more thiamin and iron than they needed.

Many seniors believe that these megadoses will prolong life, cure ailments, improve sexual performance, counteract stress, and boost their immunity. In reality, megadoses of vitamin and mineral supplements can have serious consequences, Dr. Williams says. Excess amounts of vitamin C, for instance, can spark kidney stones and gastrointestinal problems. Too much vitamin A can cause liver damage and disrupt your immune system. And megadoses of vitamin B_6 can damage nerves in your arms and legs. Too much vitamin E can make you more prone to bleeding.

So while supplements are important, it's also vital to not overdo them. Taking a multivitamin daily should fill most of the nutritional gaps in your diet, according to Dr. Rosenbloom.

Whetting Your Appetite

Eating can lose much of its appeal as you get older, simply because food doesn't seem to taste and smell as good as it once did, Dr. Rosenbloom says. Beginning at about age 60, your tastebuds lose much of their sensitivity and your nose doesn't detect mouthwatering aromas as well. In fact, you probably need 2½ times more flavor to make food taste as good as it did when you were in your twenties.

As food becomes less appealing, you're likely to eat less, lose weight, and be more prone to malnutrition, a problem that affects about one in four older Americans. Dr. Rosenbloom recommends these ways to boost your appetite and increase your enjoyment of food.

• Get more exercise, like walking or gardening. Regular physical activity can rekindle your appetite.

• Try new recipes and foods. Enliven familiar ones with crunch and color. Add orange slices to salads, for instance.

• When using vanilla or other extracts, double the amount called for in the recipe. It will enhance the flavor of the dish.

• Use bacon bits, grated Parmesan cheese, and butter-flavored sprinkles to enhance the taste of your food.

• Add fruit like crushed or chunked pineapple or sliced apples to meats while they cook. The fruit will add texture as well as flavor.

• Make a tasty sauce for meat or rice by cooking the nectar from juice-packed, canned peaches or apricots until it is reduced by half. Then thicken the sauce with a tablespoon of flour.

• Switch foods as you eat. Take two or three bites of a food, then try something else. Doing this will make all of the foods on your plate seem more flavorful and inviting.

• Combine foods with different temperatures—chilled cottage cheese and hot cooked pasta, for example—to create a variety of dining sensations.

• Take a drink—in moderation. Moderate amounts of alcohol can stimulate hunger. So if your physician approves, enjoy a 4-ounce glass of wine, a 12-ounce glass of beer, or 1½ ounces of distilled spirits before dining.

• Appearance counts. Use colorful plates and napkins—orange seems to spark hunger pangs best.

• Carry a small pocket alarm clock or electronic timer and set it to go off every three to four hours as a reminder to eat. Even if you only have a piece of bread, the alarm may tweak your appetite and help you establish regular mealtimes.

Dine Out Smart

A typical person over age 65 dines out more than two times a week and spends about $1,021 a year in restaurants. But often, these meals are laden with fat and are far less healthy for you than you might expect, Dr. Rosenbloom says. Here are some ways to choose wisely when you're eating out.

• Eat something before you go. The worst thing you can do is go to a restaurant absolutely starved. You'll be so hungry that you won't make wise food choices. So have a banana, three graham crackers, or another light snack to pacify your stomach before you dine out.

• If you eat at a restaurant frequently, ask for a copy of the menu to take home with you. That way you can plan your food choices wisely and feel less tempted to order less healthy options. At fast-food restaurants, where many foods are 40 to 55 percent fat, try salads, plain hamburgers, or grilled chicken, or ask for a copy of their nutritional information so you can make wiser selections.

• Ask your server to bring a doggie bag when your meal is served. Before you take your first bite, you can cut the meal in half and put half in the bag to take home. You'll have a meal for the next day and you'll slash the amount of fat and calories in each serving.

• Split a meal with a friend. Ask your server if you can order soup or salad à la carte with one entrée. It will save you money and reduce the fat in each meal.

PREVENT ACCIDENTS

A ccidents are constantly on the prowl. They lurk in a loose throw rug waiting for someone to slip or in a stray telephone cord looking for someone to trip. They roam the highways hoping to transform a missed turn signal or blown stop sign into a smashup worthy of the 10 o'clock news. Or at least it can seem that way.

No, accidents aren't out to get you. But they seldom "just happen," either, and many can be prevented.

In fact, accidents of all kinds become more common as people reach their sixties, seventies, and eighties, says Jan I. Maby, D.O., director of the Geriatric Medical Home Care program at Mount Sinai Medical Center in New York City. As you get older, it becomes a little bit harder for you to hit the brakes quickly or stop yourself from falling.

Preventing accidents will take a bit more foresight than it did when you were younger. But you can do it. Here's how.

Stay Safe in the Driver's Seat

Driving is freedom. Driving is self-reliance. Driving is the American way. But driving is also one of the most dangerous activities an older person does, Dr. Maby says.

Traffic accidents injure 139,000 and kill more than 7,600 Americans over age 65 each year, according to the National Safety Council. Crashes are the leading cause of accidental deaths among people 65 to 74 and the second most common cause of these deaths (falls are first) after age 75.

In fact, for every mile behind the wheel, a typical 75-year-old is four times more likely to be involved in a fatal traffic accident than other American drivers.

But there's no reason that you can't be among the safest of the 24.8 million drivers over 65 who are still on the road, says Michael Seaton, manager of the American Association of Retired Persons (AARP) 55 ALIVE/Mature Driving program in Washington, D.C. Here are a few reminders that, he says, can help you safely get where you are going.

• The driver's seat is hardly the best place for you to daydream. Don't drive when you're upset, depressed, angry, drowsy, or not feeling well.

• Back pain, neck pain, and arthritis all can contribute to fatigue, which can make you less safety conscious. When traveling, take frequent breaks to stretch and walk around.

• Medium-size cars may be better for older drivers. In smaller cars, the drivers sit lower and can't see out of the vehicle as well. Power steering and brakes, automatic transmission, and adjustable seats and steering wheel can all cut driver fatigue.

• Wear your seat belt. When used, lap and shoulder safety belts slash the risk of serious injury or death nearly in half, according to the National Highway Traffic Safety Administration, an agency of the U.S. Department of Transportation in Washington, D.C.

• Keep a three-second safety cushion between you and the car in front of you. As you're driving along, notice a tree or other stationary object along the roadside. Once the rear of the car ahead passes the object, you should be able to count "one-thousand one, one-thousand two, one-thousand three" before reaching the same point.

• Plan your route before you start out. You need to concentrate on driving rather than on navigating. If you're headed someplace unfamiliar, ask a passenger to navigate for you.

• Watch out for left turns. Seventeen percent of accidents among older drivers involve left-hand turns, compared to 11 percent among younger drivers. To avoid a left turn at a traffic light, go a block beyond your turn, then turn right around the block until you cross the intersection. For safety's sake, you will be making three right turns instead of one left turn.

• If you will be taking an unfamiliar route at night, try to make a trial run in daylight.

• Look down the road far enough ahead to get a big picture of what's ahead. Heed what passengers are saying. They may spot a problem before you do.

• Check your mirrors frequently. There is a tendency to focus on what's going on ahead of us. Traffic, however, comes from all directions.

ARE YOU SAFE AT ANY SPEED?

Honest responses to the following questions, prepared by the American Association of Retired Persons (AARP), could help you make a decision about whether you should continue driving or become a passenger.

• Have you had a citation for a moving violation, a warning from a police officer, or more than one minor accident or near miss in the past two years?

• Do you ever have trouble making left-hand turns across traffic?

• Do you have trouble following directions from one place to another? Or have you gotten lost for no apparent reason while driving in a familiar area?

• During the past two years, have you occasionally missed a red light or stop sign?

• During the past year, have passengers in your car told you that your driving sometimes makes them nervous?

• Do you take antianxiety or antidepressant drugs, painkillers, sleeping pills, or antihistamines?

• Do you suffer chronic pain in your lower body, particularly in your back or feet?

• During the past year, have you experienced brief numbness, loss of function on one side of your body, or slurred speech?

• Do you have any known medical problems, particularly heart disease, diabetes, Parkinson's disease, or epilepsy?

• Do you have trouble seeing at night? Do the roads seem darker, or do oncoming headlights seem brighter and more blinding?

If you answer "yes" to any of these questions, you should have a talk with your doctor about these problems and perhaps take steps to modify your driving behavior.

Fall-Proofing the World around You

About 40 percent of people over age 65 fall each year. In most cases, these falls just cause minor bruises, scrapes, and a bit of embarrassment. But up to 1 in 10 falls among seniors leads to broken bones and other serious injuries that can result in permanent disability, social isolation, and the loss of the ability to live independently, Dr. Maby says. Falls are the second leading cause of all accidental deaths in the United States and the leading cause of accidental death in people over age 75.

Even if a fall doesn't cause serious harm, it can shatter your self-confidence, according to Dr. Maby. In fact, up to 25 percent of seniors who have fallen report that they avoid certain daily tasks like shopping or housekeeping, because they fear falling again. Ironically, without these activities, muscle and bone can gradually weaken and you can actually become more prone to falling.

Another reason that falls become more likely as you age is that your sense of balance declines and your reaction time slows. Arthritis, cataracts, and other diseases that affect your ability to see, hear, or move also can make you more susceptible to falls, Dr. Maby says. In addition, sedatives, diuretics, high blood pressure medication, and other drugs can make you feel wobbly.

Since three out of every four falls involving seniors occur at home, Dr. Maby offers some suggestions to reduce the risk of taking a tumble there.

Throughout the House

• Avoid wearing open-backed shoes or sandals, which make you shuffle and make it difficult to maneuver, especially on stairs.

• Keep telephone and electrical cords tucked out of the way so you won't trip on them. If possible, tack them up over doorways.

• Make sure your home is lit brightly enough that there are no shadowy areas and you can always see where you are going.

• Place night-lights throughout the house, especially on stairways and along the route you take from the bedroom to the bathroom. Install illuminated light switches in the area that you frequently use at night.

• Get rid of all throw rugs in your home. They're a major cause of household falls.

• Remove any clutter, including excess furniture that could cause a fall.

• When you are sitting, keep a telephone within arm's reach so if it rings, you won't have to rush across the room. A cordless phone may be your best bet because you can carry it with you from room to room.

• As you walk through your home, evaluate the furniture you lean on for support. Avoid putting weight on pedestal tables, items on wheels, or other furniture that cannot withstand much weight.

Kitchen

• Use a step stool if you need something that's on a high shelf, or consider moving items to a lower shelf where you can reach them easier.

• Clean up all spills as soon as possible to prevent slipping.

• Stay off freshly waxed floors until they are thoroughly dry.

Bathroom

• Install nonskid strips or use a rubber mat on the floor of the tub and shower.

• Install grab bars beside the toilet and around the bathtub to help balance yourself. Avoid using towel bars for support. They simply aren't designed to withstand heavy pressure.

• Use nonskid mats, adhesive nonskid strips, or carpet in areas that may get wet.

• If you have difficulty getting in and out of the bathtub, consider installing a shower seat and a portable, hand-held showerhead to let you sit while showering.

Bedroom

• Place a light source within easy reach of your bed. A flashlight may be helpful.

• If you like to wear long pajamas or a nightgown, make sure your sleepwear is short enough that you won't trip over it.

• Be sure to have a telephone that you can reach from your bed without having to scramble for it in the dark.

Stairways

• Install handrails on both sides of all stairs.

• If possible, apply brightly colored tape on the top and bottom steps so it's easier for you to see where the steps begin and end.

• Install nonskid strips on all steps.

• Make sure all carpet edges are tacked down securely.

• Put light switches at both the top and bottom of the stairwell.

Outside the Home

• Wear low-heeled, rubber-soled shoes to prevent slips and falls.

• Use a cane or walking stick to keep your balance on uneven or unfamiliar ground. Be especially wary on wet or icy pavement.

• Like medication, assistance devices come in various forms and sizes. Never use a friend's cane. An improperly issued assistance device can do more harm than good. Although you can purchase such equipment without a prescription, see a physiatrist or trained primary-care physician for proper sizing and instruction.

• Remove loose rocks, boards, and other tripping hazards from your yard and walkways. Fill in any holes in your lawn. Put away gardening tools and hoses when they're not in use.

• Make sure your walkways are shoveled and cleared of ice and snow in the winter to prevent slips and falls. If possible, use salt or an ice-melting product to keep surfaces clear of slippery ice.

Fire-Proof Your House

Americans over age 65 account for one in four fire-related deaths each year. In fact, people over age 65 are twice as likely to die in fires as any other age group, says Sharon Gamache, executive director of the National Fire Protection Association's Center for High Risk Outreach in Quincy, Massachusetts.

But seniors can do plenty to prevent household fires and survive one if disaster strikes, Gamache says. Here are a few pointers.

• Install smoke alarms outside all sleeping areas on each floor of your home, including basements and bedrooms. If you have hearing problems, get smoke alarms that are specially designed for people with severe hearing impairments. These trigger a strobe light or sound with an extra-loud alarm.

• Test your smoke alarm once a month by pushing the test button. Change batteries on the same days each year that you change your clocks and whenever the detector is "chirping" or signaling in some other way to indicate that the battery is low.

• Plan two escape routes out of each room. If a fire starts, smoke or flames may block your primary way out, forcing you to use an alternate escape route.

• Windows should open fully and easily to allow you to escape. Make sure there is no furniture or clutter in the way that might obstruct your exit. If you have security bars on your windows, they should be equipped with quick-release devices that every person in your house can operate.

• If you have difficulty using stairways, sleep on the first floor. Never use elevators during a fire.

• If you live in an apartment building, count the number of doorways between your apartment and the two nearest exits.

• Keep portable space heaters at least three feet from everything—including you. Just brushing up against one could set your clothing on fire.

• If you smoke, use large, deep nontip ashtrays. Empty your ashtrays often, wetting the contents before dumping them into wastebaskets. Never smoke in bed.

• Sleeping with your bedroom door closed will provide you with extra minutes of protection from smoke, toxic fumes, and fire. (If you do sleep with the door closed, make sure you can hear the smoke alarms from inside your room.) For added protection, install a smoke alarm in your room.

• Never leave cooking unattended. Use oven mitts and wear tight-fitting, short-sleeved shirts or rolled-up sleeves when you cook.

• Use a timer to remind you to turn off stove burners and the oven.

• Don't cook if you've been drinking alcohol or are taking medication that makes you drowsy.

STAY MENTALLY SHARP

Y ou can teach an old dog new wits.

In fact, with patience and perseverance, a typical person over 60 can maintain and possibly even improve his mental sharpness, says Michael Chafetz, Ph.D., clinical psychologist in New Orleans and author of *Smart for Life*.

"The brain is pliable at any age. It just slows down a little bit as you get older," Dr. Chafetz says. "But research shows that you can stimulate blood flow to the areas of the brain that are responsible for certain functions like mental calculations, language, learning, and memory, just by exercising your mind." To make the most of your mind's potential, you need to challenge it, stay socially active, and believe in yourself. Here's a closer look at these three mind-building tools.

Seek Out Challenges

Even at age 60, 70, or 80, the brain is a work in progress. It needs constant stimulation to stay mentally sharp. That's why challenging activities are your brain's best friends. In fact, the more you can keep your brain doing things—reading, writing, traveling, learning new information—the more resistant your brain will be to the effects of aging, Dr. Chafetz says. Here's what he suggests to keep your mind challenged.

• Turn off the television. TV really is mindless. Researchers at Kansas State University in Manhattan found that people who watched just 15 minutes of television had diminished brain-wave activity, an indication that their minds were turning off.

• Flip open the nearest book. Reading is a time-tested brain booster that helps improve language skills while keeping your memory strong.

• Turn your head into a calculator. Your brain will stay sharper if you trust it to add, subtract, and multiply.

• Anytime you pick up a pen instead of the telephone, you help keep your mind sharp. Writing clarifies thoughts, improves logic, and strengthens memory. Take a few minutes to write at least one letter a week to a friend or relative. Or write a letter to the editor or a note to a manufacturer, evaluating a product you recently bought.

• Take part in civilized debate. Debate is a terrific way to strengthen your logic, particularly if you can practice arguing both sides of an issue. For fun, ask a friend to debate a controversial issue like Medicare reform with you. Each of you can take a few minutes to jot down 10 statements supporting or opposing the issue. Swap lists and take turns trying to find logical gaps in the other person's argument.

• Tongue twisters not only improve speech but also help improve concentration by exercising circuits between brain cells. At least once a day, take a minute to practice your favorite tongue twister. Try saying this one five times in a row: Fresh fried fish don't flip like fresh fish flip.

• Puns and other types of humor spark creativity and encourage your mind to look at problems in new ways. Take a moment to really think about words you hear, and then see what odd twists you can come up with. For example, dumbbell—a bell that's not too bright.

• Clip funny cartoons, photos, and stories from newspapers and magazines and put them up in a "humor gallery" in your home. Whether you're making your own humor or enjoying someone else's, you need to look at the world from odd angles. This change in perspective will help keep your mind active.

• Doing crosswords and other puzzles creates new pathways in the brain, literally exercising the brain cells involved in word retrieval, vocabulary, and comprehension.

• Put a new twist on old games. When playing Scrabble, for example, require that each word have a minimum number of letters. When doing a jigsaw puzzle, try turning over all the pieces and then put it all together from the blank side. These added challenges will stimulate your imagination, focus your concentration, and put your logic skills to the test.

• Take up an instrument. Playing music brings an enormous number of skills into play, from improving coordination and concentration to fostering your creative instincts. Just playing an instrument for 10 to 15 minutes a day can give your brain a good workout.

• Allow yourself to shift gears. If your favorite hobby seems a bit stale, your mind may be getting weary, too. So try something new. If you tire of woodworking, why not try sculpting with clay? Certainly, different hobbies require different skills, but you need to be open to change if you want to stay mentally sharp.

• Sharing your accumulated lifelong learning with others is a tremendous challenge and great for the mind. Many community centers and civic organizations are eager for volunteers who can teach hobbies, languages, or other skills.

Dare to Connect

Loneliness kills. In fact, compared to those with strong social networks, older Americans who have few relationships are at two to four times greater risk of premature death, regardless of weight, alcohol use, and other lifestyle factors, says Robert L. Kahn, Ph.D., professor emeritus of psychology and public health at the University of Michigan in Ann Arbor and co-author of *Successful Aging*.

"The impact of social isolation on mortality is even stronger than cigarette smoking," Dr. Kahn says. "Talking, touching, and relating to each other is essential to our well-being. The bottom line is that we do not outgrow our need for others."

A typical American, regardless of age, has a personal network that includes 8 to 11 close friends or relatives. Certainly, there are losses as you age—mainly through death, changes in residence, and retirement. But most of these lost relationships are replaced by others. In fact, filling the social gaps in your life is vital for healthy aging, according to Dr. Kahn.

Older Americans who get strong emotional support—expressions of affection, respect, liking, and encouragement—from their circles of friends are more physically active and mentally alert, he explains. Intimacy appears to lower the risk of arthritis, depression, and alcoholism among people over 60. And people—including seniors—who say that they have strong social support also need less pain medication after surgery, recover faster, and follow their doctors' orders more faithfully. Here are a few things that Dr. Kahn suggests to widen your social circle.

• Dive into your community. Help out at your local library. Tutor at an elementary school. Volunteering is an excellent way to meet interesting people.

• Get a part-time job. Even if you don't need the money, the social contacts that you'll make with your co-workers can be priceless.

• Hang out in places where you are likely to meet people who share your interests. Churches, museums, flea markets, and bookstores are good starting points.

• Accept every invitation you can to social events like parties, graduations, and weddings.

• At a party, recreation center, or other gathering, make a conscious effort to meet new people. After you introduce yourself to someone, try to keep the conversation focused on that person's interests. You'll probably make a new friend.

• Pamper a pet. Caring for dogs, cats, and other pets has been shown to help many older people live longer, and animals are an instant icebreaker among strangers.

• If you have difficulty getting out, call your local geriatric social service agency or area agency on aging and ask for a list of others who are interested in developing a network of phone pals. If the organizations in your area haven't started such a list, volunteer your services to get one going.

Believe in Yourself

Self-doubt can erode your sense of independence. "If you're feeling insecure and incapable of coping effectively in the world, I think it really will begin to adversely affect your mind and body," says Elizabeth R. Mackenzie, Ph.D, director of the Wellness, Healing, and Ongoing Learning for Elders (WHOLE) program at the University of Pennsylvania Health System in Philadelphia. WHOLE is designed to include exercise and fitness programs, gardening projects, arts and music therapy, and education classes aimed at promoting health, boosting self-worth, and helping seniors stay connected to the world around them.

Believing in yourself and feeling that you can successfully do things is vital to staying mentally sharp, Dr. Kahn says. Seniors who have a strong sense of self-efficacy—a can-do approach to tasks or challenges—are more likely to view memory as something that can be learned and improved. The belief that memory is controllable encourages them to make an effort to do things like playing mental exercises and games that strengthen recall. Without this sense of self-efficacy, you may accept memory loss as a normal part of aging and let memories slip away without a fight, he says.

But there are plenty of ways that you can restore your self-confidence and regain your motivation to keep your mind sharp as you age, explains Dr. Mackenzie. Here's how.

• Take an adult education class. Whether the subject is French, calligraphy, or dancing, the classroom is a great place to learn new skills that will boost your self-confidence and improve your memory. Plus, classes are a wonderful way to meet new people.

• Involve yourself in activities that include people of all ages. Join a hiking club, become a foster grandparent, or participate in a public-speaking group like Toastmasters. You'll probably discover that not only do you have wisdom to share but also you can still do some things as well as or even better than younger people.

• Do at least one new thing a month. Go to a museum, attend a lecture at a local college, eat at a new restaurant, or walk through a different neighborhood. The bottom line is that monotony destroys optimism and ultimately undermines your mental health.

• Spend a moment each day to take a fresh look at something in nature and marvel at it. Observing nature will help you get in touch with your spirituality—reminding you that you are part of a larger whole—and can spark hope for your future.

• Meditation, contemplation, or prayer can help you cleanse out of your body anxiety, hopelessness, depression, and other negative emotions associated with disease.

• Keep a journal and every day write down at least 20 wonderful things that happen to you. Even small things, such as finding a dollar under the sofa, count. Doing this regularly will help you feel more positive about yourself and life in general. This, in turn, will make you more likely to take on new challenges, keeping your brain active.

• Adopt a plant. Houseplants make people feel calmer, more optimistic, and more self-assured. So starting a garden or tending to a houseplant may help you forget problems, boost your self-worth, and improve your health.

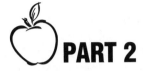 **PART 2**

HOME
REMEDIES
FOR SENIORS

ACHES AND PAINS

Between arthritis and the hard-knock experiences of a life well-lived, aches and pains seem to be an inevitable part of aging. But they're not.

In fact, everyday aches and pains in your joints aren't necessarily due to arthritis. Sometimes, pain can simply occur from an afternoon of really brisk walking or a morning spent out in the garden. Those are the pains that you can alleviate or easily prevent.

First, you have to know your trouble zones. Men and women over 60 tend to be most prone to pain in the lower joints—the hips, knees, ankles, and feet—according to Dale L. Anderson, M.D., coordinator of the Minnesota Act Now Project in Minneapolis and author of *Muscle Pain Relief in 90 Seconds*. These are the areas that you'll especially want to protect and pamper.

If you have occasional joint pain and inflammation, you can do a number of things to feel better and prevent them from returning. If your pain frequently returns, it could be the result of arthritis.

Try This First

Make it right with RICE. If you have joint pain, then RICE might be the answer, says William Pesanelli, a physical therapist and director of Boston University's rehabilitation services. In this case, we're not talking about Uncle Ben's latest concoction. RICE is an easy way to remember the pain-relieving sequence of rest, ice, compression, and elevation.

1. Until you notice that the pain has decreased, rest the affected area and avoid the activity that caused the pain, Pesanelli says.

2. Put ice on the injured area to help narrow the blood vessels and limit swelling. Keith Jones, trainer for the Houston Rockets

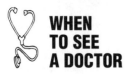

WHEN TO SEE A DOCTOR

Everyday minor aches and pains are just a part of life for most people. But if the aches and pains in your joints worsen after three or four days or if you have pain that doesn't subside at all after proper rest and other home remedies, then it's time to see a doctor, says David Richards, M.D., orthopedic surgeon at the Lexington Clinic Sports Medicine Center in Lexington, Kentucky.

basketball team, recommends applying ice wrapped in a towel or cloth to the area at least three times per day for 20 minutes.

3. Use compression, which means wrapping an elastic bandage, such as an ACE bandage, around the injured area to help limit the swelling and to allow you to resume your everyday activities, recommends Pesanelli. However, remove the bandage at once if the area below the bandage feels numb or tingles like it is falling asleep, if it changes color, or if it feels cooler than the rest of your body. Wait for those symptoms to subside and then rewrap it more loosely.

4. Elevate the affected area above the level of your heart. This will prevent blood and other fluids from collecting at the injury, thereby reducing the swelling, says Pesanelli. If you have a history of impaired circulation in the injured area, however, skip the elevation step because limiting blood flow to an area of the body with impaired circulation can be dangerous, says Dr. Anderson.

Other Wise Ways

Mix RICE with peas. An ice pack is good, but frozen peas are better, at least when it comes to icing a sore joint, says Pesanelli. A bag of frozen peas won't leak the way some ice packs do, he points out. "And because the peas are so small, you're able to bend the package to conform to the painful area, whether it's your shoulder or your kneecap." He suggests applying the bag of peas wrapped in a thin towel every couple of hours as part of the RICE sequence.

After you've used the peas once, you can just toss them back in the freezer compartment, get them iced, and use the same bag again. But since bacteria can quickly multiply in food that has been thawed and refrozen, make sure to clearly label the bag so that you don't accidentally try to serve the peas for dinner.

Lose some weight. "If people lose 5 to 10 pounds, it considerably lightens the load on all of their lower joints—hips, knees, ankles, and feet," according to Dr. Anderson. "One of the main causes of these joint-related pains is that people are simply overweight. They're carrying a Mack truck frame on Volkswagen tires, and eventually their joints wear out from the stress."

Alter your walking style. If your ankles, feet, or knees are aching, you may be walking too hard. Hard walkers suffer from more aches and pains in their feet, ankles, and knees because their heels strike the ground with greater force than soft walkers' do, says Dr. Anderson. But he points out that it's never too late to alter your walking style.

Just try this exercise: Imagine that you're a puppet with threads lifting you up at the head and shoulders. Visualize yourself lightening up and walking on a layer of air, with your feet gliding as though on imaginary ice skates.

Shoe away the pain. If you do a lot of walking, boot out any hard leather-soled shoes or high heels that are in your closet, recom-

MANAGING YOUR MEDS

Taking 600 milligrams of a nonsteroidal anti-inflammatory drug (NSAID), such as ibuprofen or aspirin, four times per day for a week to 10 days should help ease inflammation pain in your joints.

But if you have certain pre-existing abdominal conditions, these medications can make them worse, says David Richards, M.D., orthopedic surgeon at the Lexington Clinic Sports Medicine Center in Lexington, Kentucky. Ask your doctor for another kind of pain relief if you've been previously diagnosed with ulcers or any inflamed bowel disorder. And of course, you never want to take aspirin if you know you're allergic to it.

mends Dr. Anderson. "Opt instead for a shoe with a cushioned sole and heel and proper arch supports to save some wear and tear on your legs, ankles, feet, and hips."

Stand up straight. It turns out that your mom—or your drill sergeant—was right all those years ago when she told you to stand tall like a soldier. Stand up straight, push your shoulders back, arch your back slightly, and keep your chest out when sitting and walking. If you walk with your shoulders slouched, your chin forward, and your back rounded, it can lead to back, shoulder, or neck pain.

Stay active. To prevent joint aches and pains, get yourself on an exercise program, says Pesanelli. Joint surfaces naturally wear down over time, and this is complicated by the fact that your body usually produces less lubricating fluid as you get older. Since movement helps get vital nutrients into your joints, you can keep the joints better lubricated if you keep them warm and moving, he adds.

Pesanelli suggests a thorough warm-up routine with plenty of gentle stretching, followed by low-impact activities such as brisk walking or lap swimming for at least 20 minutes at a time three or four times per week. This is a sound form of exercise for seniors, he says, not only to keep your joints in good shape but also to keep your heart and lungs in working order. Just be sure to check with your physician before you begin an exercise regimen.

AGE SPOTS

A ge spots are not caused by age, nor are they a sign of aging. "Age spots are caused by overexposure to sunlight," says Debra Price, M.D., dermatologist and clinical assistant professor at the University of Miami's department of dermatology.

When continuously assaulted by the sun's ultraviolet (UV) rays, the skin protects itself by stepping up production of a chemical hormone called melanin. Melanin makes the skin more pigmented, or darker, which blocks the dangerous UV light from penetrating too deeply into the vulnerable cells below the skin's tough, outer surface. Unlike a suntan, however, age spots don't fade away naturally.

Try This First

Screen your skin. Since exposure to sunlight is the primary cause of both age spots and melanomas, you need to get away from those damaging rays.

"Your first and most important line of therapy is to use a broad spectrum sunblock every day," says Seth L. Matarasso, M.D., associate clinical professor of dermatology at the University of California School of Medicine in San Francisco. "Sunblock not only will protect you against future spots but also it can lighten existing ones by preventing the sun from darkening them the same way it would the rest of your skin. This reduces the color contrast between your skin and the age spots."

Your sunscreen should have a sun protection factor (SPF) of at least 15, dermatologists advise. Anything less will allow too many UV rays to penetrate.

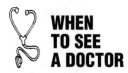

WHEN TO SEE A DOCTOR

Have any suspicious-looking spots checked by your dermatologist, says David Margolis, M.D., assistant professor of dermatology at the University of Pennsylvania in Philadelphia. You want to be sure that the spot isn't a melanoma, a potentially life-threatening form of cancer. That advice is especially important if the spot suddenly changes shape, becomes raised, or starts to bleed.

Other Wise Ways

Try fading them away. Lightly pigmented spots can often be made even lighter, or sometimes removed, by bleaching preparations—what many people refer to as fade creams. Such products, which typically contain hydroquinone, interfere with your skin's production of melanin. For many, hydroquinone can lighten spots to the point that they are either barely visible or easily hidden with a small amount of makeup, says Dr. Price.

Hydroquinone may irritate sensitive skin, so apply it to a small area beneath your chin the first day to see what reaction, if any, you might have. If you notice signs of redness, itching, or irritation, stop using it and contact your physician, she says.

Raze them from the surface. Exfoliating agents containing alpha hydroxy acid (AHA) can loosen and remove darkened dead cells at the surface of your skin and promote the growth of new flesh-colored tissue. The most widely used AHA is glycolic acid, says Dr. Matarasso. It works for many people who have light brown spots.

Still, be careful when you apply such products. Even more than hydroquinone, glycolic acid can be irritating to sensitive skin. Start out by applying the exfoliant to a small area beneath your chin or some other less visible part of your neck or face. Wait a day to see if there is any sign of irritation or redness. If not, apply the lotion to your entire face, keeping it an inch or so away from your eyes. Very often, the lotion causes tingling of the skin that passes away within minutes, says Dr. Matarasso. Once it dries, apply a moisturizer and then a sunscreen with a moisturizing base.

Color them away. People often use AHAs for about two months before they see significant results. Some doctors recommend that while you are waiting for the glycolic acid to work, you can cover up the spots with a heavy foundation, such as Dermablend. They are available at many department stores. Salespeople can help you find the right shade to match your skin color.

ANEMIA

You expect to slow down a little as you grow older, but if you're feeling overly tired, maybe even dizzy or breathless, the cause may be more than natural aging. It could be anemia.

A disorder that your doctor can detect with a single blood test, anemia most often results from a shortage of the red pigment in your blood known as hemoglobin. This red pigment helps your red blood cells carry oxygen to your body. If you don't have enough hemoglobin, your body tissues don't get enough oxygen. Without enough oxygen, your body reacts in a number of ways: In addition to the symptoms mentioned above, anemia can produce chest pain and rapid heart beat.

While anemia isn't just an older person's problem, you are at greater risk if you're over 60, says Paul E. Stander, M.D., medical director of the Good Samaritan Regional Medical Center in Phoenix.

Causes of anemia include dietary problems, blood loss or bleeding, or exposure to toxic drugs such as hydroxychloroquine (Plaquenil), which is prescribed for rheumatoid arthritis. It's also associated with chronic diseases such as kidney disease, cancer, and certain forms of arthritis or infection, says Dr. Stander.

If you have anemia, you should be treated by a doctor. But meanwhile, there are things you can do to prevent some cases of anemia or supplement your doctor's treatment.

Try This First

Eat enough protein. Eat two to three servings of protein a day, says Marvin Adner, M.D., director of the division of hematology at the Metro West Medical Center in Framingham, Massachusetts. A serving is as little as two eggs, ½ cup of cooked dry beans, or a small piece of meat. Many foods that are high in protein also contain vitamin B_{12}, which you need to keep your blood healthy and protect it from anemia. You should get a Daily Value (DV) of 6 micrograms of B_{12}. Foods high in B_{12} include shellfish and fish.

Other Wise Ways

Go for the greens. Fill your plate with a couple servings of spinach, broccoli, turnip greens, or asparagus. These green vegetables as well as others are loaded with the B vitamin folate, Dr. Adner says. Folate helps make the red blood cells that carry hemoglobin, and if you have anemia, it could be because you aren't getting enough folate. The DV of folate is 400 micrograms. You'll get about one-fourth of that amount in ½ cup of cooked spinach. Greens aren't the only sources. Try breakfast cereals fortified with folic acid (the synthetic form of folate) as well as chickpeas, lima beans, beets, and orange juice.

Cover the bases with a multi. Pick up a bottle of multivitamins the next time you are at the pharmacy or supermarket. Find one that offers the DV of most vitamins and minerals, but especially look for 400 micrograms of folic acid and 6 micrograms of vitamin

MANAGING YOUR MEDS

The type of medicine prescribed for anemia depends on what's causing the condition. If you have iron-deficiency anemia, your doctor may prescribe high-dose iron supplements. For vitamin B_{12} deficiency, you might need injections of the vitamin on a regular basis. Although both nutrients are available in over-the-counter (OTC) supplements, you need a higher dose than you'd get from OTC medications, says Paul E. Stander, M.D., medical director of the Good Samaritan Regional Medical Center in Phoenix.

Some medications may cause internal bleeding, which could make anemia worse. Discuss your anemia with your doctor before being prescribed blood thinners such as warfarin (Coumadin). And check with your doctor before taking aspirin or nonsteroidal anti-inflammatory drugs (NSAIDs) such as ibuprofen.

WHEN TO SEE A DOCTOR

Be on the lookout for the following symptoms.

• You feel weak, dizzy, fatigued, or appear pale.

• You lose a significant amount of blood.

• You notice blood in your vomit, stool, or urine.

• You experience sudden weight gain or loss.

Any of these could be signs that you have health problems, according to Bruce Leff, M.D., assistant professor of medicine at the Johns Hopkins Bayview Medical Center Geriatric Center in Baltimore. Call your doctor immediately.

B_{12}. By taking a multivitamin once a day, you'll ensure that you get the nutrients you need to nourish your blood and help prevent anemia, Dr. Adner says.

Skip your teatime. Both hot tea and iced tea contain tannic acid, which can hinder iron absorption, says Dr. Adner. A glass once in a while won't hurt, but you shouldn't use tea as a substitute for water, he says.

Go easy on the iron. When you check out that bottle of multivitamins, remember that you only need 18 milligrams of iron to meet your Recommended Daily Allowance, which you're probably getting in your diet anyway, says Richard J. Wood, Ph.D., chief of the mineral bioavailability laboratory at the Jean Mayer USDA Human Nutrition Research Center on Aging at Tufts University in Boston. Don't take iron supplements unless your doctor tells you to.

ANGINA

When you have angina, your heart has to go begging for fresh oxygen—a task that it hates. This heart complaint occurs because your pumper isn't receiving enough blood and, therefore, is not getting all the oxygen it needs. If you have what doctors call stable angina, challenging activities like fast walking or digging in the garden may cause your overworked heart to start up the protests.

But there's another kind of angina, called unstable angina, in which the heart doesn't get enough blood even when you're doing something as simple as kicking back in a lounge chair or crossing the room.

If you're in your sixties or seventies, don't count on the usual type of chest pain if you have angina, says Gary Francis, M.D., director of the coronary intensive care unit at the Cleveland Clinic Foundation. Instead, you might just feel pressure. Or suddenly, for no apparent reason, you find you're short of breath. And some people experience angina in the form of a squeezing sensation in the chest, as if someone diabolical is tightening a belt around their ribs. Oddest of all, you might have pain in some area that seems completely unrelated to your heart, for instance, in your jaw or even one of your elbows.

The tips below are all about stable angina because the unstable variety is no candidate for home remedies. Here are some steps to stop the pain quickly or prevent it from starting at all.

Try This First

Stop. If angina comes on during an activity, stop whatever you are doing. Sit down and prop up your feet, says Michael A. Brodsky, M.D., professor of medicine in cardiology at the Univer-

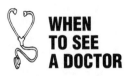

WHEN TO SEE A DOCTOR

If you've had angina pain before and are under a doctor's care, be alert to changes, says Robert March, M.D., associate professor of cardiovascular surgery at Rush-Presbyterian–St. Luke's Medical Center in Chicago. If the pain comes on more frequently with less activity, see your doctor.

Call for immediate medical help if you have pain that lasts more than 10 to 15 minutes and you get no relief from nitroglycerin.

If angina comes on in the middle of the night or when you haven't been doing anything active, you should call your doctor or go to the emergency room.

sity of California, Irvine, Medical Center. Don't try to work or push through the pain. Take a few minutes to relax.

"If you stop the activity, the pain should go away," adds Robert March, M.D., associate professor of cardiovascular surgery at Rush-Presbyterian–St. Luke's Medical Center in Chicago.

Other Wise Ways

Don't take it lying down. If you are lying down or sleeping when you have angina pain, sit up or stand up. "Standing up takes the pressure off your heart," Dr. Francis says. When you take the pressure off, your body demands less from your heart, giving it time to recover from the angina episode.

Breathe deeply. It's not a coincidence that many angina episodes get started when someone's in a tense situation. Stress often precedes a bout with angina, Dr. Francis says. When in the midst of an angina attack, calm down by taking slow, deep breaths. That may help control your stress and stop the pain. Deep breathing, experts explain, is when your abdomen expands outward as you inhale rather than your chest or shoulders rising.

Can the cigarettes. If you are a smoker, you are making it that much harder on your heart, Dr. March says. Cigarette smoke absorbs oxygen out of your blood and nicotine constricts your blood vessels. That triggers angina because your arteries shrink and less blood makes it to your heart.

Keep aspirin on hand. Take one adult aspirin tablet a day, Dr. March says. The adult dose is about 325 milligrams. Aspirin is thought to decrease heart damage during an angina episode. While the drug may not prevent an attack of angina all the time, studies show that men with angina who take aspirin are less likely to have heart attacks or die of heart problems than men who don't take aspirin.

Make it a slow morning. Take your time when you get up in the morning, Dr. Francis suggests. Don't hop right out of bed. Stretch, get acclimated to being awake, and give yourself enough time to eat a nice breakfast and read the paper.

Why the early morning slow down? Because the early hours of the day are the most dangerous for your heart, Dr. Francis says. As people get older, their bodies can't handle the jump-out-of-bed-grab-a-quick-bite-rush-to-work routine, he points out. If you force

MANAGING YOUR MEDS

The key medication for angina is nitroglycerin. It is available in two forms: one reduces the number of attacks, such as the patch (Nitro Dur), or the other relieves an attack in progress, like the under-the-tongue tablet (Nitrostat). Your doctor may advise you to keep the tablet form of nitroglycerin with you at all times and may give you a list of a few precautions.

Nitroglycerin works by dilating blood vessels, which reduces the workload for your heart. But while it's doing this, the medication can also lower your blood pressure very rapidly. When that happens, you're at risk of fainting. So the medication should only be taken while you're sitting down, says Robert March, M.D., associate professor of cardiovascular surgery at Rush-Presbyterian–St. Luke's Medical Center in Chicago. If you feel dizzy or faint, there's no harm done as long as you're not standing or walking around.

And talk to your doctor before mixing nitroglycerin and any of the following medications.

- High blood pressure medication like beta-blockers such as metoprolol (Toprol-XL)
- Sildenafil (Viagra), a drug used to treat impotence

it in the morning hours, you might put a lot of unnecessary pressure on your heart, and that additional pressure could jumpstart an angina attack. "Get up a little more slowly and don't rush around," Dr. Francis says.

Put one foot in front of the other. Walk as much as you can every day. "Walking is the best exercise," Dr. Francis says. The activity keeps your heart healthy, which may help offset angina. Unlike other activities, walking won't put much strain on your heart. If you like other forms of exercise such as swimming or bicycling, go ahead as long as it doesn't bring on angina, Dr. Francis says. "I encourage physical activity as long as you feel good doing it." Strive for at least 20 minutes three times a week.

Eat light before exercise. Don't have a heavy meal before taking your walk. If you're hungry, munch on a light snack such as an apple, Dr. Francis suggests. If you eat a big meal and then exercise, you are more likely to experience angina pain.

Leave heavy lifting to others. If you have to move something heavy, find someone else to do the job, Dr. March says. Heavy lifting is a common trigger for angina pain in many people, he adds. Even something as simple as lifting a suitcase and carrying it up a flight of stairs can cause angina pain.

Stay by the fireplace. When the weather is ice cold, make it a point to stay inside and stay warm. Below-freezing days provoke angina in some people, Dr. Francis says. "On extremely cold days, it's dangerous for people with angina to go out."

Identify your triggers. What triggers angina is different for each person. "People should learn to identify the activities that provoke angina, then they should avoid those activities," Dr. Francis says. If you can't see an obvious cause, write down the circumstances around each angina episode or just think about exactly what was happening. Over time, you will probably find a pattern, and once you're familiar with that pattern, you may be able to offset future angina attacks. "Listen to your body. It will tell you when angina is going to happen," he says.

ARM FLAB

Perhaps the real reason that the Venus de Milo is now armless is because she had jiggly arm flab—and art patrons of the Hellenistic period just couldn't stand it.

A combination of factors cause arm flab as you become older, says Alan Mikesky, Ph.D., director of the human performance and biomechanics laboratory at Indiana University–Purdue University in Indianapolis. First, he says, many people exercise less as they age, causing a loss of muscle mass.

At the same time, people tend to continue with their regular eating habits. Since they are not burning as many calories as they used to, their bodies tend to store more fat. Some of that fat goes underneath the arms.

"Finally, skin loses some of its elasticity as people grow older, which means it tends to stretch out," says Dr. Mikesky. These three factors result in loose, flabby skin that hangs underneath the arms.

But this process isn't as inevitable as it may sound. " A person can't get rid of the fat in just one area, but a good diet and regular physical activity can make a huge difference with arm flab," Dr. Mikesky says.

Try This First

Tone at home. "Working the triceps muscles—the ones that run along the back of the upper arms—improves muscle tone and counters the loss of muscle mass that contributes to arm flab," says Dr. Mikesky. One of his favorite exercises to work the triceps is called the wall pushup. Here's how it works.

• Face a wall, standing with your feet together, toes 18 inches away from the wall. Place your palms against the wall about 6 inches apart and at chest-level.

• Lower your chest toward the wall, bending your elbows but keeping the rest of your body straight. ("Make sure your elbows are close to your body and pointing downward, not sideways," cautions Dr. Mikesky.)

• Slowly push yourself back up to the starting position, again making sure to keep your elbows pointed downward.

Repeat this exercise 10 to 12 times, emphasizing proper form over speed. "Do this two times a week on nonconsecutive days," says Dr. Mikesky. "Start with one set of 10 wall pushups, then add an additional set every three or four weeks until you're doing three sets every workout session."

Other Wise Ways

Tri, tri again. Triceps kickbacks are another exercise that will target the area that you want to tone, says Billy Corbett, a certified strength and conditioning specialist and owner of Inside Out Fitness in Denver. You can do the following with a light dumbbell. Start with a weight between one and five pounds; you should be able to handle it easily. Here's what to do.

• Gripping the weight lightly in your right hand, stand with your right foot a few inches behind your left foot. Bend forward slightly, resting your left hand on your left knee to provide support.

• Bring the dumbbell up and toward your body, bending your elbow at the same time. This motion brings the dumbbell close to your right chest muscles, with your right arm close to your ribcage and your elbow pointing backward.

• Slowly extend the dumbbell out and away from your body with your right arm, using your elbow as the hinge, says Corbett. Your arm at your elbow should form a 90-degree angle, slowly straightening to 180 degrees. As your arm straightens, feel the pull in your triceps—the muscle on the outside of your arm. When your arm is fully straight, hold for a beat, then return to the starting position.

Repeat 10 to 12 times, then switch the dumbbell to your left hand and repeat, exercising the left arm. "This can also be done standing up straight or using a gym bench for support," says Corbett. When 15 repetitions of the exercise becomes easy, add a bit more weight. "But if any of those positions cause pain, either stop immediately or ask for help."

Boost the biceps, too. Biceps exercises will also help, says Walter M. Bortz II, M.D., former president of the American Geriatrics Society and clinical associate professor at the Stanford University School of Medicine. The more muscle that you have filling the area underneath the skin, the less the skin can sag. So it helps to bulk the biceps as well as the triceps.

Corbett suggests dumbbell curls as a simple, effective exercise for your biceps. Stand straight with your arms at your sides, choose a weight you can lift easily, and grip a dumbbell lightly in each hand. Turn your hands so your palms face forward.

Keeping your elbows close to your body, curl the dumbbell in your right hand up toward your right shoulder. To keep the pressure on your biceps, be sure to keep your wrist straight throughout the motion, and don't rock or sway to gain momentum. Lower your right hand back to the starting position, then repeat the motion with your left hand—again, with the concentration on "pulling" with the biceps. Do 10 to 12 repetitions on each side.

ARTHRITIS

Arthritis is basically a packaging problem. Your joints, remarkable and elaborate hinges, are cushioned by cartilage. They're held together with various other tissues, including muscles and tendons. Lubrication is in the form of some oily goop called synovial fluid, which is released by the synovial lining of the joints.

If you have osteoarthritis, the kind that most frequently coincides with aging, the cartilage around the joints starts to thin down or disappear. That's not your fault. What's more, it's not always preventable, either. Overuse may be the root of the problem. "It is caused by years of wear and tear or overuse of the joints," says Arnold Katz, M.D., rheumatologist at the Overland Park Regional Medical Center in Overland Park, Kansas. Obesity may contribute to the development of osteoarthritis in weight-bearing joints.

The runner-up, rheumatoid arthritis, is far less common, more mysterious, and equally pain producing. Rheumatoid arthritis is an inflammatory disease. With some people, the onset begins between the ages of 30 and 40, but more often it starts when people are between the ages of 40 and 60. For reasons that aren't fully understood, your body's immune system attacks your own joints, which start to suffer dire consequences.

For osteoarthritis, there are many tactics that can help hold off pain and maintain mobility. Some of these strategies might help people with rheumatoid arthritis as well. It all hinges on staying active, Dr. Katz emphasizes.

Try This First

Move those joints. To keep the pain of arthritis from getting an even tighter grip on you, get yourself on an exercise program, says

Dale L. Anderson, M.D., coordinator of the Minnesota Act Now Project in Minneapolis and author of *Muscle Pain Relief in 90 Seconds*. "Folks who are suffering from osteoarthritis must stay active; otherwise, the already-affected joints will get weaker and the people's overall aerobic capacity will drop," he says.

If you're over 60, start with low-impact aerobic activities such as 20-minute walks or exercises in a swimming pool at least three or four times per week, says William Pesanelli, physical therapist and director of Boston University's rehabilitation services. Any aerobic exercise program should be matched to your physical capacity, says Pesanelli. "If a person has been inactive for a period of time, then we're not suggesting that he go out and try to run the Boston Marathon. Instead, start with something like a five-minute walk a couple times per week, and then slowly start to increase your distance as you feel more comfortable."

Other Wise Ways

Pepper yourself. You may not like hot peppers on your sandwich, but you might like hot-pepper cream for arthritis relief. Capsaicin cream, made from the active ingredient in hot peppers, has been shown in studies to ease arthritis pain when used regularly, according to Jeffrey R. Lisse, M.D., professor of medicine and director of the division of rheumatology at the University of Texas Medical Branch at Galveston. You can buy this cream over the counter. Follow instructions on the label, wash your hands thoroughly after application, and keep this stuff away from your eyes and other mucous membranes. It can really burn.

Take the plunge at your local Y. The Arthritis Foundation sponsors water exercise programs in community centers, YMCAs, and YWCAs all over the country. "Many senior citizens enjoy the social interaction and camaraderie of participating in a group setting," says Dr. Katz. "And if an exercise program is made to be fun, then people are more likely to stick with it."

Ease the burden. Arthritis gets worse more rapidly in overweight individuals, according to Dr. Anderson. "If you lose 5 to 10 pounds, it considerably lightens the load on all of your weight-bearing joints—hips, knees, ankles, and feet," he says.

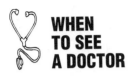

WHEN TO SEE A DOCTOR

If any of the joints in your body appear red or swollen or if tenderness in them persists for several weeks, you should see a doctor, suggests Robert Swezey, M.D., medical director of the Arthritis and Back Pain Center in Santa Monica, California. Also, be sure to schedule an appointment if your hands are bright red and swollen and you can't grab things properly. "Whatever you do, don't put off seeing a doctor if you're in pain," says Dr. Swezey. "An early, accurate diagnosis will help you immensely."

Vary your terrain. Walking is always recommended but it's important to not get into a rut. "If you walk the same exact path every day, then you're landing on the same part of your foot each and every day and you're putting stress on your knees and hips the exact same way every day," says Dr. Anderson. For the sake of interest as well as exercise, seek out new terrain like hills, fields, and pathways as well as flat road or sidewalk.

Walk softly. Dr. Anderson believes that there are two types of walkers in this world: soft walkers and hard walkers. Soft walkers glide across a room like Gene Kelly and don't put their heels, ankles, feet, or knees through much stress. Hard walkers are in the habit of hitting the ground with their heels or the soles of their feet.

If you suffer from arthritis and are a hard walker, try out a softer, more gliding style. Try to *place* your feet when you walk, rather than *plunk* them. Or imagine that you're gliding on a layer of air or that attached to your head and shoulders you have puppet-like strings that straighten you up. "You'll feel like you're walking on air, and it will save serious wear and tear on your weight-bearing joints," promises Dr. Anderson.

Go fish. Eat more salmon or other cold-water fish such as herring and sardines, and you just may take some of the sting out of rheumatoid arthritis, says Dr. Katz. That's because these fish are high in omega-3 fatty acids, a type of fat that actually eases the aches and swelling of an arthritic joint.

Ask for alternative oils. If you're not a fish-eater, Dr. Katz recommends a visit to the nearest health food store. Look for either evening primrose oil, flaxseed oil, or fish oil. All contain the same omega-3 fatty acids found in cold-water fish. If you take one teaspoon of any of these each day, it may lightly ease some of the inflammatory aspects of arthritis, Dr. Katz says. If you decide to take capsules, follow the manufacturer's instructions on the label.

Try a cold pack. If you have swelling, especially after any physical activity, put some ice with a thin towel wrapped around it on the area around the affected joint, says Keith Jones, head trainer for the Houston Rockets basketball team. "Ice the area for 15 to 20 minutes after exercise to reduce the discomfort and also minimize the amount of swelling," Jones says.

Or as an alternative to ice packs, Pesanelli recommends applying a package of frozen peas to the affected area because they can contort to the shape of the hurting joint. After you've used the peas once, you can just toss them back in the freezer compartment, get them iced, and use the same bag again. But since bacteria can quickly multiply in food that has been thawed and refrozen, make sure to clearly label them so that you don't accidentally try to serve them for dinner.

MANAGING YOUR MEDS

Anti-inflammatory drugs can certainly help you deal with arthritis pain. But anti-inflammatory medicines like aspirin and ibuprofen may aggravate certain pre-existing gastrointestinal conditions, notes David Richards, M.D., orthopedic surgeon at the Lexington Clinic Sports Medicine Center in Lexington, Kentucky. Be sure you talk to your doctor about taking these medications if you have the following symptoms.

- Ulcers or intestinal bleeding
- Any inflamed bowel disorder
- Aspirin allergy

Also, exposure to toxic drugs such as hydroxychloroquine (Plaquenil), which is prescribed for rheumatoid arthritis, can cause anemia.

Give yourself a hot wax. A hot-wax treatment can provide soothing relief if your hands are aching from arthritis, says Dr. Katz. The treatment is available at many hospitals, he points out, but it's less expensive to treat yourself at home. A professional therapist should instruct you on its appropriate use before you try this at home.

For a hot-wax or paraffin treatment kit, call an orthopedic supply store to check availability. These units are also available from mail-order companies, such as Comfort House, 189-V Frelinghuysen Avenue, Newark, NJ 07114-1595. "Heat the wax in the heating unit, apply it to your hands, and wrap them in plastic gloves for 10 minutes. You should feel some relief," says Dr. Katz. Professional units are also available for home use.

The beauty of the at-home hot-wax treatment is that the wax can be reused for several weeks. Just be careful when you're using it around children, cautions Dr. Katz. "You don't want to do a hot-wax treatment with lots of kids around, because they could quite easily knock over the heating unit and burn themselves," he says.

Immobilize the achy area. Buy a splint and use it to immobilize the joints affected by arthritis. The splint will keep the area from being bumped or moved, says David Richards, M.D., orthopedic surgeon at the Lexington Clinic Sports Medicine Center in Lexington, Kentucky. But Dr. Richards cautions that a splint, sling, or other protective device shouldn't be used for more than a couple of days. If you start to rely on the splint, your muscles could weaken quickly. If the symptoms persist after a couple of days, see your doctor.

Give high heels the boot. To ease the impact on your hip, leg, ankle, and foot joints, invest in a pair of walking shoes, advises Dr. Anderson. Because these shoes have softer heels, walking will be easier on your arthritis. Leather-soled shoes and high heels are out if you do a lot of walking, he says.

Plan for weather changes. Unless you live in a climate that's balmy throughout the year, plan for weather changes before they occur. If you start a walking program in summer, for example, consider how you will modify it before winter sets in. With some planning, you don't have to miss a single day. That's important because once you stop, it is much harder to start up again, says Alice G. Friedman, Ph.D., associate professor of psychology at Binghamton University in New York.

ASTHMA

Of the 13 million Americans who have asthma, 1.5 million of them are 65 or older. Asthma in the over-60 set doesn't pose any more health dangers than it does for the rest of the population. In fact, when asthma is controlled with medication and lifestyle changes, people of any age should be able to lead full and active lives.

But the risk that asthma poses to older folks is that it can mimic and complicate other serious health problems. The symptoms of asthma—wheezing, coughing, shortness of breath, and chest tightness—are similar to symptoms of emphysema, bronchitis, and even heart disease, which may also cause breathing problems.

Without tests, it may be difficult for the doctor to diagnose asthma in people over 60. One tip-off is that the symptoms occur after someone is exposed to a trigger, says Henry Gong Jr., M.D., professor of medicine in the division of pulmonary and critical-care medicine environmental health service at the University of Southern California School of Medicine in Downey. A trigger is something that irritates the airways, causing them to get inflamed and swell, which narrows the air passages.

Try This First

Know your enemy. Strong odors and exposure to chemicals tend to cause more problems for older people with asthma. Whatever aggravates your asthma, stay away from it, says Karin Pacheco, M.D., physician in the division of occupational and environmental medicine at the National Jewish Center for Immunology and Respiratory Medicine in Denver. Although every person may have a different set of triggers, some common potential problems include cold air, tobacco and wood smoke, perfume, paint, hairspray,

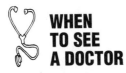

WHEN TO SEE A DOCTOR

People with asthma usually develop a sense of what is normal and what needs attention, says Joe W. Ramsdell, M.D., head of the general internal medicine and geriatrics division at the University of California, San Diego, School of Medicine. But get in touch with your doctor if:

• Your symptoms become more intense or frequent than they used to be.

• You wake up almost every night with attacks.

• You find that you need to use your inhaler or any short-acting medicine more than four times a day.

• Your inhaler doesn't seem to be working for you.

room deodorizers, cleaning chemicals, and talcum powder.

Other Wise Ways

Follow pollution reports. For older people with asthma, pollution is more likely to trigger an episode, explains Dr. Pacheco. Many television and radio stations now track pollution and air quality. Use these reports and then plan your day accordingly.

If the pollution is high, stay indoors and keep the air conditioner on (weather permitting), says Dr. Pacheco. You may not get asthma symptoms on the very day that pollution is high, she warns. Pollutants can take two to three days to trigger an asthma attack.

Roam the produce aisle. Eat at least five servings of fruits and vegetables a day. Have one or two servings with each meal, and you'll reach five easily. Fruits and vegetables are loaded with antioxidants including vitamins C and E, chemicals that may protect your lungs from an asthma attack, says Gary E. Hatch, Ph.D., researcher and pharmacologist in the U.S. Environmental Protection Agency Pulmonary Toxicology Branch in Research Triangle Park, North Carolina.

Seek supplements for extra protection. To be sure you keep those antioxidant levels up, take 500 milligrams of vitamin C and 400 international units (IU) of vitamin E a day, Dr. Hatch says. These supplements may be especially beneficial as you get older, especially if you have asthma, according to Dr. Hatch. Researchers at the University of Washington in Seattle found that taking 500 milligrams of C and 400 IU of vitamin E helped people with asthma breathe easier when exposed to pollutants. Although vitamin E is generally sold in doses of 400 IU, one small study showed a possible risk of stroke in dosages higher than 200 IU. Consult with your doctor if you are at high risk for stroke.

Deactivate the acid. When stomach acid backs up into the esophagus in a process called acid reflux, it causes heartburn. It

MANAGING YOUR MEDS

Many medications can help treat asthma. The key approach to treatment of persistent asthma is the use of anti-inflammatory agents, especially corticosteroids. These include triamcinolone (Azmacort) and beclomethasone (Vanceril), drugs that prevent the asthma attack and the airways from closing up. But these medications have many possible side effects, says Michael S. Stulbarg, M.D., professor of clinical medicine and director of the clinical pulmonary center at the University of California, San Francisco.

For some people, the medications may speed up the onset of osteoporosis—bone loss—and also glaucoma. Two other classifications are leukotriene antagonists such as zafirlukast (Accolate), and mast cell inhibitors such as cromolyn (Intal). These medications do not have significant side effects and may be used over the long term to manage asthma. But they are not useful to stop an asthma attack.

Another group of medicines are inhaled bronchodilators such as albuterol (Proventil) and salmeterol (Serevent), which are used during an asthma attack to open the airways by relaxing the bronchial muscles. Some people may experience nervousness or trembling with these medications.

Other kinds of medications can actually make asthma worse. Talk to your doctor before taking the following:

- Aspirin
- Blood pressure medications known as beta-blockers, such as propranolol (Inderal)
- Beta-blocker eyedrops such as betaxolol (Betoptic) and carteolol (Ocupress) that are used to treat glaucoma

may also cause an asthma attack. The esophagus contains nerves that connect to your lungs and airways. Researchers think that those nerves may send signals that unleash an asthma attack when the reflux triggers the symptoms. "If you take care of acid reflux, asthma gets better," Dr. Gong says. To keep acid reflux to a minimum, follow these simple tips.

- Eat smaller but more frequent meals throughout the day.
- Don't eat heavy late-night snacks before bed.
- Put bricks underneath the bed legs near your head so you lie at a 45-degree angle while sleeping. Lying flat causes acid to work its way back into your esophagus.
- Ask your doctor about over-the-counter acid-suppressing drugs such as famotidine (Pepcid AC) and ranitidine (Zantac).

Dust out dust mites. Among older people, allergies caused by dust mites aren't a common problem, yet they can still trigger asthma in some cases, Dr. Gong says. These barely microscopic bugs thrive on dust and humidity. To keep their numbers down, follow these basic tips.

- Clean often with a damp mop or cloth.
- Wash your bedding in water that is at least 130°F.
- Encase pillows and mattresses in airtight covers that keep dust mites out.
- Use window shades or blinds instead of curtains.

While you'll never be able to completely get rid of the dust mites, these practices can help keep them under control and may rescue you from an attack of asthma.

Vacuum into the light. When trying to figure out what triggered his own asthma, Dr. Hatch suspected that his old vacuum cleaner might be a culprit. So he turned his vacuum cleaner upside down under a strong light in a dark room and hit the power switch. Clouds of dust and irritants spewed out. "Under the light, you can see all of the dust blowing out into the air," he says.

Try this light test with your own vacuum. If you see dust spurting out, change the bag. If that doesn't help, it may be time to invest in another vacuum cleaner. Look for one that has anti-allergenic features like special bags or a HEPA filter, says Dr. Hatch.

BACK PAIN

If you've experienced back pain, you're in good company because 8 out of 10 people experience back problems sometime in their lives. And when they feel back pain, it's often in the lower back because it gets so much use. This part of the spine links your upper body (chest and arms) to your lower body (pelvis and legs). It lets you turn to greet a friend or stoop to kiss a baby, and it gives you strength to stand, walk, or lift a box. Most lower-back problems, though painful, are not caused by serious medical conditions. Poor muscle tone and improper movement often are the culprits.

After 60, you may end up with a hodgepodge of reasons for back pain, says Anthony Wheeler, M.D., neurologist in private practice in Charlotte, North Carolina. But whatever the cause, there are lots of ways you can help yourself feel better today or prevent back pain tomorrow.

Try This First

Go mobile. Resist the urge to rest in bed, especially for more than two to three days, says Steven Mandel, M.D., clinical professor of neurology at Thomas Jefferson University Hospital in Philadelphia. Studies show that light activity actually hastens healing. If you feel that you need bed rest, take it, but try walking around every few hours, even if you have a little pain, he says. A stroll around the house or yard will help strengthen muscles and keep them limber.

Until you're feeling better, though, avoid activities that may strain the lower back, such as vacuuming or gardening, Dr. Wheeler says.

63

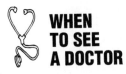

WHEN TO SEE A DOCTOR

Nearly everyone gets a twinge of back pain now and again. But if your pain is severe, lasts more than three days, or radiates to your hips or legs, see your doctor. Sudden pain in someone who's never had backache also is reason to make that visit, says Steven Mandel, M.D., clinical professor of neurology at Thomas Jefferson University Hospital in Philadelphia. Your doctor can rule out serious injury and prescribe a course of action that can have you up and about quickly.

Other Wise Ways

Pack some ice. To relieve backache, reach for an ice pack, says Sheila Reid, therapy coordinator at the Spine Institute of New England in Williston, Vermont. Apply it for 5 to 10 minutes at a time. Alternately, fill a paper cup with water, freeze it, peel back the paper, and rub the ice on sore spots, Dr. Wheeler says. Don't hold the ice on the area for more than 20 minutes, and keep a thin towel between you and the ice to prevent damage to your skin.

Or pack some heat. After the first couple of days, you may get more comfort from the warmth of a heating pad, bath, or shower. Try moist heat, Dr. Wheeler says. Rinse a small towel under hot water and wring it to near dry. Apply heat for up to 15 minutes at a time. If you use a heating pad on a medium setting, be careful not to fall asleep or leave it on too long, he says. You could burn your skin.

Reach for the home stretch. As soon as you're able, add some gentle stretches to your daily routine. This will speed healing and increase flexibility, says Dr. Mandel.

Try this exercise. Lie on the floor on your back and hug your knees to your chest. Hold for 15 seconds. Relax. Repeat two times. Go to the point of stretch, not to the point of pain, Reid says.

If you can't get down on the floor, you can still stretch, Reid says. Sit in a sturdy chair with your feet flat on the floor. Lean forward from your waist, bringing your chest slowly toward your thighs. Breathe in on the way down, and let the air out with a sigh as you lower yourself. Hold the stretch for 15 seconds. Do this stretch as often as you like.

Or try this standing stretch, Reid suggests. Stand with your feet shoulder-width apart, with your hands on the small of your back. Lean backward as you breathe out, then ease off and repeat several times. This promotes a backward motion of the spine, Reid says.

Give yourself a lift. Bending and lifting incorrectly are major causes of back pain, says John E. Thomassy, D.C., chiropractor in private practice in Virginia Beach, Virginia. "Even if you're not lifting anything, 70 percent of your body weight is above the waist." That means a 150-pound person lifts about 100 pounds every time he bends.

Don't lift with your back, Dr. Thomassy says. The next time you reach for a suitcase in your car trunk, bend your hips and knees, keeping your back straight.

Hold on tight. When you're carrying luggage, keep it close to you. The farther away you hold an object, the heavier it feels, Dr. Wheeler says. And avoid lifting loads of more than 5 to 10 pounds, he advises.

Be straight. If you're moving a box, don't pick it up and twist your body. "Never bend and twist," Dr. Thomassy says. Instead, grasp the box diagonally from the bottom, keeping it close to your body. Lift with your legs and buttock muscles while keeping your back straight. Then face squarely to where you set it down.

MANAGING YOUR MEDS

If it's not poor muscle tone or improper movement that has your lower back in knots, you may want to peek into your medicine cabinet. A few drugs can cause backaches, says W. Steven Pray, Ph.D., R.Ph., professor of nonprescription drug products at Southwestern Oklahoma State University in Weatherford. They include:

- Temazepam (Restoril), a central nervous system depressant that is prescribed to relieve tension
- Sumatriptan (Imitrex), which is used to treat severe migraine headaches

Also, Vitamin D, especially when taken in high amounts, can cause muscle and joint pains, including backache.

To ease your pain, your doctor may recommend that you take acetaminophen or nonsteroidal anti-inflammatory drugs (NSAIDs) such as ibuprofen, or aspirin. These medicines may interact with other drugs.

Please don't be seated. Sitting can actually aggravate back problems, Dr. Thomassy says. Sleeping or sitting for long periods on soft, cushy sofas or recliners can cause your back to slouch or your neck and head to be held forced forward, he says.

Get out of a slump. When you're sitting at your desk, try not to slouch, Reid cautions. Tuck a pillow or rolled towel behind your lower back for extra support. Or invest in a high-end office chair with a seat height and seat pan (the forward-back tilt of your seat) that can be adjusted to meet your needs, Reid says.

Stand safely. When you're standing for long periods of time, that, too, can aggravate back pain. Vary your position, Reid says. While standing, keep one foot on a low stool. Or keep a taller stool nearby so you can sometimes sit while you work, Dr. Wheeler suggests. And run errands during off-peak hours so you won't have to spend as much time standing in line.

Sleep right. To prevent or minimize back pain at night, keep your spine in a neutral position, Dr. Thomassy says. Don't prop your head and neck on a big pillow. Instead, choose one that keeps your head and neck in line with your upper back. "Sleep only on your side or your back, but never on your stomach," he says. Sleeping on your stomach twists your neck and back. Also, avoid extremes in surfaces, such as saggy mattresses or bare floors. A good mattress and pillow will maintain your neck and back in the correct posture even while you sleep. Pillows between your knees or along your back or sides may provide further comfort to your back and shoulders.

Or, Dr. Wheeler says, if you're on your back, prop a pillow under your knees.

Ease into the driver's seat. To get safely into your car, lower yourself backward onto the seat, keeping your feet on the ground. Bring one leg and then the other into the car, "even if you have to use your hands to pick up your legs," Dr. Thomassy says. To get out of the car, do the opposite. If you need to, carefully support yourself on the back of the seat as you rise.

Ride in style. If you're driving or riding in the car on a long trip, use a small pillow and vary its position on your back for comfort. Take a break about every two hours and walk a bit. Your back will thank you for it, says Dr. Thomassy.

BAD BREATH

First, God made Adam. Then, He made Eve. And when the couple awoke the next day and got a whiff of each other's morning breath, they discovered that the serpent wasn't the only evil thing in the Garden of Eden.

The culprits were bacteria that live mainly in difficult-to-clean areas of the mouth such as between the teeth and on the top of the tongue. These bacteria like to feast on stagnant saliva or dying epithelial (surface) cells. As a result, they give off volatile sulfur compounds as a by-product. When the environment of the mouth becomes dry, these compounds, which smell like rotten eggs, evaporate and become airborne. Here's how to ground them for good.

Try This First

Get in a scrape. Scrape that film of bacteria off your tongue with one of the spoon-shaped devices that are designed for this purpose, which are available in drugstores. Or just use a plastic spoon.

At first, you need to scrape the very back one-third of the tongue 12 to 15 times, says Jon Richter, D.M.D., Ph.D., director of the Richter Center for Breath Disorders in Philadelphia. But if you do it on a regular basis, 4 or 5 scrapes twice a day should help. Just relax your tongue, grasp it with a gauze square that you hold with your fingers, and pull it out gently, rather than just sticking it out. To reduce gagging as you scrape, breathe deeply through your nose to relax. "Scraping the tongue is the simplest approach and will produce the most dramatic short-term relief," says Dr. Richter.

Other Wise Ways

Go for gargling. Gargle with a mouthwash for about 30 seconds every morning. It helps flush out those vile bacteria in a way that

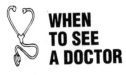

WHEN TO SEE A DOCTOR

It is rare, but bad breath can be a sign of more serious disease. If bad breath happens abruptly or is suddenly getting worse, it may be caused by a respiratory infection, and you should seek a doctor's help. Bad breath can also be caused by other chronic illnesses in their advanced stages, such as a serious liver dysfunction, says Jon Richter, D.M.D, Ph.D., director of the Richter Center for Breath Disorders in Philadelphia.

Seeing a dentist to make sure that you are free of periodontal disease can also be important, says Dr. Richter. Periodontal disease often means there will be more blood in the mouth and therefore more protein. And odor-causing bacteria just love to eat more protein. So take care of periodontal disease and help starve the bacteria.

you might not be able to if you can't overcome gagging with a scraper. "With gargling, you're able to get quite far back. You really get to the back of the throat," says Israel Kleinberg, D.D.S., Ph.D., professor and chairman of the department of oral biology and pathology at the School of Dental Medicine, State University of New York, in Stoneybrook. Look for products that contain zinc (the longest acting), sodium chlorite, or other formulations that kill bacteria.

Practice the basics. If you don't clean your teeth, then you provide more of an environment for odor-causing bacteria to lodge, feed, and give off their noxious fumes, says Clifford W. Whall Jr., Ph.D., director of product evaluation for the American Dental Association. So brush your teeth at least twice a day and floss at least once a day to remove plaque and bacteria. It's also important to make room in your schedule for regular visits to your dentist for professional cleanings and checkups. This will ensure that both your breath and your oral health are at their best, says Dr. Whall.

Don't stop short. Brush for at least two minutes. "Most people don't brush long enough," says Dr. Whall. "You don't have to brush hard, just thoroughly." Make sure to brush the fronts and backs of your teeth, especially along your gumline. When you floss, gently scrape the sides of each tooth, pulling away from the gums.

Do right by your dentures. Dentures can absorb bad odors in the mouth, says Mel Rosenberg, Ph.D., secretary general of the International Society of Breath Odor Research and a researcher and associate professor at the Maurice and Gabriela Goldschlelger

School of Dental Medicine at Tel Aviv University in Israel. Unless your dentist tells you otherwise, always soak your dentures overnight in an antiseptic solution.

Clean your dentures every day, brushing them with a commercial denture cleaner, recommends Ken Yaegaki, Ph.D., clinical professor in the department of oral biological and medical sciences at the University of British Columbia in Vancouver. If you don't have denture cleaner on hand, use toothpaste instead for one to two minutes. It's not as good, but it will help remove odor-causing bacteria, Dr. Yaegaki says.

Keep those juices flowing. If dry mouth is contributing to your bad breath, you'll need to kick your salivary glands into gear. One way to get your salivary glands going is to eat an orange or have some orange juice. The citric acid in the orange prompts the flow of saliva, says Dr. Kleinberg.

Even occasionally spritzing a little water in your mouth can help, adds Dr. Kleinberg. And be aware that although the acid in diet

MANAGING YOUR MEDS

Because medicines often affect the way that water is transported through your body, there are hundreds of medicines that can contribute to dry mouth and bad breath, says Israel Kleinberg, D.D.S., Ph.D., professor and chairman of the department of oral biology and pathology at the School of Dental Medicine, State University of New York, in Stoneybrook. Some common over-the-counter drugs that can dry the mouth are antihistamines such as diphenhydramine (Benadryl) and decongestants like pseudoephedrine (Sudafed).

Over-the-counter diet medicines are very similar to decongestants and can contribute to dry mouth, warns Charles Lacy, Pharm.D., drug information specialist at Cedars-Sinai Medical Center in Los Angeles.

Antidepressants such as fluoxetine (Prozac), antipsychotic drugs, and drugs for high blood pressure can also parch the mouth. But if you suspect that one of these drugs is aggravating your bad breath problem, be sure to check with your doctor before changing your regular course of medication.

sodas can stimulate saliva flow, they can also erode tooth enamel. In some individuals with gum recession and exposed roots, this can result in erosion of some of the cementum (the covering over the roots), causing sensitive teeth.

Break the fast. Make sure you eat three meals a day. "Skipping meals is bad," says Dr. Richter. The very process of eating helps scrape bacteria off the tongue and stimulates the washing action of saliva. Also, as the time lengthens between meals, the mouth gets a chance to dry out and bacteria builds up.

Favor odor-free eating. Maybe bacteria isn't your problem. Maybe it's your love of garlic or curry. As you may know from personal experience, some foods can linger for days because their oils are absorbed in the bloodstream and then released when you breathe. Munching on the pungent herb parsley can help mask their smell, says Laurent Chaix, doctor of naturopathy and supervisor of the teaching clinic at the National College of Naturopathic Medicine in Portland, Oregon. You can also do the sensible thing: If you know that you have an important meeting or social event coming up and you know that a specific food lingers, avoid it. Or, says Dr. Chaix, try to persuade whoever you're with to partake in the garlic experience with you.

BEDSORES

A bedsore, otherwise known as a pressure ulcer, starts as just a red spot on the skin. It occurs when you sit or lie in a single position for so long that the sheer weight of your body pinches off blood flow to a certain area.

Usually, the danger spots are bony areas of the body, especially the hips, buttocks, and heels. If blood flow is cut off long enough, the affected skin can blister, deteriorate, and die. Left untreated, the sore can break through the skin and then extend through fat, into muscle, and finally expose bone.

Anyone who is confined to a bed or wheelchair, especially someone who has suffered paralysis or a stroke, is in danger of developing a pressure ulcer, says Mitchell Kaminski Jr., M.D., staff surgeon at Thorek Hospital and Medical Center and clinical professor of surgery at the Finch University of Health Sciences/The Chicago Medical School. But you can minimize that danger.

Try This First

Get a good pressure-relieving mattress. Try to keep the person on a mattress or cushion that distributes his weight more evenly, such as an air mattress, says Dr. Kaminski. "There are many kinds available, but a regular air mattress that you use at a lake or the beach can be used to help support a person who is bedridden." Be sure it's thickly covered with an airy cotton blanket and sheets to prevent sweating. Sponge mattresses and water beds are also good choices.

Other experts recommend using cotton padding or wool to soften the mattress. The extra padding should be evenly distributed, however, to prevent it from bunching and increasing the likelihood of pinched blood vessels.

WHEN TO SEE A DOCTOR

Bedsores can develop into infection. Be alert to common signals such as odor, pus, drainage from the wound, or fever. If you note any of these, check with your doctor. He may want to prescribe antibiotics to assist healing. The doctor may also want to remove, or debride, dead tissue that surrounds a bedsore, says Mary Ruth Buchness, M.D., chief of dermatology at St. Vincent's Hospital and Medical Center in New York City and associate professor of dermatology and medicine at New York Medical College in Valhalla.

Other Wise Ways

Move around in bed. "You have to rotate the person's body throughout the day," says Dr. Kaminski. "The person should be shifted at least once an hour, just to relieve the pressure on any area of the body." Not only is this an essential way to keep bedsores from worsening once they start but it's also one of the best ways to prevent them. Be sure to reposition the person so that pressure is relieved from any reddened area on the body.

Maintain good nutrition. "In a scientific study of nursing home patients, we have never found a pressure ulcer in anyone who was well-nourished," Dr. Kaminski said. "Along with pressure, malnutrition is the single biggest co-factor in the creation of bedsores."

Keep that from happening by getting your loved one the minimum daily requirement for protein, which is two to three servings of meat, poultry, fish, or eggs a day. A serving is two to three ounces of meat, poultry, or fish (which is a piece that's about the size of a deck of cards), or two or three eggs, says Dr. Kaminski.

In addition, doctors recommend that people eat 6 to 11 servings of unprocessed whole grains, 2 to 4 servings of fresh fruits, and 3 to 5 servings of vegetables a day.

Choose your oils wisely. If you're preparing food for someone who is bedridden, be careful about the kinds of oils that may be in the foods, according to Dr. Kaminski.

"Omega-3 oils, which are found in fish, canola oil, and flaxseed oil, lower blood cholesterol and support good circulation," Dr.

Kaminski says. Avoid using corn or safflower oil in your cooking, because such oils can enhance inflammation, which decreases blood circulation and can increase bedsore risk, he adds.

Supplement against sores. Dr. Kaminski encourages people who are at risk for bedsores to take a multivitamin that contains vitamins C and E and beta-carotene. These are antioxidants that can speed healing.

Maximize blood flow to existing pressure ulcers. Make sure there is no pressure on any area where a pressure ulcer already exists, warns Mary Ruth Buchness, M.D., chief of dermatology at St. Vincent's Hospital and Medical Center in New York City and associate professor of dermatology and medicine at New York Medical College in Valhalla. If an ulcer appears on the heel, suspend the heel by raising the lower leg with pillows or soft blankets, she recommends. Once pressure is relieved, blood will flow to the existing wound and aid healing.

Make the wound moist. To help speed healing, cover any existing sores with gauze bandages coated in petroleum jelly or similar moist, thick ointment. This encourages tissues to grow rapidly, says Dr. Buchness. There are special dressings such as Duoderm and Vigilon, which are available through your pharmacist, that dissolve into the wound and create a good environment for healing.

Keep the healthy skin dry. "Keep the wound moist and the surrounding skin dry," suggests Dr. Kaminski. Healthy skin that is allowed to remain moist is more susceptible to developing a sore and an open wound. For patients who are incontinent, undergarments must be changed when needed in order to keep skin dry.

Keep the wounds clean. Pressure ulcers have to be kept clean in order to avoid infection and to heal properly. "Rinse the wound and surrounding skin with soap and water," says Dr. Kaminski. Do not use cleansing solutions containing disinfectants, such as povidone-iodine. Disinfectants generally slow the healing process.

BODY ODOR

D espite the many fragrant locker rooms that give sweat a bad name, our basic cooling system doesn't really deserve its malodorous reputation. "Actually, most of the sweat that we produce does not have any smell," says Norman Levine, M.D, professor and chief of dermatology at the University of Arizona Health Sciences Center in Tucson. Eccrine glands, found in most of the exposed areas of the body, produce a watery sweat that usually evaporates quickly, leaving behind only dry skin, which does not attract much odor-producing bacteria.

Apocrine glands produce sweat that bacteria love, and the odor created from the combination of eccrine and apocrine sweat can be a humdinger. The apocrines are located in parts of the body where moisture can collect and thus attract bacteria.

So if your daily shower doesn't seem to be enough to keep your body odor at bay, our experts offer these suggestions.

Try This First

Select an antibacterial soap. Since body odor is the result of apocrine secretions combining with bacteria, an antibacterial soap can temporarily eliminate the source of the most offensive odors, says Dr. Levine. Some antibacterial soaps, however, can dry out or irritate your skin. In that case, use a soap substitute like Dove or Cetaphil to help add moisture when washing the less odor-producing parts of your body.

Other Wise Ways

Take a powder. Odor-producing bacteria hate dry places. You can keep your body dry by applying talcum powder or methylcellulose powder such as Zeasorb to any odorous areas, says Dr. Levine. If you suffer from yeast infections, or candidiasis, avoid products that contain cornstarch, as they can exacerbate the problem. "Cornstarch contains sugars that may support the growth of candida," Dr. Levine explains.

Wipe 'em out. Baby wipes are not just for babies. They're especially handy when you're under stress and your sweat glands are secreting more odor-producing moisture than usual. So if you find yourself sweating even the small stuff, use a premoistened towelette (a feminine-hygiene wipe or baby wipe) to wash away odor instantly, suggests Mary Ruth Buchness, M.D., chief of dermatology at St. Vincent's Hospital and Medical Center in New York City and associate professor of dermatology and medicine at New York Medical College in Valhalla.

Watch what you eat. Certain foods, particularly spicy foods and those made with garlic, can increase body odor. If you suspect that a food or spice is causing your body odor problem, eliminate it from your diet to see if that helps, says Dr. Buchness.

Be smart about socks. Make sure your socks are absorbent so that they can soak up and draw moisture away from the foot. One of the best materials to look for in socks is a synthetic called polypropylene. And make sure you change your socks frequently, especially after any type of strenuous activity or if you are prone to foot odor.

MANAGING YOUR MEDS

Just as some foods can cause body odor problems, so can certain medications. Ones to be wary of include bupropion (Wellbutrin) and venlafaxine (Effexor), which are prescribed for depression, and pilocarpine (Salagen), which is used to treat dry mouth, says W. Steven Pray, Ph.D., R.Ph., professor of nonprescription drug products at Southwestern Oklahoma State University in Weatherford. If you suspect that one of your medications is at the bottom of your body odor problem, check with your doctor to see if there is an alternative medication available that won't cause you the same troublesome side effect.

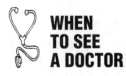

WHEN TO SEE A DOCTOR

While occasional body odor is certainly not a serious health concern, you should see a doctor if nothing seems to help, says Norman Levine, M.D, professor and chief of dermatology at the University of Arizona Health Sciences Center in Tucson. Some diseases actually have particular scents that accompany them as a symptom. Or you could have hyperhidrosis (excessive sweating) or another problem that requires a prescription-strength deodorant or antiperspirant.

Air out the tootsies. For as many hours as possible, go barefoot. Let your shoes air out for at least 24 hours between wearings.

Step up the attack. Entrenched fungus that causes foot odor and chronic athlete's foot may require stronger measures. Over-the-counter products containing miconazole nitrate (Desenex spray) or clotrimazole (Cruex or Mycelex cream) can kill the source of such irritation and may save you from further distress. Use as directed on the label.

BONE SPURS

Just like the spurs that cowboys sport, bone spurs are projections capable of causing great pain.

Older people are prone to heel spurs because as you age, there is an increasing likelihood of developing heel trouble, according to Glenn Gastwirth, D.P.M., executive director of the American Podiatric Medical Association and executive editor for the *Journal of the American Podiatric Medical Association*. High heels, flimsy sandals, and wing tips without shock-absorbent soles all encourage heel spurs, says Dr. Gastwirth.

In addition, as you grow older, the natural fat pads that cushion the sole of your foot including your heel can wear down, like pads under a carpet. They don't provide the shock absorption they once did, says Dr. Gastwirth. Here's how you can blunt heel spurs.

Try This First

Reduce inflammation. Acute pain can be reduced by applying ice to the inflamed area four or five times a day, says Terry Spilken,

MANAGING YOUR MEDS

On occasion, patients taking isotretinoin (Accutane) may develop bone spurs, says W. Steven Pray, Ph.D., R.Ph., professor of nonprescription products at Southwestern Oklahoma State University in Weatherford. Since isotretinoin is most commonly used to treat acne, the side effects of this drug are mainly limited to the younger population. However, isotretinoin is sometimes used to treat psoriasis and tumors for research purposes, so it might be prescribed to an older person, says Dr. Pray.

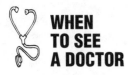

If you have chronic pain for three to four weeks in your heel, or if the pain is acute and severe, you should contact a doctor immediately, says Terry Spilken, D.P.M., podiatrist and adjunct faculty member at the New York College of Podiatric Medicine in New York City. You may actually have a certain type of arthritis.

D.P.M., podiatrist and adjunct faculty member at the New York College of Podiatric Medicine in New York City. Hold an ice pack wrapped in a towel or cloth on the area for 10 minutes, then remove the pack for another 10 minutes. Repeat this procedure several times, or until the throbbing subsides.

Other Wise Ways

With a chronic problem, apply heat. Keep inflammation in check with daily heat applications. Hold a heating pad or a hot-water bottle, as warm as can be tolerated and wrapped in a towel, on the affected area for 10 to 15 minutes four or five times a day, says Dr. Spilken.

Get help from OTC drugs. Doctors recommend over-the-counter anti-inflammatory painkillers such as ibuprofen to reduce pain caused by bone spurs and reduce further inflammation. Be sure to take these with a meal to prevent stomach distress, says Dr. Spilken.

Eschew flat shoes. Unless you find that they really provide adequate support and shock absorption, steer clear of flat shoes. They stretch the ligament on the bottom of the foot even farther, says Dr. Gastwirth. Canvas tennis shoes are a bad choice for people with heel spurs, he says, as are sandals and sling-backs. These styles provide little to no heel support and control.

Put your foot in a padded cell. When you're buying new shoes, select supportive, well-padded shoes—the kind with shock-absorbing insoles and a rigid heel support, says Dr. Gastwirth. In addition, shoes with laces will provide more support than slip-on shoes or sandals.

Make like an athlete. The American Podiatric Medical Association recommends well-supported walking or running shoes. Laced shoes with stiff, closed-in heel counters (the part of the shoe that surrounds the heel itself) keep the feet from rolling and provide stability, says Dr. Gastwirth.

Toss the worn ones. Shoes should be replaced every 300 to 350 miles, Dr. Gastwirth says. You don't have an odometer on your shoes, of course, but the mileage is pretty easy to figure out. If you wear one pair of shoes twice a week and walk 3 to 4 miles each day you wear them, you'll want to consider buying a new pair of shoes once a year.

Try massage. Gently massaging the heel really helps, says Dr. Spilken. Stroking the pained area brings up extra blood, further reducing inflammation, he says.

Sitting in a chair, support the sore heel on the knee of your opposing leg, says Dr. Spilken, then stroke the aching area with your thumb, applying gentle pressure in a circular motion. He recommends doing this for five minutes whenever your heel hurts.

BRITTLE NAILS

Think of your fingernails as brick and mortar, says Paul Kechijian, M.D., clinical associate professor of dermatology and chief of the nail section at New York University Medical Center in New York City. As you age, the "bricks" that are your nail cells and the "mortar" that holds them together gradually break down. Your nails become brittle. That's why the problem is more common among people over 65. Everyone has brittle nails to some extent, some more than others. "A lack of moisture doesn't cause the problem but it can worsen an already brittle condition," says Dr. Kechijian. Here's how to make things better.

Try This First

Reach for hand cream. Apply a moisturizing hand cream to your nails and hands frequently. The cream traps the moisture in your nails and keeps them from drying out, says Dr. Kechijian. "This is a wise step for any person who constantly wets and dries his hands during the course of a day." Nails expand when they absorb water then contract like an accordion when they dry, so he suggests applying a hand cream immediately after you dry your hands.

Any over-the-counter cream should do the trick, says C. Ralph Daniel III, M.D., clinical professor of dermatology at the University of Mississippi Medical Center in Jackson.

Whatever hand cream you pick, buy several small tubes of it and leave them all over the place—in your pocketbook, in your desk drawer, beside the kitchen sink. That way, you'll always have some on hand, says Dee Anna Glaser, M.D., associate professor of dermatology at St. Louis University School of Medicine.

Other Wise Ways

Horse around with biotin. Years ago, Dr. Daniel says, researchers found that the B vitamin biotin increased the toughness of horses' hooves. Doctors saw the positive results in horses and concluded that biotin might have the same effect on human nails. Biotin may thicken nails and can prevent cracking and splitting, Dr. Daniel says. To get biotin in your diet, fill your glass with milk and your plate with servings of corn, barley, cauliflower, and legumes such as peanuts and soybeans. But you'll have to take biotin supplements to get the amount you need for brittle nails, Dr. Daniel continues. For four to six months, take 300 micrograms four times a day with food. This should provide the necessary amount of biotin and could increase your nail thickness over a six-month period.

Keep them short and sweet. If you're bothered by brittle nails, Dr. Kechijian advises that you trim them shorter. Shorter nails are much less likely to be injured or get caught on something and tear. To keep nails strong, they should be cut straight across and rounded slightly at the edges. Use sharp nail scissors or clippers. He also recommends cutting your nails after washing, when they're softer, less brittle, and less likely to break. File away any rough edges by stroking the nail file in one direction—not back and forth. "And don't use your nails like a screwdriver or crowbar," he adds.

Glove 'em or leave 'em. If washing dishes is one of your daily chores, Dr. Daniel sug-

WHEN TO SEE A DOCTOR

Brittle nails aren't much more than a nuisance. If after two weeks of applying moisturizer you haven't seen any improvement, and they still bother you, you may want to see a doctor to rule out certain types of infections or vitamin deficiencies, says Paul Kechijian, M.D., clinical associate professor of dermatology and chief of the nail section at New York University Medical Center in New York City.

gests investing in several pairs of vinyl gloves with cotton liners. The vinyl outside keeps the water off your nails, while the cotton liner absorbs sweat so that your nails won't get wet inside the gloves.

Watch your washing. Good hygiene is certainly important, but if you're prone to brittle nails, don't wash and dry your hands any more than you have to, says Dr. Daniel. Although you'd think that wetting your hands would keep them moist, frequently washing and drying them actually strips away the moisture in and around your nails. That may also cause them to dry out and become brittle.

Go acetate, not acetone. Take a look at the ingredients list of your nail polish remover. It should be made with acetate, not acetone, Dr. Daniel says. "Acetone nail polish removers are stronger, but they can take much-needed moisture out of your nails and can perhaps lead to the nails becoming more brittle. I recommend nail polish removers with acetate because they are less likely to dry out a person's nails," he says.

BRUISES

If you studied the history of your bruises over the last 60 years or so, it would be a book with many black-and-blue pages. And if you're somewhat older and more bruise-prone than you were in your youth, it may seem like you're adding a page a day. And maybe you are. That's because you tend to bruise more as you grow older.

When we start to get up there in years, we simply have less protection under the skin than we did in the past, says Mitchell Kaminski Jr., M.D., staff surgeon at Thorek Hospital and Medical Center and clinical professor of surgery at the Finch University of Health Sciences/The Chicago Medical School. "As we age, the layers of fat and connective tissues beneath our skin become thinner," he says. And that means those layers provide less of a cushion for blood vessels, making the vessels more susceptible to injury.

Most bruises do not pose a serious health risk and do not require any special treatment, says Dr. Kaminski. Still, there are ways to prevent bruising and several things you can do to promote healing once you suffer a bruise.

Try This First

Curb the blues with RICE. The quickest way to control bruising is with a combination of four methods. RICE is an easy way to remember the pain-relieving sequence of rest, ice, compression, and elevation.

- Rest.
- Ice the injured spot.
- Apply compression.
- Elevate the limb.

WHEN TO SEE A DOCTOR

Sometimes, bruises are indications of serious illnesses such as blood disorders, says Mitchell Kaminski Jr., M.D., staff surgeon at Thorek Hospital and Medical Center and clinical professor of surgery at the Finch University of Health Sciences/The Chicago Medical School. If you have bruises that appear without any seeming cause, you should talk to your doctor.

Also, see your doctor if:

• The bruise occurs at a joint and is accompanied by swelling.

• The bruise occurs above the ear on the side of your head, which is an area that is susceptible to fractures.

• The bruising is accompanied by a fever.

Rest gives injured tissues a better chance to heal, ice constricts the blood vessels around the injury so less blood leaks into the tissues, and compression and elevation help drain blood from the injured area.

Apply ice as soon as possible after the injury occurs. Wrap the ice pack in a towel to keep it from contacting your skin directly, and keep it in place for about 15 minutes. Then let your skin warm before you reapply the ice. You can ice the bruise four or five times the first day, then after 24 hours, switch to heat to improve circulation to the bruised area, says Arthur K. Balin, M.D., medical director of the Sally Balin Medical Center for Dermatology and Cosmetic Surgery in Media, Pennsylvania, and co-author of *The Life of the Skin*.

Gently but securely wrap the bruise with an elastic bandage as soon after you injure yourself as possible, advises Dr. Balin. Then elevate your limb as much as possible for the first 24 hours. The pressure and elevation will help stop the blood from flowing into the tissues and will minimize the size of the bruise.

Other Wise Ways

Sprinkle on some parsley. Crush some fresh parsley leaves, then spread them directly on the bruise, advises James Duke, Ph.D., botanical consultant, author of *The Green Pharmacy*, and a former ethnobotanist with the U.S. Department of Agriculture who specializes in medicinal plants. Parsley can promote healing and clear up black-and-blue marks within a day or so, he says. Hold the leaves in place with an adhesive bandage or with gauze and tape.

Reach for the citrus. Vitamin C and substances called bioflavonoids that are in oranges and other citrus fruits strengthen capillary walls. As the blood vessels get stronger, they're less prone to leakage, so there's less bruising, says Dr. Duke. Also, he says that both vitamin C and bioflavonoids promote more rapid healing of capillaries after they are damaged. To help prevent bruises, make sure you eat some citrus fruit every day.

Try a multivitamin. If bruises show up without much apparent cause, maybe you're just not getting enough vitamin C from your diet, says Dr. Kaminski. If so, be sure you get a supplement, he advises. "I recommend that people take a multivitamin to ensure that they're getting the basic requirements for the vitamins they need."

Go easy on aspirin. If you take aspirin for any reason, it could be contributing to the number of bruises you're getting, says Dr. Balin. "There is evidence that an adult aspirin, which is 325 milligrams, will thin the blood too much and cause blood to leak through the vessels. Among other things, that will lead to more bruises. It's good to take aspirin but only the smaller dose."

If you're taking aspirin to help reduce your risk of heart attack, as some doctors advise, you shouldn't stop taking it without talking to a physician. But your doctor might recommend another solu-

---

MANAGING YOUR MEDS

Besides aspirin, there are several medications that can contribute to excessive bruising, says Arthur K. Balin, M.D., medical director of the Sally Balin Medical Center for Dermatology and Cosmetic Surgery in Media, Pennsylvania, and co-author of *The Life of the Skin*. These include:

- Anticoagulants like heparin (Heparin Flush) and warfarin (Coumadin)
- Nonsteroidal anti-inflammatory drugs such as ibuprofen
- Certain antibacterials, including nitrofurantoin (Macrodantin)
- Certain heart drugs, such as verapamil (Isoptin)

Check with your doctor to see if a medication you may be taking is contributing to weakened blood vessels, excessive bleeding, or bruising.

tion, such as switching to baby aspirin, which has only 81 milligrams. That much aspirin will not cause the same problems as the stronger adult dose, so it's safer and more appropriate for daily consumption, recommends Dr. Balin.

Try some special K. A deficiency of vitamin K can prevent normal blood clotting, says Dr. Kaminski, and you need some clotting action to help prevent bruising. "Some people who bruise excessively and have a lot of broken blood vessels below the skin should eat more vegetables rich in vitamin K," he says. Vitamin K is abundant in leafy greens and members of the cabbage family, such as broccoli, brussels sprouts, cabbage, and spinach, among others. "You might consider a supplement of K as well."

Protect your vulnerable spots. Be sure to wear protective clothing, especially over those areas where you tend to repeatedly bruise yourself, suggests Dr. Balin. Wear long sleeves and long pants, sweaters that fall below your waist and cover your hips, and shoes that protect your feet. If you repeatedly bruise your thighs or forearms, ask your pharmacist about protective pads that you can easily slip on to guard those areas.

BUNIONS

Shoes, especially tight shoes, use high-pressure tactics that can make life miserable for the area right next to your big toe. If there's too little room and too much pressure in that area, chances are, you'll form a bunion. And not just a dull, insensitive bump, either. A bunion that's been nudged and budged all day is a real complainer. By day's end, you'll be only too glad to get your shoes off and give that howling mound of pain some much-needed relief.

What happens is this: When you wear shoes that are too tight, the constant pressure starts to push your big toe slam-bang against the neighboring toe. Eventually, the joint that holds your toe to your foot starts to accommodate this lateral action. It changes position until a bump starts to form and the big toe points to the small toe.

If it's any consolation, about one out of every three people you pass in the street has bunions. So it definitely qualifies as shared misery.

You can't banish bunions without surgery. But you can reduce the redness and swelling and keep them from getting worse. Here's how.

Try This First

Take a painkiller. For immediate relief, try an over-the-counter anti-inflammatory medication such as ibuprofen, which will reduce pain and swelling, says Mark Caselli, D.P.M., supervisor of podiatric services for the New York City Marathon and professor of orthopedic services at New York College of Podiatric Medicine in New York City. Follow the package directions. But make sure you don't rely on the painkiller as your only fix, Dr. Caselli advises.

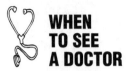

WHEN TO SEE A DOCTOR

If you have chronic, recurring pain that interferes with your daily life and you've already tried all the tips in this chapter, it's time to consult your doctor. Podiatrists and orthopedic surgeons are qualified to do a procedure called a bunionectomy. It's a commonly performed procedure, but you'll need to stay off your foot for up to six weeks following the surgery. To find an orthopedic surgeon who is a foot and ankle specialist, write to the American Orthopedic Foot and Ankle Society, 1216 Pine Street, Suite 201, Seattle, WA 98101.

Follow the rest of the tips in this chapter to prevent pain from popping up and stop the bunion from getting worse.

Other Wise Ways

Buy shoes that fit. If your foot hurts when you have shoes on, it's a pretty good bet that your shoes don't fit properly. So pitch out those ill-fitting pumps and get shoes that are just your size. This will keep your bunion from getting worse as well as prevent pain. When shopping, says Stephen F. Conti, M.D., associate professor of orthopedic surgery and chief of the division of foot and ankle surgery at University of Pittsburgh Medical Center, make sure to:

• Shop in the afternoon or evening when your feet have swollen to their widest, and wear your thickest pair of socks.

• Get your feet measured. Your feet get longer and wider with age. So your shoe size at age 60 should not be the same as it was at age 20.

• Have someone measure the length and width of your feet while you're standing up. And get them measured every single time you buy shoes.

• Have a friend or the clerk check to make sure that you have at least a thumb's width of space between your longest toe and the end of the toe box (the front of the shoe) when you are standing.

• Get shoes that are wide enough to accommodate your feet. You need a shoe that fits narrow in the heel and wide in the forefoot. In shoe store lingo, this is called a combination last. Only a few companies make them. Easy Spirit is one example, says Dr. Conti. You'll know the shoe is a combination last if the sizing information looks like a fraction such as D/B or C/A.

• When buying athletic shoes, ask for shoes that come in different widths. Not all brands do but Dr. Conti recommends New Balance and Saucony as good choices.

• If you're a wide-footed woman, consider trying on men's sneakers. Most men's sneakers have a D width, making them wider than most women sneakers, which usually have a B width.

• Check to see if the widest part of your foot fits into the widest part of the shoe. This will ensure that the shoe will bend in the proper place when you walk.

• Keep the heel height 1½ inches or lower. Studies show that when your heel lifts off the ground more than 1½ inches, the force you put on the front of your foot goes up exponentially, says Dr. Conti. This is another way of saying that wearing heels higher than 1½ inches is really bad.

• Look for a rounded toe box.

• Look for shoes made from soft leather.

Fit the larger foot. If you have two different size feet, buy shoes that fit your larger foot and use padding and inserts to keep the smaller foot from sliding around, says Robert Schwartz, certified pedorthist (professional shoe fitter) and founder of Eneslow Pedorthic Institute in New York City.

Get an arch support. People who pronate (whose feet roll inward as they stand or walk) put pressure on their big toes and create bunions. An arch support bought over the counter will prevent this rolling in and alleviate the pain that accompanies walking, says Dr. Caselli.

Stretch your heel. If your foot rolls inward when you walk, you may have a tight Achilles tendon. That crucial tendon connects your heel to your calf muscle, and if it's too tight, the tension can flatten your arch, leading to pressure on your toe during walking. To remedy this situation, stretch your Achilles tendon a few times a day, suggests Dr. Caselli. Place the balls of your feet flat on the floor and lean forward against a wall. Hold the stretch for 5 to 10 seconds. Perform this exercise 20 times on each side, alternating legs. Just be sure you don't bounce and injure the tendons or leg muscles.

Pad the bump. Athletic-shoe stores and medical supply stores sell padding that you can put on the bump to cushion it from rubbing against the side of your shoe, says Schwartz. The padding will shield the bunion and keep the toe from sliding.

BURNS

Irons, microwaves, coffeemakers, stoves—our households are teeming with items that make life easier but that can also cause burns if you're not careful.

Every year, about two million Americans are burned or scalded badly enough to need some medical attention. Many of these burns occur in the home, the majority befalling children and older people, says Randolph Wong, M.D., plastic and reconstructive surgeon and director of the burn unit at Straub Clinic and Hospital in Honolulu.

If the burn is serious enough, you'll want a doctor to look at it. If you aren't sure whether you have a first- or second-degree burn, call your doctor. But minor singes and small burns are easily treated with these simple methods.

Try This First

Cool it. As soon as you can, immerse the burned area in cool water and keep it there for 5 to 10 minutes, says Dr. Wong. Cool water stops the burning process and helps ease pain. Don't use ice to cool a burn, though. That's too cold and could further injure already-damaged skin.

If you're not near water, use whatever is convenient to cool a burn quickly—even a glass of milk or cold can of soda wrapped in a clean towel, says D'Anne Kleinsmith, M.D., staff dermatologist at William Beaumont Hospital in Royal Oak, Michigan.

Other Wise Ways

Deflame the pain. If you take an anti-inflammatory medication within an hour of getting the burn, you'll not only ease the pain but

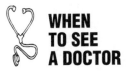

WHEN TO SEE A DOCTOR

See a doctor for any burn that isn't first- or second-degree, says Randolph Wong, M.D., plastic and re-constructive surgeon and director of the burn unit at Straub Clinic and Hospital in Honolulu.

• First-degree burns like sunburns and scalds are painful and red, but the skin sur-face is unbroken.

• Second-degree burns ooze, blister, and are painful. If the burn is smaller than a silver dollar, you can treat it at home.

• Third-degree burns leave skin charred and can turn white or cream-col-ored. They may not hurt, because nerve endings are damaged. That's all the more reason to seek imme-diate medical help, says Dr. Wong.

also you might actually prevent the burn from getting worse, says Evelyn Placek, M.D., dermatologist and doctor of internal medicine in private practice in Scarsdale, New York. Aspirin or ibuprofen works best. Dr. Placek recommends taking two 200-mil-ligram tablets or capsules of ibuprofen every six hours for one to two days to re-duce inflammation and swelling and to help decrease the severity of the wound.

Cool with a compress. To further reduce pain, apply a washcloth or towel soaked in cool, not icy, water on and off for several hours, says Dr. Placek.

Use antibacterial ointments. Over-the-counter salves like Neosporin or Bacitracin will help kill germs and prevent infection, says Dr. Wong. Sealing the wound with greasy folk remedies such as butter or pe-troleum jelly can keep nerve endings from drying out, he says, but they do little to con-trol bacteria that can get into a wound after a burn.

Bandage the burn. For small burns, place an adhesive strip over the antibacterial oint-ment, making sure the strip is large enough that it doesn't stick to the traumatized skin, explains Dr. Wong. For larger burns, you'll need a sterile piece of gauze dressing over the injured area, held down with medical adhesive tape. Be certain that it is loose enough to allow for some swelling and loose movement without compromising blood flow.

Say aloe. Aloe vera gel can speed the healing process, according to Dr. Wong. Whether fresh from the cleaned and sliced leaf of the plant or out of a tube, aloe vera gel seals and protects the burn, says Dr. Wong, and encourages healing with minimum scarring.

Take the sting out with honey. When applied as a lotion, raw honey, which is available in natural food stores as opposed to the processed variety sold in the supermarket, can be spectacularly effective against burns. Recent Chinese research shows that honey has soothing antiseptic properties that help speed healing, according to Andrew T. Weil, M.D., director of the program in integrative medicine and clinical professor of internal medicine at the University of Arizona College of Medicine in Tucson.

Think zinc. To encourage healing from within, Dr. Wong suggests taking 220 milligrams of zinc sulfate in pill form once or twice a day until the burn dries up. But if you develop some gastrointestinal upset, discontinue its use immediately. This mineral helps the regeneration of new skin, he says, especially when taken with 10,000 international units of vitamin A or 10,000 international units of beta-carotene.

Keep it moist. Once the wound has healed over, keep it supple with a thin layer of moisturizing lotion. This will help restore elasticity to the skin and reduce dryness, itching, and scaling, according to Dr. Wong. Fragrance-free lotions are best, but anything that traps moisture will be effective, says Dr. Wong, including vegetable shortening. However, don't use lanolin, he says, because it can cause a burning sensation.

Don't be a flame magnet. Something as innocent as putting a teakettle on the stove can have serious consequences if you're wearing a housecoat with dangling sleeves, which can easily catch fire. When you're cooking, don't wear loose-fitting clothing, especially garments with wide, dangling sleeves. Look for flame-retardant fabrics and avoid clothes made of cotton, cotton/polyester blends, rayon, and acrylic, which ignite easily and burn quickly.

BURSITIS
AND TENDINITIS

ursitis and tendinitis sneak up on unsuspecting people all the time. Often, it happens something like this: After months of being trapped indoors because of frosty winter temperatures and snowstorms, you head outside as soon as the weather finally breaks. And suddenly you see 1,001 things to do: repaint the garage door, reseal the driveway, dig a new flower bed, or give the house a thorough spring cleaning.

Then after spending three to four hours doing chores in the to-do list, it happens. You may start to notice swelling in and around your joints, plus a pain that just won't quit. One of the all-too-common "-itises"—either bursitis or tendinitis—has claimed another victim.

But what exactly is going on? "With tendinitis, you get an inflammation that develops in your tendons, which connect muscle to bone," says David Richards, M.D., orthopedic surgeon at the Lexington Clinic Sports Medicine Center in Lexington, Kentucky. "And it can be quite painful."

Bursitis is equally painful but begins from different origins. It's caused by an inflammation of a bursa, a fluid-filled sac surrounding joints or tendons, says Keith Jones, head trainer for the Houston Rockets basketball team. These home remedies can help you ace either "-itis."

Try This First

Give it a rest. This might sound obvious, but because bursitis and tendinitis are often triggered by using a body part in a way that it's not used to, rest is one of the first steps on the road to recovery. "Complete rest is necessary in order for the pain to subside," says Jones. Whatever activity triggered the bout of bursitis or tendinitis, avoid it for three to six weeks, if possible. Even multimillion-dollar athletes take a break when they have bursitis and tendinitis—you should, too.

Other Wise Ways

Try some ice. In addition to rest, Jones recommends putting ice wrapped in a thin towel on the area that ails you. "If you suffer from bursitis or tendinitis, make sure you apply ice to the sore area for 20 minutes at least three times per day," says Jones. "The combination of the rest and the ice should pay noticeable dividends within days."

Beat the heat. If you're suffering from bursitis or tendinitis, avoid the urge to apply a heating pad to the affected joint, says William Pesanelli, physical therapist and the director of Boston University's rehabilitation services. "It's like pouring lighter fluid on an already existing fire," he cautions. "If you're suffering from bursitis or tendinitis, the tissues in the sore area are already inflamed and will feel warmer to touch than the rest of your body, so adding

MANAGING YOUR MEDS

Taking an anti-inflammatory for a week to 10 days, such as two to three ibuprofen three to four times per day, depending on your weight, should help ease the pain and swelling that comes with either bursitis or tendinitis, says Dale L. Anderson, M.D., coordinator of the Minnesota Act Now Project in Minneapolis and the author of *Muscle Pain Relief in 90 Seconds*. If the symptoms persist, a doctor might prescribe a different anti-inflammatory drug. All anti-inflammatory drugs should be taken with food or milk because they can cause your stomach to get upset if you take them on an empty stomach, says Dr. Anderson.

Because anti-inflammatory medicines like aspirin and ibuprofen may aggravate certain conditions, ask your doctor for another battle plan if you have ulcers or an inflamed bowel disorder, advises Dr. Anderson. Also, if you're planning to have surgery, make sure to stop taking the anti-inflammatory a week before your operation. These drugs can thin your blood, which can complicate surgery.

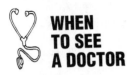

WHEN TO SEE A DOCTOR

If the pain from your bursitis or tendinitis worsens after three to four days, or if it doesn't subside at all after proper rest and other home remedies, then it's time to see a doctor, says David Richards, M.D., orthopedic surgeon at the Lexington Clinic Sports Medicine Center in Lexington, Kentucky. Besides ruling out serious injury, your doctor can prescribe medications and exercises that can alleviate pain and still give you some degree of mobility.

heat will only make matters worse." Instead, you'll find more relief by using ice until the inflammation is gone.

Limber up. To prevent bursitis and tendinitis, take time to stretch first, says Pesanelli. For example, if you are about to perform a task that your body is not used to, warm up that area of the body first. "Tendinitis or bursitis is often triggered when someone does something that his body is not used to," he says.

"If you've been playing pinochle all winter and then want to go out and garden for three hours on the first warm spring day, make sure to do some slow warm-up activities first, then a few gentle stretches to prepare for the activity," says Pesanelli. "And don't go out and do three hours worth of activity if you've been inactive for a while. You need to gradually work up to that level of activity." To get some idea of what your body can handle (before you find out the hard way), it's a good idea to sign up for a stretching class at a senior citizen center or YMCA.

Elevate your injury. If the inflammation is in the knee, foot, or ankle, Jones recommends that you elevate the affected area above your heart level. "If you put two or three pillows below your sore ankle to prop it up, it often can help reduce the swelling," Jones says. If you have a history of impaired circulation in the injured area, however, don't elevate it above your heart level, because limiting blood flow to an area of the body that has impaired circulation can be dangerous.

Wrap it up. If you need to continue to perform an activity that may cause a reoccurrence of the tendinitis in your knees, put on knee sleeves before you do anything else, says Jones. Available in pharmacies and many sports stores, the sleeves are flexible cylindrical bandages that you can pull into place over your knees.

"The knee sleeve serves two important purposes," says Jones. "First, it keeps the area warm, which helps maintain flexibility. And second, it keeps the joint from being bounced around and from causing another flare-up of the tendinitis." Similar devices for your ankles, elbows, and wrists are available at drugstores.

Keep active. To prevent injuries such as bursitis and tendinitis, get yourself on an exercise program, suggests Pesanelli. If you can get out for a brisk walk or swim three times or more per week all year round, you'll be able to keep your heart, lungs, and muscles in good condition. Many senior centers and YMCAs also offer exercise programs specifically tailored to older adults. Just be sure to consult with your physician before embarking on an exercise program, says Pesanelli.

Ease your way back into activity. After you've been treated for bursitis or tendinitis, don't jump headfirst into the activities that you were doing before the attack. "You must ease yourself back into action after you start to feel better. Otherwise, it is a vicious cycle," cautions Dr. Richards. "You'll suffer an attack of bursitis, feel better, and then be in pain again quickly if you don't slowly ease your way back into things."

CAFFEINE DEPENDENCY

In small amounts (one or two six-ounce cups of coffee), caffeine helps reduce drowsiness and fatigue, improves concentration, and aids digestion. But if you overdo it—particularly if you are over age 60—caffeine may backfire on you, says Bernard Vittone, M.D., psychiatrist and director of the National Center for the Treatment of Phobias, Anxiety, and Depression in Washington, D.C.

As you age, your body—particularly your brain—becomes more sensitive to caffeine, so you're more susceptible to many of its adverse effects, including tremors, insomnia, anxiety, panic attacks, irritability, rapid heartbeat, muscle twitching, and abdominal pain, he explains.

The amount of caffeine it takes to trigger these side effects varies from person to person, but many researchers suspect that as little as 300 milligrams (about three six-ounce cups of coffee) may be too much for some people.

On the other hand, if you regularly use caffeine, you may develop withdrawal symptoms like headaches, fatigue, and depression if you abruptly stop drinking it, says Roland Griffiths, Ph.D., professor of behavioral biology and neuroscience at Johns Hopkins University School of Medicine in Baltimore. In one small study co-authored by Dr. Griffiths, nine people had such severe caffeine withdrawal that they stopped doing household chores, canceled important social activities like birthday parties, and were more prone to mental lapses. But in most cases, weaning yourself off caffeine isn't that difficult. Here are some shrewd ways to do it.

Try This First

Coast to a stop. Even if you only drink one cup of coffee a day, you can develop withdrawal symptoms if you quit cold turkey, Dr. Griffiths says. Instead, he suggests weaning yourself off caffeine gradually over a period of two to four weeks. So if you make a 10-cup pot, for instance, try a mixture of nine parts caffeinated coffee and one part decaffeinated for two to three days. Then switch to eight parts caffeinated and two parts decaffeinated. Whether you drink a pot or a cup, keep reducing the amount of caffeine you use in this blend every two to three days until you are drinking fully decaffeinated coffee, Dr. Griffiths suggests.

If you're a tea-lover, try brewing a pot of regular and a pot of decaffeinated. Then mix the two in the same proportions as suggested for coffee, says Anthony Liguori, Ph.D., caffeine researcher and assistant professor at the Wake Forest University School of Medicine in Winston-Salem, North Carolina.

Other Wise Ways

Can the soda. Soft drinks like Mountain Dew, Dr Pepper, and most colas contain up to 55 milligrams of caffeine in a 12-ounce

MANAGING YOUR MEDS

Two lesser known sources of caffeine—guarana and kola nut—are commonly found in herbal remedies and in weight-control products like Fast Burner and Diet Now, which are sold in some health food stores, says W. Steven Pray, Ph.D., R.Ph., professor of nonprescription drug products at Southwestern Oklahoma State University in Weatherford. Caffeine also is an ingredient in many over-the-counter (OTC) medications, including pain relievers. So read the labels on these preparations carefully. Consult with your physician before using any product containing caffeine if you have heart disease, high blood pressure, ulcers, or are allergic to any stimulant. In addition, avoid using caffeine if you are taking:

- Any OTC diet, allergy, or decongestant preparation containing phenylpropanolamine (Acutrim 16 Hour, Dimetapp, Robitussin-CF)
- Monoamine oxidase (MAO) inhibitors for mental problems, such as phenelzine (Nardil)
- Antianxiety medications such as alprazolam (Xanax)

WHEN TO SEE A DOCTOR

Whenever you discuss your medications with your doctor, be sure to mention how much coffee, tea, cola, or other caffeinated beverages you are consuming, suggests Max A. Schneider, M.D., clinical professor of psychiatry specializing in addictive behaviors at the University of California, Irvine, College of Medicine. This is particularly important if:

• You develop a rapid heartbeat.

• You feel jittery, "charged up," or anxious most of the time.

• You have insomnia.

• You have panic attacks.

• You have high blood pressure.

Simply eliminating caffeine from your diet may resolve many of these symptoms, Dr. Schneider says.

serving, according to the Center for Science in the Public Interest in Washington, D.C. Read labels carefully or stick with drinks that are clearly labeled caffeine-free, suggests Max A. Schneider, M.D., clinical professor of psychiatry specializing in addictive behaviors at the University of California, Irvine, College of Medicine.

Watch those midnight snacks. Any dessert made with chocolate or coffee, like fudge, ice cream, or frozen yogurt, is probably going to contain caffeine. Some coffee-flavored desserts, in particular, contain as much caffeine as a small cup of instant coffee, says Dr. Griffiths.

Keep water, water everywhere. Hot water with a twist of lemon is a terrific substitute for coffee or tea, Dr. Schneider says. Not only does it taste good, you're still going through the ritual of drinking a hot beverage, which may ease your psychological yearnings for caffeine, he says. Be wary, however, of using some bottled waters like Aqua Blast and Java Water, which contain up to 125 milligrams of caffeine per serving. Read the labels.

Stay on course. Once you have shaken the caffeine habit, stick to decaffeinated drinks, Dr. Liguori advises. Decaffeinated beverages like coffee still have trace amounts of caffeine, but you'd have to drink about 50 cups of decaffeinated coffee to get the same buzz that you would from 1 cup of regular java.

CANKER SORES

O f all the great medical mysteries, the run-of-the-mill canker sore is among the most baffling. "Canker sores continue to frustrate oral pathologists," says Brad Rodu, D.D.S., professor in the department of pathology at the University of Alabama School of Medicine in Birmingham. "Researchers have looked for the reasons that mouth ulcers develop in the first place, and nobody has been able to get a handle on them."

Canker sores begin as small white swellings and develop into open ulcerlike wounds in the mouth, says Flora Parsa Stay, D.D.S., dentist in Oxnard, California, and author of *The Complete Book of Dental Remedies*. Most of these painful sores heal within 10 days.

If you are among those who continue to get these pesky mouth ulcers, here are several swift ways to cope with them.

Try This First

Soothe with aloe or E. Dab a bit of aloe vera gel or juice from the inside of a cut aloe leaf directly onto the sore, Dr. Fischer says. Or poke a hole in a vitamin E capsule, squeeze the liquid out, and apply it directly to the sore. Be sure to dry the sore off first, Dr. Fischer says. Either of these remedies will speed up the healing process and reduce the stinging. You can use these remedies as often as you like until your sores heal, Dr. Fischer says.

Other Wise Ways

Slip in some supplements. L-lysine, an amino acid that is available in health food stores, may help, Dr. Fischer says. Take 1,000 milligrams three times each day with meals. Continue this

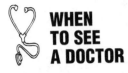

until the sores are gone. After they disappear, take 500 milligrams three times a day with meals for a week. People with recurring canker sores may try taking 500 milligrams each day as a maintenance dose, he adds.

Supplement some more. Try taking 500 milligrams of vitamin C with bioflavonoids three times a day and 15 milligrams of chelated zinc two times a day. These supplements can help boost your immune system and speed healing of canker sores, Dr. Fischer says. Continue to take these supplements until a week after your sores are gone, he says.

Note: Excess vitamin C can cause diarrhea in some people and this amount of zinc should be taken under medical supervision.

In addition, try taking 400 micrograms of folic acid, 18 milligrams of iron, and 200 micrograms of B_{12} daily, Dr. Stay suggests. Deficiencies of these nutrients may cause canker sores. With any of these doses, take them just until the canker sore improves—then stop.

Disinfect it. To help cleanse your mouth and prevent a canker sore from becoming infected, gargle three or four times a day with a solution made with three parts water and one part hydrogen peroxide, Dr. Fischer says. But be sure to avoid swallowing the solution.

Try flower power. To try an herbal remedy, make a solution of 1 part calendula tincture and 10 parts water. Rinse your mouth with it, then spit the liquid out, Dr.

Fischer says. It's a good disinfectant and you can use it as often as necessary until your sores heal.

Watch what you munch. Allergies to foods like chocolate, nuts, and citrus fruits can trigger canker sores, says Richard D. Fischer, D.D.S., dentist in Annandale, Virginia, and past president of the International Academy of Oral Medicine and Toxicology. If you suspect that a particular type of food is causing your canker sores, eliminate it from your diet for two weeks. Then try a small amount. If a mouth sore develops, you may have found your culprit, Dr. Fischer says.

CLUMSINESS

Everyone is occasionally fumble-fingered, less than graceful, or downright klutzy. In all probability, you are no more clumsy today than you were when you were in your twenties or thirties.

"Getting older doesn't necessarily mean that you'll drop more things or trip and fall more often," says Daniel Fechtner, M.D., assistant professor of rehabilitation medicine at Albert Einstein College of Medicine of Yeshiva University in New York City. "There are plenty of active people in their seventies and eighties who have never been tremendously clumsy and probably never will be." But if you do feel clumsier than usual, try these simple solutions.

Try This First

Take a seat. Sit down at a table or on a counter-high stool when you do chores like peeling vegetables or washing dishes, Dr. Fechtner says. That should help you become less accident-prone, because you can concentrate on what your hands are doing without having to worry about tripping over your own two feet.

Other Wise Ways

Tone up. The more physically fit you are, the less clumsy you'll be, says Jan I. Maby, D.O., director of the Geriatric Medical Home Care program at Mount Sinai Medical Center in New York City. Strong bones and muscles will help you maintain your balance and enhance your ability to reach and grasp.

Activities like gardening and walking that use the majority of your muscles are among the best exercises for older Americans, Dr.

Maby says. Try to exercise at least 30 minutes a day three times a week, she suggests.

Eyeball your spectacles. Poor eyesight can make you seem more clumsy. Have your vision checked at least once a year or if you find yourself more fumble-fingered than usual, Dr. Maby suggests.

Take your time. You'll be more accident-prone when you are in a rush, Dr. Maby says. So allow yourself plenty of time to do chores, drive across town, or prepare for special occasions like Thanksgiving. If you feel more comfortable taking just a step or two at a time and pausing for a couple of moments before moving on, do it, she says. It's better than taking a tumble or bumping into a wall.

Make a grip. Wrap cork tape around the handles of your spoons, knives, and other eating utensils to reduce your risk of dropping these items, Dr. Maby says. A coarse, spongy material commonly used on bicycle handlebars, cork tape is available at most bicycle shops.

Select chunky handles. Thicker-handled coffee mugs and other specialized products also can make it easier for you to maintain a solid grasp on things, Dr. Maby says. Visit a medical supply store to

MANAGING YOUR MEDS

Virtually any drug that can cause drowsiness also can make you a bit more clumsy, says W. Steven Pray, Ph.D., R.Ph., professor of nonprescription drug products at Southwestern Oklahoma State University in Weatherford. In particular, be wary of over-the-counter (OTC) sleeping pills like diphenhydramine (Sominex) and prescription antianxiety medications known as benzodiazepines, including alprazolam (Xanax). In addition, consult your doctor or pharmacist if clumsiness develops when you are taking the following medications.

* OTC and prescription antihistamines that include diphenhydramine (Benadryl)
* Antipsychotics such as phenothiazines, including chlorpromazine (Thorazine)
* Diuretics and other high blood pressure medications, including prazosin (Minipress) and methyldopa (Aldomet)

WHEN TO SEE A DOCTOR

Even if you have only an occasional clumsiness or balance problem, do not pass it off as a natural sign of aging, says Francis X. J. Bohdiewicz, M.D., specialist in physical medicine and rehabilitation at Youville Hospital and Rehabilitation Center in Cambridge, Massachusetts. "Let your doctor know about the problem and let him decide what the most appropriate next step is. A problem related to clumsiness, balance, coordination, or weakness could be a sign of treatable, underlying diseases such as stroke, arthritis, complications of diabetes, or even cancer," he says.

see all the options available or check home health-care catalogs for major department stores.

Make nonskid fingers. Wear rubber gloves when washing dishes, Dr. Fechtner says. The rubber helps you grasp and hold slippery glasses and plates.

Spot your weakness. Often, clumsiness is caused by poor depth perception, says Jim Buskirk, physical therapist at the Balance Centers of America in Wilmette, Illinois. But he says that you can learn to focus your eyes by moving your head toward a stationary object. The following exercise will help improve your depth perception and hand-eye coordination. Hand-eye coordination is dependent on good depth perception by the eyes and the ability to judge distances. Here are the steps.

1. Mark a dot on a wall at about eye level.

2. Stand opposite the dot with your hands pressed up against the wall.

3. Lower your upper body toward the wall as if you were doing a pushup. As you do this, keep your eyes focused on the dot.

4. Slowly push your body back to the starting position, again keeping your eyes focused on the dot.

Do this exercise for one minute three times a day, Buskirk advises. It may take awhile, but gradually you'll be likely to notice an improvement in your ability to lay your hands on objects more quickly and smoothly.

Take time to melt down. Some people who are prone to stress or who are suffering from anxiety can become more fumble-fingered, says Marc L. Gordon, M.D., chief of neurology for the Hillside Hospital Division of Northshore–Long Island Jewish Health System in New Hyde Park, New York.

Movement meditation is a terrific stress buster that also may help you overcome clumsiness, says Eileen F. Oster, occupational therapist in Bayside, New York, and author of *The Healing Mind*. Here's how to do it.

1. Stand if you can, or sit in a comfortable chair if you're concerned about falling. Take several deep, cleansing breaths.

2. Center yourself by visualizing your feet connected to the soil.

3. Visualize the center of the Earth, from which we draw our energy.

4. Gently move your body in an undulating, snakelike, swaying motion.

5. See yourself as a flower opening up or as an animal gracefully moving through the brush.

6. If it pleases you, use music to focus your attention on the movement and on the vibration.

7. Allow yourself to get lost in the sense of movement and the beauty of your body as it moves. Feel the areas of your body that are tight and let the movement loosen them.

Practice movement meditation at least twice a day for five minutes a session, Oster suggests.

COLD HANDS AND FEET

At one time or another, everyone gets caught in the chilling grip of Old Man Winter. It's inevitable. However, some of us get the chills even after the winter months are in the rearview mirror. Believe it or not, some folks suffer from cold hands and feet just by setting foot in the frozen-food section of the supermarket or by entering an air-conditioned room.

If this happens to you, there's a good chance that you have Raynaud's syndrome. Raynaud's is a common disorder that causes your fingers and toes to become very cold and numb, says Jay D. Coffman, M.D., chief of peripheral vascular medicine at Boston University Medical Center.

A bout with cold fingers and toes is usually temporary and is mostly just uncomfortable. And if you do have this disorder, you aren't sentenced to a lifetime of cold hands and feet. Doctors have come up with things you can do to prevent rampant Raynaud's or even fight off the chilly numbness when it nips your fingers and bites your toes.

Try This First

Get relief at arm's length. If you start to feel a chill and see your fingers begin to turn white, quickly place your cold hand in a warm place, Dr. Coffman says. Your armpit, for example. "By sticking your hand under your arm, you can stop the cold and numbing sensation of Raynaud's quickly," he says.

To reverse or help prevent the cold-feet problem, try wearing thermal socks, using warming chemical packs obtained at a sports or ski shop, or purchasing boots that can be heated, suggests Dr. Coffman. "Remember not to stamp your feet when they are cold, to avoid injury to them," he says.

Other Wise Ways

Freeze out your triggers. The next time your fingers and toes go cold, take note of what you just did that triggered it. Were you holding a cold can of soda? Did you reach into the freezer? Now you know what to avoid. "Triggers can be everyday things like holding a frozen beer mug at a party, walking into an air-conditioned room from the sweltering heat, or emerging from a heated pool into a cooler environment," says Dr. Coffman.

Warm up to wearing mittens. Of course, if cold days are the trigger, you can't take a flight to the tropics every time winter sets in. But you can protect your hands.

If gloves don't put your fingers in a tropical mode, try wearing mittens. "They do a better job of trapping the heat from your entire

MANAGING YOUR MEDS

The most commonly prescribed medication to treat Raynaud's is a vasodilator that acts as a calcium blocker, such as nifedipine (Procardia). Calcium blockers dilate the blood vessels in your body and allow blood to flow freely to your extremities, says Jay D. Coffman, M.D., chief of peripheral vascular medicine at Boston University Medical Center.

The most common side effect of taking calcium blockers is occasional headaches, but they are less common as your body adjusts to taking the medication, according to W. Steven Pray, Ph.D., R.Ph., professor of nonprescription drug products at Southwestern Oklahoma State University in Weatherford.

There are a number of medications that may *trigger* Raynaud's, except if you already have primary Raynaud's, in which case you won't be effected. Even if you aren't prone to cold fingers and toes, talk to your doctor before taking the following:

- Migraine headache medications such as ergotamine preparations (Wigraine)
- Heart and blood medications such as beta-blockers, like propranolol (Inderal)

hand," Dr. Coffman says. Wear them whenever you go out on a cold winter day.

And you might need mittens inside the house, too. "I have patients that wear mittens every time they reach into their freezer," says Dr. Coffman.

Wear a head-heating hat. When you warn your kids and grandchildren not to leave the house without a hat on, remember to take that advice yourself. You lose much body heat from the top of your head, so cover that head of yours with a hat, says Donald McIntyre, M.D., dermatologist in private practice in Rutland, Vermont. By keeping the heat in your body, you're protecting your hands and feet from a bout of Raynaud's.

Swing into action. Suffering from cold fingers? You can warm up those ice-cold digits with a simple arm-swinging exercise, says Dr. McIntyre. Pretend you're about to pitch a softball, but keep your fingers, wrist, and elbow straight while swinging your arm in a windmill fashion. "Living in Vermont, I borrowed this idea from people whom I watched up here on the ski slopes," says Dr. McIntyre. "I noticed that they kept their hands and arms warm by whirling them around when they are on top of the mountain. And I found out that it not only works on the mountain, it works in everyday life." Dr. McIntyre recommends a swinging speed of 80 whirls per minute, but notes that any windmill speed will boost the blood flow to your cold digits.

COLDS

A simple cold isn't so simple for seniors. Now, it's true that by adulthood you've been exposed to so many cold and flu bugs that you're immune to many of the sniffles that your grandchildren are likely to develop in a given winter. But that hard-won immunity does little to protect you from the scores of new strains of cold viruses that develop every year. What's more, the older you get, the less vigorously your immune system responds, so while your body is busy fighting off a cold, another infection can slip in, says Katherine Sherif, M.D., assistant professor of medicine at the Medical College of Pennsylvania/Hahnemann University School of Medicine in Philadelphia.

Colds occur more often during the winter months but cold weather doesn't cause colds. "It mainly happens because people are close together," says Michael Fleming, M.D., doctor in private practice in Shreveport, Louisiana. "During cold weather, we can't get outside a lot. We tend to be close to each other. And so with coughing and sneezing and all those other things we tend to do when we have colds, it's easier for viruses to be passed." Even though colds are more common in the winter, don't think that you're immune in the spring, summer, and fall. Because colds are caused by viruses, not bad weather, you can get them anytime.

Will there ever be a cure for the common cold? Not likely, experts say. So don't hold your breath. Instead, here are some tips to help get through colds with a minimum of suffering.

Try This First

Crush a cold with vitamin C. While it may not be a cure-all, research seems to indicate that vitamin C does bolster the body's im-

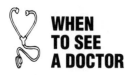

mune function, says Elson Haas, M.D., director of the Preventive Medical Center of Marin in San Rafael, California, and author of *Staying Healthy with Nutrition*. And at high doses, vitamin C seems to help stop viruses from growing. Take 1,000 milligrams six to eight times a day for up to a week, suggests Dr. Haas.

Note: Excess vitamin C may cause diarrhea in some people.

Other Wise Ways

Pump up your immune system. There's pretty good evidence that aerobic exercise does increase the effectiveness of the immune system, Dr. Sherif says. And you don't have to train for a triathlon for your workouts to be effective. "You're so much less likely to get sick if you walk five days a week for 30 to 45 minutes," Dr. Sherif states.

Get more rest. When your cold leaves you feeling wiped out, it's just trying to tell you something. To fight the cold and recover your health, you need the restorative powers of sleep and rest, advises Dr. Fleming. It helps a lot to get to bed on time when you're fighting the germs. But even during the day, try to lie down and take it easy whenever you can.

Suck on a zinc lozenge. Zinc has also shown some ability to lessen a cold's severity, Dr. Sherif says. Three or four times a day, suck on a zinc gluconate throat lozenge until it dissolves in your mouth. Or take up to 50 milligrams of zinc in supplement form at least once every day. Zinc can make you feel nauseous, so take it on a full stomach. Also, doses of zinc over 20 milligrams a day should be taken under medical supervision.

Add some echinacea. Otherwise known as the purple coneflower, echinacea is a North American plant of which the roots were used by Native Americans and early settlers to treat colds and flu. Most health food stores sell echinacea in a liquid form known as a tincture. Add one-half dropperful of tincture to a few ounces of water and drink it three times a day the first day that you feel cold symptoms coming on. If you don't experience any side effects the first day, from the next day on, add one full dropperful of tincture to the water each time, instead. Don't take echinacea if you have an autoimmune condition such as lupus, tuberculosis, or multiple sclerosis or if you're allergic to plants in the daisy family, such as chamomile and marigold.

Sip some soup. "Hot soups are helpful," Dr. Haas says. "They open you up, they warm you, and they nourish you." Of course, chicken soup is the old standard that many doctors recommend when their patients have colds. Dr. Haas also suggests making a big

MANAGING YOUR MEDS

If you have heart disease or high blood pressure, don't take an over-the-counter (OTC) cold medicine that contains the decongestant ingredient pseudoephedrine (Sudafed), warns Michael Fleming, M.D., doctor in private practice in Shreveport, Louisiana. This is a potent stimulant and can have effects on the heart.

Older men also need to beware that some OTC antihistamines, like chlorpheniramine (Chlor-Trimeton) and pseudoephedrine (Sudafed), can aggravate prostate problems and cause difficulty with urination, says Dr. Fleming.

Do not take acetaminophen with over-the-counter or prescription painkillers such as aspirin or nonsteroidal anti-inflammatory drugs (NSAIDs), for example, ibuprofen, ketoprofen (Orudis KT), and naproxen (Aleve, Naprosyn), for more than a few days, says W. Steven Pray, Ph.D., R.Ph., professor of nonprescription drug products at Southwestern Oklahoma State University in Weatherford.

pot of vegetable soup including onion, garlic, carrot, potato, cabbage, zucchini, and a little pressed or sliced ginger.

Eat the stinking rose. Sure, you could take garlic capsules, even the popular odor-free ones sold in stores. But because no one will want to get too close and risk catching your cold, why not try a little bit of garlic, straight, fresh, potent, and in a palatable form? Make it a final addition to your soup, Dr. Haas suggests. "When you put your bowl of soup on the table, you actually press a clove or two of fresh garlic right into your bowl so you're not cooking it at all, but it gets to be dispersed into the warm soup."

Relieve your pain. For the aches and pains and headache that accompany a cold, take acetaminophen or ibuprofen according to the bottle's instructions, Dr. Fleming says.

Humidify your world. If a lot of congestion accompanies your cold, help loosen it and move it on its way with a damper environment, says Penelope Shar, M.D., internist in private practice in Bangor, Maine. Use a humidifier, keep a pot of water simmering on the stove, or put a pot of water on the radiator.

Try a Tabasco tonic. When you have a cold, you're often fighting the discomfort caused by a buildup of mucus and secretions that your body is producing to help conquer the cold virus. That means a lot of hacking, coughing, and nose blowing.

Spicy foods can be a great way to cut through those secretions, thin them out, and help you expel them, says Marshall Postman, M.D., allergist in private practice in Reno, Nevada. He recommends using Tabasco sauce because it's readily available, cheap, and easy to measure. Just shake the bottle well, put 10 drops of Tabasco into a full glass of water, and drink it. Do this three times a day for as long as your symptoms persist. You can increase this up to 20 drops, but cut back to 10 if your stomach starts burning and bothering you.

"Most people are surprised," Dr. Postman says. "It's really not as spicy as people imagine. It's like a moderately spicy Bloody Mary."

Water your cold down. Drink as much clear liquid as you can—at least eight glasses a day—whether you feel thirsty or not. "When you have a cold, you become dehydrated," says Dr. Sherif. "People don't realize that's happening. By the time they feel thirsty, it's much too late. They need that water to fight off the infection." Keep in mind that even when you're getting over a cold, the weakness you still feel can be a sign that you're dehydrated. And whatever fluid you drink, make sure it doesn't have caffeine in it. Steer clear of coffee and colas. They'll only dehydrate you more.

Get gargling. A sore, scratchy throat and cough caused by a cold can make you feel miserable. Gargle with salt water—that's a pinch of salt in one-quarter of a glass of warm water—three or four times a day. It can help you feel a little better, according to Dr. Shar.

Sip hot lemonade. It's not lemonade in the traditional sense, but it can ease the pain of a sore throat. "Hot lemonade is half lemon juice and half tea. You add enough honey so that you can stand drinking it and it coats your throat. It makes your throat feel good," Dr. Shar says.

COLD SORES

If you're over age 60, you stand a better chance of seeing a blizzard in Phoenix than of getting a cold sore, dentists say. "As you get older, cold sores tend to burn themselves out," says Michael Siegel, D.D.S., associate professor of oral medicine and diagnostic sciences at the University of Maryland School of Dentistry in Baltimore.

Why cold sores, which appear on the outsides of your lips and are also known as fever blisters, subside as you age is a mystery. But some researchers suspect that the body, in a process that can take decades, gradually becomes more resistant to herpes simplex, the virus that causes cold sores, Dr. Siegel says.

If you are among the few older Americans who continue to get cold sores, you probably have years of experience in dealing with them and know a number of ways to ease an outbreak. But here are a few reminders.

Try This First

Drop a tannic bomb. Over-the-counter drops (such as Zilactin-L) that contain tannic acid can, if applied soon enough, prevent a cold sore from forming or, at the very least, help to reduce its size, says Brad Rodu, D.D.S., professor in the department of pathology at the University of Alabama School of Medicine in Birmingham.

The key is to start using the drops as soon as your lip begins tingling. That's an early warning sign that a cold sore may appear in the next 4 to 12 hours, Dr. Rodu says. Reapply the drops every hour while you feel the tingling. It will help keep the sore small.

Other Wise Ways

Have a tea party. Like some over-the-counter (OTC) drops, nonherbal tea contains tannic acid, too. The OTC medications are more effective, but you may want to try putting a wet tea bag on the sore for a few minutes every hour to provide temporary relief until you can get to the drugstore, Dr. Rodu says.

Give it a frosty reception. If your lip starts tingling, put ice on it to slow the growth of the virus that causes cold sores. That should lessen the severity of an outbreak, Dr. Rodu says. Wrap an ice cube in a towel and apply it to the affected spot for 5 to 10 minutes, repeating about once an hour.

Lube up. Moisturizing ointments such as petroleum jelly can soothe the pain and prevent cracking and bleeding skin, Dr. Rodu says. Apply them as needed.

Play it safe in the sun. Sun exposure can trigger a cold sore outbreak. To prevent it, be sure to wear a lip balm that contains a sun protection factor of at least 15, Dr. Rodu suggests. Reapply it every hour, as necessary.

Bundle up on blustery days. Cold, windy weather is a well-known trigger for cold sores. Always wear a ski mask or cover your mouth with a scarf when the wind kicks up and temperatures tumble, Dr. Rodu advises.

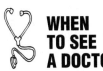

WHEN TO SEE A DOCTOR

Most cold sores heal within 10 days with or without treatment. If a mouth sore persists beyond this time, see your doctor or dentist, urges Brad Rodu, D.D.S., professor in the department of pathology at the University of Alabama School of Medicine in Birmingham. He can determine if an underlying infection is causing the problem and can prescribe medication to solve the problem.

CONSTIPATION

To understand constipation, it helps to gain a basic grasp of the normal workings of the gastrointestinal tract. The tract's primary purpose is to nurture the body by extracting energy, nutrition, and chemicals from food for later use. This extraction process takes place among the twists and turns of a long, winding path. After its sojourn in the stomach and the area just below—called the duodenum—digested food travels through the small intestine to the colon (also known as the large intestine). Once through the colon, waste is stored in the rectum as individual stools, before being passed through the anus. "The process is kind of like making mulch out of grass," says Sam Sugar, M.D., doctor in private practice in Evanston, Illinois.

Constipation is a common problem, especially among people over 60, says Dr. Sugar. While your toilet-going patterns may not change much as you age, some shifts in lifestyle patterns can affect the state of your intestinal tract.

Though it's likely that at some point in our lives we will all feel blocked, it's generally not a cause for great concern, experts say. A sensible regimen of diet and exercise can often return you to normal.

Try This First

Add fiber. The root of the word constipation means "to press or crowd together." Think of the freeway at rush hour with cars just inching along. Your listless gastrointestinal tract, if constipated, moves slower unless you help it out. The best way to do this is to consume more fiber. Both soluble and insoluble fiber play a role in preventing constipation. Soluble fiber, which dissolves easily in water, takes on a soft texture in the intestines, helping to prevent dry, hard stools. Insoluble fiber passes almost unchanged through the intestines and adds bulk to the stool. "Try to get from 25 to 40 grams of fiber in your diet a day," says Christopher Lahr, M.D., director of Complete Colon Care in Charleston, South Carolina, and the author of *Shining Light on Constipation*. High-fiber foods include beans, whole grains like buckwheat, bran cereals such as Kellogg's All-Bran, fresh fruits like avocados, and vegetables such as artichokes.

MANAGING YOUR MEDS

The medications you take to treat an existing condition may occasionally cause constipation. Pain medications, especially narcotics like codeine (found in products like Tylenol with codeine) and morphine (Duramorph), can induce the gut to slow down its normal functioning, says Christopher Lahr, M.D., director of Complete Colon Care, in Charleston, South Carolina, and the author of *Shining Light on Constipation*.

Here are other drugs that could lead to constipation.

- Over-the-counter (OTC) antacids, for example, aluminum hydroxide (Alu-Cap) and calcium carbonate (Tums)
- Antidyskinetics, which are prescribed to treat Parkinson's disease; for example, benztropine (Cogentin) and trihexyphenidyl (Artane)
- Tricyclic antidepressants, for example, amitriptyline (Elavil)
- Lithium (Lithane), which is prescribed for manic-depressive illness
- Calcium channel blockers, especially verapamil (Isoptin), used to control high blood pressure
- OTC diarrhea products such as loperamide (Imodium A-D)
- OTC and prescription iron supplements, for example, ferrous fumarate (Femiron)

If you're taking these medicines under a doctor's direction, don't stop without checking with your doctor first. Just let your doctor know that you're having a problem with constipation, and maybe he can recommend some substitutes.

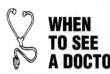

WHEN TO SEE A DOCTOR

Usually, you can treat constipation at home, says Sam Sugar, M.D., doctor in private practice in Evanston, Illinois. But if you can't, he advises that you should make a doctor's appointment urgently if constipation is accompanied by:

• Bleeding
• Pain, especially far removed from the bowel or anus, such as the right upper quadrant of your abdomen, under your rib cage

Other Wise Ways

Go slow. Adding too much fiber too quickly to your diet may solve your constipation but replace it with gassiness, bloating, and diarrhea. But you can avoid these side effects by introducing fiber slowly. Each week, increase your daily intake by no more than five grams, the amount of fiber in one cup of cooked carrots, suggests Dr. Lahr.

Wash it down. While fiber provides the bulkiness of fecal matter, it alone cannot ensure adequate passage of stools through the body. To complete the job, the bowel needs water. Without it, stools dry out and become difficult to pass.

"The simplest way to influence your BM ability is to increase your intake of water," says Dr. Sugar. To maintain good bowel movements, he advises drinking six to eight glasses of water a day.

Move around. As we get older and cut back on vigorous exercise, more sitting around directly affects the colon by making it work more sluggishly. "We generally recommend just walking," Dr. Lahr explains. "Try to walk up to three miles a day." He says that bedridden people, who frequently experience constipation, should at least stand up as often as possible (if their doctors say that it is safe for them to do so), letting sheer gravity aid the digestive process.

Go when you have to. On occasion, according to Dr. Lahr, people simply ignore the urge to defecate. This may happen for a variety of reasons, but a primary one has to do with habit. "Some people don't want to go anywhere other than their own homes," he explains.

While he sympathizes with that desire, he warns that ignoring the urge to move the bowels could lead to constipation. So wherever you are, try to go to the bathroom when you get the urge.

Use your fingers. Overall, women report more constipation than men. Dr. Lahr says that some women experience constipation because of a rectocele—a bulge of the lower rectum into, over, or behind the vagina. A rectocele sometimes forms after a hysterectomy, as the rectum falls into the place of the uterus. Rectoceles trap stool and make evacuation extremely difficult. However, a woman can insert a finger or thumb into her vagina to spur defecation.

Pushing on the rectocele bulge through the wall of the vagina helps to push the stool out of the rectum. "There is nothing dangerous about using the fingers to aid defecation," he says. "We manage a lot of people with rectoceles. We just tell them, 'Put your finger in your vagina and empty out the stool.' "

Buy in bulk. Bulk-forming laxatives, available in pharmacies and grocery stores, absorb water in the intestine and make the stool softer. Well-known brands include Metamucil and Citrucel—and you can select flavors that make them easier to swallow, says Dr. Lahr. Follow the instructions on the package. And be sure to drink as much water as recommended: The fiber in the laxative needs that liquid to "bulk up" and do its job.

Add a little more. For his part, Dr. Lahr observes that underdosing on fiber additives could be a problem for many consumers. "The label recommends one tablespoon one to three times a day," he says. He agrees with the amount but has found that the dose is often more effective if taken all at once. "I have come upon this through trial and error over 10 years with thousands of patients. Start at the recommended level, but work up to three heaping tablespoons of the additives once a day. That will dramatically improve most people's bowel regularity," he observes. Just be sure that you have one 10-ounce glass of water when you take those three tablespoons.

Take a dose of encouragement—but not too often. Popular stool-moving remedies such as enemas, stool softeners, and castor oil have all shown positive effects. They mildly irritate the colon into action and slow down water absorption from the gut. Don't use any of these habitually, though, says Dr. Sugar. Used long term, these powerful remedies can damage your colon.

Go to extremes. An alternative approach to constipation is to stimulate the central nervous system and blood flow. People can do this in their own homes using hot and cold foot baths, says Thomas Kruzel, naturopathic physician in private practice in Portland, Oregon. Spend five minutes with your feet or legs in a hot foot bath and then plunge them into cold water for a minute. As a general rule, the temperature should not be greater than 105°F, and the greater the contrast between the hot and cold temperatures, the stronger the reaction. "That really gets the circulation going," Dr. Kruzel says. (People with diabetic neuropathy should use a thermometer to check the temperature to avoid being burned, advises Dr. Kruzel.)

Heed warning signs. According to Dr. Lahr, some people accept constipation as a fact of life, ignoring symptoms or habitually treating them with quick-acting laxatives. Either approach could have serious consequences. "Those over age 65 are at high risk for colon cancer," he says, "and constipation can be a sign of colon cancer." So keep your doctor informed about your bowel movement patterns—and give him a call immediately if constipation is accompanied by abdominal pain or if you see blood in your stool.

CORNS AND CALLUSES

They're just dead skin. A bunch of hardened skin cells with no better job than to cushion the bone underneath. Corns and calluses form on parts of your feet where there is excessive friction due to underlying bony deformities. Extra layers of skin form in these areas, creating calluses on the bottom of your feet and corns on the top. They're annoying, to be sure, but you can ease the discomfort with a few simple steps.

Try This First

Get fitted. Corns and calluses are your first warning sign that your shoes don't fit properly, says Donna Astion, M.D., associate chief of foot and ankle service for the Hospital for Joint Diseases, Orthopaedic Institute in New York City. Go to a shoe store that has professionals who will carefully measure your feet—both length and width—before you start trying on shoes. Avoid shoes that rub corns or calluses.

Other Wise Ways

Have patience with a pumice. The best way to make a painful corn or callus smaller is to rub it with a pumice stone or abrasive pad, says Dr. Astion. Soften your feet by soaking them in plain luke-warm water for 5 to 10 minutes. Then use the stone to rub off dead skin a little at a time. Finally, massage some moisturizing cream onto your feet.

Get them wet. To keep your feet soft, try this natural remedy. Buy a foot soak containing the herb calendula, which is available in many health food stores or drugstores. Following package directions, mix the calendula with water and give your feet a good

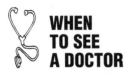

WHEN TO SEE A DOCTOR

If you continue to use home treatments but your corn or callus keeps getting worse, see a doctor to make sure you don't have an infection. A doctor can also shave that corn or callus for you.

Also, if you have persistent calluses and corns, your foot doctor may talk to you about surgical options to correct your particular problem, says Ernest Levi, D.P.M., podiatrist in private practice in New York City.

long soak. This herbal soak, done once a week or so, will loosen up dead skin and help new skin cells grow, says James J. Berryhill, Ph.D., naturopathic doctor in Decator, Georgia.

Use padding. On that pharmacy rack that offers dozens of foot-care supplies, you'll find protective pads for your feet. The package directions will tell you what to do. Every morning before you put on your shoes, put the pads around those areas where you tend to form corns or calluses, says Ernest Levi, D.P.M., podiatrist in private practice in New York City.

Avoid the medicated products. The word "medicated" may seem like a guarantee that your foot won't get infected if you use protective foot pads carrying that label. But in fact, the acids contained in those medicated pads can actually irritate the skin of older people and possibly lead to infection, according to Dr. Levi. Choose the unmedicated kind instead, he advises.

COUGHING

No matter how hard you try to stifle it, medicate it, or otherwise circumvent it, a cough is one of your body's defense mechanisms. A cough usually means that something is bothering your airway, whether it's a buildup of phlegm from a cold or pollutants from your environment.

But if you have a run-of-the-mill, bothersome cough that could stand to be muffled, try these methods to calm it down.

Try This First

Huff and cough. To minimize a coughing spell, try coughing in a rhythm that begins with several smaller, gentler coughs and then one large one. When you start with several little coughs,

MANAGING YOUR MEDS

Coughing may be a side effect of a class of drugs called angiotensin-converting enzyme inhibitors used to treat high blood pressure and congestive heart failure.

These drugs, such as captopril (Capoten) and enalapril (Vasotec), cause coughing in about 20 percent of people who take them, says Anne L. Davis, M.D., associate professor of clinical medicine at New York University in New York City. Other drugs that may cause coughing include beta-blocker drugs for high blood pressure, such as propranolol (Inderal); drugs for hyperthyroidism, such as methimazole (Tapazole); and beta-blocker eyedrops for glaucoma, for example, timolol (Timoptic).

But even if these drugs make you cough, don't stop taking them without seeing your doctor, who may be able to prescribe a substitute.

WHEN TO SEE A DOCTOR

According to Anne L. Davis, M.D., associate professor of clinical medicine at New York University in New York City, see your doctor if:

• The cough doesn't improve after three or four days.

• You develop a fever.

• You start coughing up more mucus instead of less.

• You start coughing up mucus that's puslike.

• You start coughing up blood in your mucus.

• You develop sharp pains in your chest.

you move things up toward the upper part of your air passage, the trachea, explains Anne L. Davis, M.D., associate professor of clinical medicine at New York University in New York City. "Then it can be coughed out." If you use this gradual technique instead of coughing with all of your might, you'll run less of a chance of straining a muscle or further irritating your throat.

Other Wise Ways

Have a nice cup of tea. Hot tea with a little bit of honey can be just the thing to settle down a cough. As the tea is brewing, breathe in the steam to open air passages and ease the cough. Then drink the tea and let the honey coat your throat, says Dr. Davis. Just be sure to keep your eyes closed while you're breathing in the steam, and don't get so close that you burn your skin. Steam for 5 to 15 minutes. This remedy is more likely to help a dry, irritative cough.

Kill the pain carefully. Sometimes, coughing can leave you with a raw feeling in the upper part of your chest and your throat, notes Dr. Davis. Taking a painkiller such as acetaminophen can help. Follow the instructions on the label, though, and don't take any more than the recommended daily dosage, she advises. Gargling with warm salt water also can help.

Shun smoky environments. Chemicals and smoke can irritate airways, which will trigger coughing. So if you're sick and already coughing, don't smoke. "Ideally, you should also avoid other people who are smoking and smoky environments such as bars," Dr. Davis says.

Humidify your world. If you're coughing because of a buildup of mucus from a cold, help clear your passages with some humidity. "Steam does tend to open up airways," according to Dr. Davis. Using a humidifier or even taking a warm shower can help get your secretions flowing and make your cough more productive. It is important to keep humidifiers clean because they can be a source of other infectious agents, she adds.

Keep liquids flowing. You can also help your cough by thinning your secretions with liquids. Water is by far the best, Dr. Davis says. Keep a glass handy and sip from it throughout the day, aiming for eight glasses.

CROW'S-FEET

Let's revise this term, right off the bat. Those little charming wrinkles around the eyes that we all get when we're older? They're not, emphatically, not, crow's-feet. They're laugh lines.

We had to do a lot of eye-crinkling laughing to win those lines, and now that we have them, why disparage them? They are associated not with crows, but with good humor, kindness, and wisdom.

Your drugstore and department store probably offer an array of wonder creams, all claiming to remove wrinkles and make your skin look 20 years younger. Forget the hype. Only a few products are widely recommended by dermatologists, and most doctors tell their patients to expect only modest results.

Try This First

Pour on the cream. The best skin products that help are skin creams containing glycolic acid, a fruit-derived form of alpha hydroxy acid (AHA), cause new, healthy cells to replace old, wrinkled tissues. AHAs usually come in a moisturizing base that prevents the creams from drying your skin, says Debra Price, M.D., dermatologist and clinical assistant professor at the University of Miami's department of dermatology.

Other Wise Ways

Try topical vitamin C. Dermatologists are increasingly impressed with vitamin C–containing skin creams, especially when they are used in tandem with glycolic acid or the more powerful, doctor-prescribed tretinoin (Retin-A) emollient cream.

Vitamin C smoothes the skin and rebuilds the underlying tissue somewhat. More research is needed before scientists know for sure the full effect that the vitamin C is having, says Dr. Price.

In a pinch, try egg white. If you don't want to alter the turnover rate of your cells with AHAs and have no interest in the stronger peels or surgery, try beating an egg white and then applying it over your wrinkles.

The egg white temporarily tightens and flattens the appearance of wrinkles, says Seth L. Matarasso, M.D., associate clinical professor of dermatology at the University of California, San Francisco, School of Medicine. It hydrates the skin somewhat and is a lot cheaper than any skin cream you'll find in a drugstore. Use a fresh egg white for each application. One is enough to cover your entire face.

Take cover from the sun. Ultraviolet light is the source of not only crow's-feet but also most other wrinkles, especially on the face and hands. Cover up your skin with a broad spectrum sunblock, a form of sunscreen that protects against both ultraviolet A and ultraviolet B light. Most high sun protection factor (SPF) products identify themselves as sunblock. Use a sunscreen with a strength of at least SPF 15 protection, applying it carefully around your eyes.

Wear all forms of shades. With more UV light hitting your skin than at any other time in recent history, sunglasses and wide-brimmed hats are more than a fashion statement, they're a necessity, says Dr. Price. Ultraviolet light can also lead to skin cancer, including the potentially fatal melanoma.

CUTS AND SCRAPES

The rough-and-tumble years may be behind you, but somehow you never fully outgrow your vulnerability to cuts and scrapes. In fact, the chances of minor wounds can increase once you're over 60, because your skin isn't as protective as it once was.

"Ultraviolet rays make the skin more fragile and thin, especially as you grow older," says Frederic Haberman, M.D., assistant clinical professor of medicine (dermatology) at Albert Einstein College of Medicine in New York City and director of the Haberman Dermatology Institute in Ridgewood, New Jersey. "Fragile skin is much more vulnerable to cuts and scrapes if you bump up against a hard surface."

If you have a minor wound or scrape, you can use the advice here to deal effectively with it. And once you have your cut under control, you may want to consider the tips on reducing your chances of injury.

Try This First

Stop the bleeding. Use gauze, a bandage, a clean cloth such as a towel or washcloth, or your hand to stop the bleeding, says Wyatt Decker, M.D., consultant and trauma coordinator in the department of emergency medicine at the Mayo Clinic in Rochester, Minnesota. Apply pressure directly to the wound. If the wound is on your arm or hand and it is bleeding profusely, raise your arm above the level of your heart and continue to apply pressure to the wound until the bleeding stops, he says.

Other Wise Ways

Clean the cut. Once the bleeding has stopped, clean the injured area thoroughly with ordinary soap and water, says Larry Millikan,

M.D., chairman of the department of dermatology at Tulane University Medical College in New Orleans. Keep the wound clean by soaping and rinsing it three times a day.

Keep it moist. Apply an antibiotic ointment or ordinary petroleum jelly, says Dr. Millikan. Moist wounds heal quicker and are less susceptible to scarring.

Put on a second skin. Try using a colloidal dressing, a new over-the-counter product that can cut healing time in half, according to Wilma Bergfeld, M.D., head of clinical research in the department of dermatology at the Cleveland Clinic Foundation in Ohio. Like a second skin, a colloidal dressing is a membranous, jellylike material that breathes, allowing air, but not water, to pass over your wound. This locks moisture in, which helps you to heal quickly.

Wear protective clothing. Older people who have diabetes or who are taking steroids for arthritis must be especially careful when working outdoors, says Dr. Decker. "They have skin that is prone to tearing easily," he says. "I would advise wearing gloves for any kind of manual labor outside the house." Also, when gardening or doing yardwork, wear trousers, long sleeves, and gloves.

Moisturize your skin. Cover your skin with a good moisturizer, even if the skin itself will be covered by long sleeves or pants. "Skin that is dried out is subject to more cuts, scrapes, and fissures than moist skin," Dr. Haberman says.

MANAGING YOUR MEDS

If you've just cut yourself and you want to take something for the pain, make sure you reach for acetaminophen rather than aspirin or nonsteroidal anti-inflammatory drugs (NSAIDs), such as ibuprofen, naproxen, or ketoprofen. Aspirin and, to a lesser degree, NSAIDs can inhibit blood clotting, says W. Steven Pray, Ph.D., R.Ph., professor of nonprescription drug products at Southwestern Oklahoma State University in Weatherford.

The anticoagulant drug warfarin (Coumadin) can also slow clotting time because it thins the blood, says Dr. Pray.

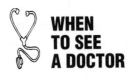

WHEN TO SEE A DOCTOR

If your cut is bleeding bright red and the blood is spurting, get to a doctor quickly. You may have punctured an artery, says Wyatt Decker, M.D., consultant and trauma coordinator in the department of emergency medicine at the Mayo Clinic in Rochester, Minnesota.

Also see a doctor if you experience these symptoms, which indicate a budding infection.

• The wound is slow to heal and there is increased pain, redness, swelling, or heat.

• The cut oozes pus or thick greenish fluid.

• Red streaks run from the site of the wound toward your torso.

• You have a fever.

Know the problem spots in your home. Be careful on stairs and never move quickly on hardwood stairs in stocking feet, Dr. Haberman advises. Hardwood stairs are slippery and you can fall easily and scrape or cut yourself. "Also, be careful getting in and out of the shower, which is where many older people injure themselves each year. Often, there's a counter that we bump into over and over again, or some object in the house that causes us trouble. That's the kind of thing that we have to change to prevent injury."

Block those rays. Use plenty of sunscreen with a sun protection factor (SPF) of at least 15 to protect any exposed area of your body from the sun, especially your face, hands, and neck, Dr. Haberman says. This will reduce the ultraviolet damage that makes your skin fragile.

CYSTS AND STIES

If you have something that looks like a pimple on or underneath your eyelid, you've turned to the right chapter. Never mind that you can't quite decide what to call that pimplelike annoyance—neither can doctors. Eye doctors frequently use both names interchangeably—cyst or sty—or even fancier terms like chalazia or hordeolum. Naming this bump can be as tricky as getting rid of it.

In plain English, here's what's going on. You have 33 oil glands per eyelid. When all is running well, these glands secrete oil to prevent your tears from evaporating. But sometimes, a gland gets clogged. The oil can't get out. So, it backs up and begins to swell and redden, becoming inflamed and sometimes painful. "It's like a blind pimple that won't come to the surface and pop," says Joseph Kubacki, M.D., professor and chairman of the ophthalmology department and assistant dean for medical affairs at Temple University School of Medicine in Philadelphia.

Sties slowly come and go on their own. If they become big enough or painful enough to inhibit your daily routine, then you should see your doctor, who may be able to drain the sty. Regardless of why you have this bump or what you decide to call it, here are some ways to get rid of it and prevent future occurrences.

Try This First

Bathe it in hot compresses. Sties can sometimes stick around for weeks, no matter what you do. But you can shorten that time with some moist heat, which stimulates blood flow, hastens the healing process, and encourages the cyst to drain, says James Gigantelli, M.D., director of ophthalmic plastic and reconstructive surgery at the University of Missouri in Columbia.

Fill your sink with the hottest water you can stand. (Don't boil

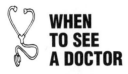

WHEN TO SEE A DOCTOR

If a sty keeps popping up in the exact same spot, if your eyeball is red or your vision blurry, or if you notice a discharge from the sty, see a doctor. These symptoms may signal an uncommon form of cancer (sebaceous carcinoma) that can affect people older than 60. If it doesn't spread to the lymph nodes, this type of cancer is curable.

water on the stove or in the microwave; you don't want to burn yourself.) Immerse two washcloths in the basin. Wring out one washcloth and hold it across your closed eyelid. When it cools, place it back in the basin and swap it for the other, says Dr. Gigantelli.

Do this for 5 to 10 minutes four to six times a day. "If you do it any less than that, you won't do any good," he says. You should notice a difference within two to three weeks. Normally, sties could last for months.

Other Wise Ways

Clean your lids regularly. To keep your glands from getting clogged, first close your eyes and place a warm washcloth over your eyelids for a minute or two. Next, cleanse your eyelids with a cotton swab dipped in "no tears" baby shampoo and gently run it back and forth along your lids, says Howard Barneby, M.D., spokesperson for the Better Vision Institute and ophthalmologist in Seattle. Then, rinse with a warm washcloth.

Keep your eyes lubricated. When you have a sty, using artificial tears that are available at the drugstore can make you more comfortable. Use one drop four to six times a day if you have dry eyes, to prevent future sties, says Dr. Gigantelli.

Throw away old makeup. Discard mascara brushes and other cosmetic items that come in contact with a sty. They could carry germs that might cause you to reinfect yourself. Also, don't share makeup with others, says Dr. Barneby.

DEHYDRATION

The desire to slake our thirsts with fresh glasses of water may seem like the most natural thing in the world, but as we age, that thirst urge diminishes, says Richard W. Besdine, M.D., professor of medicine and director of the center on aging at the University of Connecticut Health Center in Farmington. That makes older people acutely at risk for dehydration, he stresses, "because they can lose important amounts of body water without ever becoming thirsty."

But as long as you can keep up with the amount of fluid your body needs, you don't have to worry about dehydration. Here's how you can keep from going dry.

Try This First

Increase your awareness and drink frequently. "Dehydration creeps up on people. You need to be aware of the risk and take preventive measures," says Robert Kennedy, M.D., internist and director of geriatrics at Maimonides Medical Center in Brooklyn, New York.

When you're past 60, you can't depend on the usual signals to tell you that you're thirsty, says Mike Wasserman, M.D., doctor of internal medicine and chief medical officer of GeriMed of America in Denver. So you have to schedule your drinking to stay hydrated—and that often means you should drink before you feel thirsty.

The universal recommendation of doctors is to drink 64 ounces—eight 8-ounce glasses—of fluid a day. Make it simple: Just remember to drink one glass at least every other hour during the day. Plain water is best because it doesn't contain sugar, caffeine, or chemical flavorings, says Dr. Kennedy. But unsweetened fruit juice, caffeine-free soda, and milk can count toward your eight.

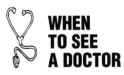

WHEN TO SEE A DOCTOR

If you or someone close to you has persistent nausea, confusion, dizziness, fainting, dry mouth, or increased heart rate, get to an emergency room or other health care facility for treatment, says Richard W. Besdine, M.D., professor of medicine and director of the center on aging at the University of Connecticut Health Center in Farmington. These are signs of serious dehydration, and you can't make the symptoms go away by providing a couple of glasses of water.

Other Wise Ways

Drink more as needed. Think about the demands on your body and up your fluid intake accordingly, says Dr. Kennedy. True, eight glasses of water is the daily requirement, but that's usually just for someone who is sitting down all day. If you're more active, you're going to need more fluids.

If it's hot or you're traveling by airplane, two particularly dehydrating situations, Dr. Kennedy recommends drinking 50 percent more than you think you need. So you might drink 12 ounces of unsweetened juice or water instead of your normal 8-ounce servings.

Drink more with exercise. When you exercise, be sure that you drink plenty of water before, during, and after. An hour before you exercise, drink 8 to 16 ounces of water, unsweetened juice, or a sports drink, says Dr. Besdine. If you exercise enough that you're breaking a sweat, you need about 20 to 40 ounces of water per hour, which is 4 to 8 ounces every 15 minutes.

When you're done exercising, slowly sip another eight ounces of water, suggests Dr. Besdine. Or, if you've had an especially taxing workout, have a sports drink. The sugar and salt in it helps the water content get absorbed into the intestines (and hence the rest of the body) faster than plain water is absorbed.

Spark the flavor. If you don't like the taste of water, dress it up with lemon slices. Buy flavored seltzer water if you like a bubbly treat or flavor up plain seltzer with cranberry juice, peach nectar, or whatever kind of juice you like.

Forget fluid flushers. Alcohol and caffeine are powerful diuretics. When you have drinks that contain these diuretics, they flush out fluid faster than they contribute it. Avoid them altogether, if you can, advises Dr. Besdine. If you can't, limit your intake. He suggests no more than two cups of coffee a day. For every alcoholic drink you have, whether it's wine, beer, or liquor, have an extra glass of water, he says. And keep in mind that many soft drinks are heavily laced with caffeine, says Dr. Besdine, even ones that aren't brown, like Mountain Dew and Surge.

Be a water carrier. Plastic water bottles are handy, easy to carry, and a constant reminder to drink throughout the day, notes Dr. Besdine. A quart-size bottle is best for day-long drinking, he says. Don't feel self-conscious carrying a bottle around: Whether you're in an office setting or a park, "water bottles have almost become part of modern dress," says Dr. Besdine.

Eat more veggies and fruits. When your body is depleted and you're trying to fill the tank, nearly any form of liquid can make a worthy contribution, recommends Dr. Wasserman. That includes the water in fresh fruits and vegetables, he notes, since the majority of these are at least 75 percent water.

Stay cool. Hot weather is another common cause of dehydration in the elderly, says Dr. Besdine. Water loss increases in a warm en-

MANAGING YOUR MEDS

Many older people take diuretics such as spironolactone (Aldactone) and furosemide (Lasix) to reduce blood pressure or to prevent congestive heart failure. While these drugs may be needed for these potentially life-threatening conditions, they all can make dehydration worse, says Robert Kennedy, M.D., internist and director of geriatrics at Maimonides Medical Center in Brooklyn, New York. Talk to your doctor about possible alternatives, but don't stop taking any prescription medication without your doctor's knowledge and consent. Also, the effect of some drugs that act on the central nervous system, such as benzodiazapines like diazepam (Valium), can be intensified if taken when you are dehydrated.

vironment, he says. Always use an air conditioner or fans in hot weather, Dr. Besdine advises. "Older adults should never stay in temperatures over 100°F, especially if they are indoors without adequate circulating air."

If you don't have air-conditioning, take frequent cool showers to keep your body temperature down, says Dr. Kennedy. Keep blinds drawn to reduce the air temperature in your home. And be very careful not to exert yourself more than you have to in warm temperatures, adds Dr. Kennedy. People with heart disease or other major health problems who are taking medication should see their doctors for advice.

DENTURE PAIN

I t's a well-worn legend that George Washington had wooden dentures. But that story, historians say, is just a load of mahogany. In reality, the Father of Our Country, who began losing his teeth at age 22, endured dentures made from an odd assortment of elephant, hippopotamus, and walrus tusks, which he called his "sea horse teeth."

He probably had a lot worse names for them.

But even modern dentures aren't perfect. Over time, your dentures may not fit as well as they once did, says Kenneth Shay, D.D.S., chief of dental services at the Veterans Affairs Medical Center in Ann Arbor, Michigan. No matter what your age, your gums continue to change over time, and as they do, dentures that once fit like a glove may begin to feel like hippo teeth. In these cases, your dentures will need to be adjusted or replaced. If you are getting dentures for the first time or having an old pair replaced, expect some discomfort. Denture pain is particularly common in the first few days after you get a new set. Here are a few suggestions that can help you adapt to new dentures.

Try This First

Stick with what is comfortable. When you first get your dentures, continue eating what you have been eating until you get accustomed to them.

"Many of my patients think, 'Boy, the first thing I'm going to do after I get my dentures is go out and eat a big, juicy steak.' That simply isn't a good idea," Dr. Shay explains. "Your mouth needs time to adjust to having two pieces of plastic inside of it. So continue eating what you were eating before you received your dentures, until you feel comfortable and confident that you can chew your food well."

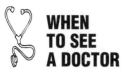

Other Wise Ways

Let a lozenge lounge around. Dentures can cause excess saliva in your mouth for a couple of weeks after you begin using them, Dr. Shay says. That's because your mouth thinks your dentures are food and produces saliva to begin digesting them. Eventually, your mouth will adapt to your dentures and saliva production will return to normal.

In the meantime, suck on sugarless candies or lozenges frequently, Dr. Shay suggests. It will help you swallow more often and get rid of some of the excess saliva.

Give your gums a rest. Don't leave your dentures in too long, especially when they are new, otherwise your gums will let you know they don't like it. If you develop sore gums, take your dentures out and set them aside for a few days while your gums heal. Then try using the dentures again, suggests Flora Parsa Stay, D.D.S., dentist in Oxnard, California, and author of *The Complete Book of Dental Remedies*.

Take your dentures out for at least six hours a day, either while you're sleeping or when you're at home doing household chores, Dr. Shay says.

Clean 'em right. Take your dentures out of your mouth before bed, brush them thoroughly with a denture cleanser, then place them in a glass of water overnight. Avoid using regular toothpastes, because they are too abrasive for most dentures, according to Dr. Shay. These pastes can damage your dentures to the point that they don't fit properly, which will cause sore gums.

Douse the ache. Take out your dentures, then rinse your mouth three times a day with a ½ cup of rinse made with goldenseal, a potent herbal remedy, to help soothe denture pain, Dr. Stay says. To prepare the rinse, add ½ tablespoon of dried goldenseal and ½ teaspoon of baking soda to ½ cup of warm water. Cool and strain before using.

Seek an herbal solution. Dab a bit of aloe vera gel or eucalyptus oil on a cotton-tipped swab and apply it directly to your gums where the dentures are causing pain, Dr. Stay suggests. These products soothe and heal sore gums. You can use them as needed, but for best results, avoid eating for at least one hour after applying these products.

Rule out allergies. Some people are allergic to denture cleansers and adhesives, Dr. Stay says. A few are even allergic to materials in the dentures themselves. In addition to a burning sensation in the mouth, these allergies can irritate the gums and cause mouth ulcers.

If you suspect that you have an allergy, ask your dentist about substitutes for the cleansers and adhesives you're using. Then try out the alternative products one by one and see whether the irritation subsides. If no change occurs after this elimination process, leave your dentures out and see what happens. If your dentures are causing the problem, you may need new dentures that are made with different materials, Dr. Stay says.

MANAGING YOUR MEDS

Any drug that dries out the mouth can contribute to denture pain, says Gretchen Gibson, D.D.S., director of the geriatric dentistry program at the Veterans Administration Medical Center in Dallas. Without enough saliva, your dentures will rub against your gums and cause discomfort.

Medications that are used to control high blood pressure, like prazosin (Minipress), and antidepressants like amitriptyline (Elavil) are among the common drugs prescribed to seniors that can dry out your mouth and lead to denture discomfort, Dr. Gibson says. Denture pain also may be a side effect of:

- Diuretics such as chlorothiazide (Diuril) or furosemide (Lasix)
- Nitroglycerin (Nitrostat) and other drugs used to control angina
- Oxybutynin (Ditropan) and other drugs used to control urinary incontinence
- Oral steriods used for asthma, like beclomethasone (Beclovent)

DEPRESSION

British statesman Winston Churchill called his bouts of gloom "the Black Dog." When President Abraham Lincoln developed melancholia, friends thought he had the gloomiest face on Earth. Novelist Nathaniel Hawthorne compared the feeling to being held captive in a dungeon. Even Sigmund Freud got the blues.

Virtually everyone slinks through an occasional period of the blues. It is as pervasive as the common cold and often no more than an annoyance, a vague feeling of self-doubt or hopelessness that quickly passes within a few days, says David Casey, M.D., geriatric psychiatrist at the University of Louisville School of Medicine in Kentucky.

Chronic illness, loss of family members and friends, social isolation, and financial worries all contribute to late-life depression. Though depression is one of the most common psychological disorders among those over 65—affecting up to 15 percent of the population over 65 years of age—it is not a normal part of aging, says Nathan Billig, M.D., geriatric psychiatrist in Washington, D.C., and author of *Growing Older and Wiser*.

To bolster your resilience, try these blues busters.

Try This First

Be a busy body. If you can keep yourself absorbed in gardening, woodworking, traveling, and other projects, it will prevent you from dwelling on whatever is making you feel unhappy. So whenever you're feeling low, ask yourself, "What am I going to do next?" suggests Isaac Tylim, Psy.D., assistant professor of psychiatry at Downstate Medical Center in Brooklyn, New York. Write down a list of goals you want to accomplish in the next week or month and dive into them. Always have something to look forward to, suggests

Dr. Tylim, and you'll be less susceptible to the blues. "Staying active gives you a sense of purpose for the future. It really is the elixir of youthfulness and hope," he says.

Other Wise Ways

Close ranks. Share your feelings with one or two close friends or relatives, suggests Richard Zweig, Ph.D., geriatric psychologist and assistant professor of psychiatry at the Albert Einstein College of Medicine in New York City. More than likely, you've helped them through many upheavals in the past and, if you allow it,

MANAGING YOUR MEDS

Although many seniors don't consider it a drug, alcohol actually is a depressant. So, far from making you happy, it will quickly bring you down, says David Casey, M.D., geriatric psychiatrist at the University of Louisville School of Medicine in Kentucky. In fact, as you get older, it takes fewer drinks to send you into an emotional tailspin, because your body can't handle alcohol as well as it once did, he says.

Here are a few other drugs that can darken your mood.

• Nytol and other over-the-counter sleeping aids containing diphenhydramine
• Diazepam (Valium), alprazolam (Xanax), and other prescription antianxiety medications known as benzodiazepines
• Medicines prescribed to strengthen the heart such as digitoxin (Crystodigin) and digoxin (Lanoxin), known as digitalis medicines
• Prescription medications for high blood pressure and angina such as propranolol (Inderal) and other beta-blocker drugs
• Reserpine (Ser-Ap-Es) and other high blood pressure medications that are prescribed to control nerve impulses

If you are taking one of these drugs and are feeling unusually sad, consult with your physician. Under no circumstances should you discontinue any prescription medications without your doctor's consent, Dr. Casey warns.

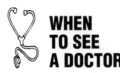

WHEN TO SEE A DOCTOR

In most instances, mild depression fades within a few days. But if you have any of the following symptoms for more than two weeks, seek immediate help from your doctor or qualified therapist, says Nathan Billig, M.D., geriatric psychiatrist in Washington, D.C., and author of *Growing Older and Wiser.*

• You feel persistently sad or empty and have lost interest in pleasurable activities, including sex.

• You feel tired or lack energy to do day-to-day chores.

• You feel restless and can't sit still.

• You either have insomnia or sleep more than usual.

• You have difficulty concentrating or making decisions.

• You have fluctuations in your appetite or weight.

• You feel hopeless, worthless, and guilty.

• You worry excessively.

they'll let you lean on them for emotional support for a while now. This doesn't mean you're asking them to solve the problem for you. It simply means you're asking them to listen, allow you to get things off your chest, and be supportive.

Plus, regular social contacts may also help keep depression away, adds Dr. Casey.

Wield the pen to trump the slump. If you're uncomfortable talking about your depression with others or have no one whom you can share your thoughts with, write down your feelings in a journal, suggests Daniel L. Segal, Ph.D., assistant professor of psychology at the University of Colorado at Colorado Springs. Writing will help you organize your thoughts and provide an outlet for your feelings that can help dissolve unpleasant emotions. Set aside 20 to 30 minutes daily to jot down your thoughts, feelings, and observations about life, Dr. Segal recommends.

Try déjà vu all over again. One terrific antidote for the blues is doing an activity you used to enjoy but haven't participated in for many years, Dr. Segal says. Bowling, camping, fly-fishing, and other long-dormant hobbies can spark fond memories that will actually uplift your spirits.

"It gets you out of a rut," notes Dr. Segal. "Let's say that you haven't been bowling for months or years because you think you're too old to do it well anymore. But don't forget, some positive things could happen, too. If you go, you might bump into an acquaintance you haven't seen in a long time and renew your friendship," Dr. Segal points out. "Or maybe you bowl better than you thought you would, and you end up feeling better about yourself. But if you just sit at home, none of those positive things are going to occur."

Step out. Regular aerobic exercise like walking, swimming, and dancing increases the production of mood-enhancing chemicals in the brain, such as serotonin, that can help pull you out of a funk, Dr. Casey says. Try exercising for at least 20 minutes a day three times a week. If you're wobbly on your feet, try this: Put a favorite piece of music on your stereo, sit in a chair, and swing your arms as if you were conducting an orchestra, Dr. Casey suggests. Doing that will give you a modest but mood-lifting aerobic workout.

Let flapjacks flip your mood. Pancakes, oatmeal, pasta, potatoes, and other foods loaded with complex carbohydrates can help a person who is 60-plus keep depressed moods under wraps, says Judith Wurtman, Ph.D., research scientist at the Massachusetts Institute of Technology and author of *The Serotonin Solution*. Complex carbohydrates elevate brain levels of serotonin. Try eating at least one meal a day that includes pasta primavera or a hearty potato soup that is very high in complex carbohydrates without lots of protein, Dr. Wurtman suggests.

Seek out seafood. Eating tuna, salmon, and other fish loaded with omega-3's, a type of polyunsaturated fat, may help bolster your mood, says Joseph Hibbeln, M.D., chief of the outpatient clinic at the National Institute on Alcohol Abuse and Alcoholism in Bethesda, Maryland. Although the research is still preliminary, Dr. Hibbeln suspects that low levels of omega-3's in your nervous system may increase your vulnerability to depression. So regular consumption of fish once or twice a week may prevent the blues, he says. Lobster, crab, shrimp, and other shellfish also contain some omega-3's.

Brew up herbal relief. For centuries, herbalists used St.-John's-wort to treat snakebites, soothe nerves, and relieve melancholy. As late as the nineteenth century, doctors studied, wrote about, and even prescribed St.-John's-wort to their patients.

But in the late 1990s, a flurry of clinical studies began re-examining the effectiveness of this lush green plant with yellow star-shaped flowers. These studies confirmed what herbalists have known all along: St.-John's-wort works, according to James Duke,

Ph.D., botanical consultant, author of *The Green Pharmacy*, and a former ethnobotanist with the U.S. Department of Agriculture who specializes in medicinal plants. In fact, some research suggests that the herb rivals the effectiveness of some antidepressant pharmaceutical drugs such as fluoxetine (Prozac), sertraline (Zoloft), amitriptyline (Elavil), and imipramine (Tofranil), Dr. Duke says.

In Germany, Commission E (the panel of scientific experts that reviews the safety and effectiveness of herbs) heaps praise on St.-John's-wort as a treatment for depression, notes Dr. Duke.

Researchers are still investigating how St.-John's-wort conquers the blues, but at least one active ingredient in the herb, hypericin, has been found to cause significant reduction in symptoms of depression and anxiety, Dr. Duke says. Several of its constituents all contribute, perhaps, synergistically to the increase in compounds that relieve depression, he says.

To try it, Dr. Duke recommends tinctures, or evening primrose infusions, in which the flowering tops have been steeped. Or use just plain old teas. He suggests steeping one to two teaspoons of the dried herb in a cup of boiling water for 10 minutes. For best results, herbalists recommend drinking one to two cups of the tea daily for four to six weeks, according to Dr. Duke.

The herb, in extremely large doses, can make the skin more prone to sunburn, so be wary of intense sun exposure, Dr. Duke warns.

Also, don't use St.-John's-wort with antidepressants without medical approval. It may affect the effective dose of prescription medication.

Keep the faith. There are no lifeguards that will keep you from getting caught in depression's undertow. But a little faith might help.

"Spirituality offers comfort in times of suffering and provides a message of hope that gives those who rely on it an extraordinary buffer against depression and other emotional upheavals," says Harold G. Koenig, M.D., author of *Is Religion Good for Your Health?* and associate professor of psychiatry and behavioral sciences at Duke University Medical Center in Durham, North Carolina.

In a study of 4,000 older Americans ages 65 to 102, Dr. Koenig found that those who attended church at least once a week were half as likely to be depressed as those who attended religious services less frequently. Other studies have shown that religiously inclined people over 60 are healthier and live longer than those who are less spiritual, Dr. Koenig says.

In particular, the Christian and Jewish faiths are therapeutic, he says, because these religions offer stellar examples of overcoming adversity and emotional suffering. "The Bible is an excellent mental health guide because it doesn't cover these issues up," explains Dr. Koenig. "It shows you lots of people, like King David, Elijah, and Jeremiah, who were extremely depressed and yet persevered."

So how do you make the most of your spirituality after age 60? "Reach up to God, reach out to others, and reach inside yourself," Dr. Koenig says. "If you actively participate in your chosen faith, help others within your community, and develop your own religious faith, it will result in personal growth and mental well-being."

DIABETES

When the ants went marching, ancient doctors watched with keen interest. They knew that ants were instinctively attracted to the unusually sweet urine of people who had a mysterious disease that caused intense thirst and dehydration. So if ants scurried toward a person's urine, it was a good bet that that person had a serious ailment we now know as diabetes.

But while diagnosis was simple, treatment was a nightmare. For thousands of years, doctors tried crude treatments like bleedings, blisterings, and drastically restricted diets consisting of 400 to 600 calories a day. Nothing worked. It wasn't until insulin was discovered in the 1920s that scientists truly began to understand how to control the disease.

"Diabetes is an eminently treatable condition these days," says Alan Krasner, M.D., assistant professor of endocrinology at Johns Hopkins University School of Medicine in Baltimore. "With the advances we've made, people who are diagnosed with diabetes today certainly can look forward to living healthier lives than others did in the past."

It's not surprising that insulin was the key to treatment, because that's the most important factor in the diabetes equation. People who have diabetes have trouble either producing or using insulin, which is an essential hormone that your cells need in order to nourish themselves. Normally, digestion breaks down some foods into glucose, a blood sugar that is your body's main source of fuel. As glucose circulates through the bloodstream, it is carried to cells throughout your body. Insulin, which is manufactured in the pancreas, is the gatekeeper. It helps glucose enter your body's cells so it can be used as fuel for growth and energy.

Without insulin—or without the ability to use it well—the cells are deprived of glucose. They'll begin to weaken. Meanwhile, glucose continues to pour into the bloodstream, building up to abnormal levels.

Diabetes becomes more prevalent with age. About half of all cases are diagnosed after 55. Nearly 6.3 million seniors—one in every five people over age 65—may have diabetes, according to Linda Morrow, M.D., medical director of Alexian Brothers Senior Health Center in San Jose, California. And another 6 million seniors who have impaired glucose tolerance are at high risk of developing the disease.

Two types of diabetes can affect seniors. Type I diabetes occurs when the body's immune system, for some yet undiscovered reason, mistakenly attacks and destroys the cells in the pancreas that are responsible for making insulin. Without insulin, blood sugars pile up and diabetes sets in. This form of the disease, which affects 5 to 10 percent of older Americans, requires insulin injections to keep blood sugars under control, Dr. Morrow says.

But 90 percent of the time when an older person gets the disease, it is Type II diabetes, says Dr. Krasner. If you have Type II, your pancreas is still doing its job. The catch is that it either isn't producing enough insulin or it is making plenty of insulin but your body has developed what is known as insulin resistance. Insulin resistance occurs when your cells snub the hormone, making it impossible for blood sugar to enter cells and be used as fuel.

Although diabetes is a chronic disease that has no cure, there are plenty of things you can do to augment the care you receive from your doctor, says Dr. Krasner.

Try This First

Know your foe. Learn as much as you can about diabetes, Dr. Morrow urges. The better you understand the disease, the more likely you are to be able to control it. Ask your doctor to recommend a certified diabetes educator in your area, or contact your local chapter of the American Diabetes Association (ADA). Books such as the *American Diabetes Association Complete Guide to Diabetes* also are terrific resources.

"Ninety-nine percent of the care and management of diabetes is in the patient's hands," says Christine Beebe, R.D., certified diabetes educator and spokesperson for the American Diabetes Asso-

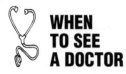

WHEN TO SEE A DOCTOR

Regular checkups are an essential part of controlling diabetes, says Alan Krasner, M.D., assistant professor of endocrinology at Johns Hopkins University School of Medicine in Baltimore. But seek immediate medical care if you:

• Have frequent or severe low or high blood sugar readings

• Notice a change in your vision

• Are confused about how to take your medication

• Have trouble following your meal or exercise plan

• Develop numbness or tingling in your hands or feet

• Have dry skin, or develop a sore

• Feel depressed or anxious about your diabetes

• Have a cold, flu, or other illness that causes dehydration, vomiting, diarrhea, or loss of appetite

ciation. "We can't move in with you, prepare your meals, and monitor your blood sugars for you. You have to know what to do and when to do it. And you can't do it if you don't have the knowledge and skills."

Other Wise Ways

Identify yourself. Wear or carry identification that will let others know that you have diabetes. If you are incapacitated, prominently displayed identification will help emergency personnel make the appropriate decisions that can save your life, Dr. Krasner says. Emergency identification tags, cards, bracelets, and necklaces are available at many pharmacies.

Step lively. Regular exercise is a vital part of any diabetes management plan, according to Dr. Morrow. Just taking a 15-minute walk every day can help lower blood sugar and can help your body use insulin more efficiently.

Some activities such as weight lifting may not be safe for you, particularly if you have high blood pressure or diabetic eye disease (retinopathy). So talk with your doctor before beginning any regular workouts, advises Dr. Morrow.

Follow your dietary blueprint. No single diet can possibly meet the unique needs of every person who has diabetes, Beebe says. So you should consult with a registered dietitian who has experience working with people who have diabetes. Jot down everything you eat and record your blood sugar readings for two to three days prior to your initial meeting with your dietitian. It will help her assess your current diet and develop a meal plan that is right for you.

"Many older people who discover that they have diabetes have very good eating habits. A lot of times, we just need to tweak the diet somewhat," Beebe says. Once your meal plan is established, meet with your dietitian at least twice a year to fine-tune it, she suggests.

Follow the pyramid. Even if you have a dietary plan specifically designed to control your diabetes, certain basics apply to everyone, says Beebe. She recommends the U.S. Department of Agriculture's Food Guide Pyramid for people who are 50-plus as an excellent starting point for any senior who has diabetes. These guidelines give you a general eating program that balances your consumption of fats, proteins, and carbohydrates in a way that should provide

MANAGING YOUR MEDS

Steroids, such as prednisone (Sterapred), that are commonly used to treat arthritis, asthma, and other inflammatory conditions can cause surges of blood sugar and make it harder for you to control your diabetes, says Linda Morrow, M.D., medical director of Alexian Brothers Senior Health Center in San Jose, California.

In addition, several other drugs commonly used by older Americans can make it more difficult to manage the disease, says Alan Krasner, M.D., assistant professor of endocrinology at Johns Hopkins University School of Medicine in Baltimore. To prevent complications, let your doctor know if you are taking any of the following medications:

- Diuretics such as hydrochlorothiazide (HydroDIURIL)
- Tricyclic antidepressants like amitriptyline (Elavil)
- Over-the-counter decongestants such as pseudoephedrine (Sudafed)

In addition, certain oral medication that is used to control diabetes, such as glyburide (DiaBeta) or glipizide (Glucotrol), can heighten your sun sensitivity, says W. Steven Pray, Ph.D., R.Ph., professor of nonprescription drug products at Southwestern Oklahoma State University in Weatherford. Consult your doctor if you suspect that one of these drugs is making you more susceptible to sunburns.

good nutrition. Here are the daily recommendations and some examples of servings.

- 6 to 11 servings of cereals and grains (examples: ½ bagel, ½ cup of cooked noodles, 2 to 3 graham crackers)
- 2 to 4 servings of fruits (examples: one orange, one banana, 1 cup of strawberries)
- 3 to 5 servings of vegetables (examples: ½ cup of corn, ¾ cup of vegetable juice, ½ cup of mashed potatoes)
- 2 to 3 servings of lean meat, poultry, eggs, dry beans, or nuts (examples: ½ cup of tuna, two ounces of meatloaf, four tablespoons of peanut butter)
- 2 to 3 servings of dairy products (examples: 1 cup of reduced-fat milk, 1 cup of low-fat yogurt, or 1½ cups of low-fat ice cream)

Fats like olive oil, mayonnaise, butter, margarine, and salad dressing should be used sparingly, notes Beebe.

Although the pyramid can help you cope with many of the dietary challenges of having diabetes, remember that you should still consult with a dietitian before beginning any meal plan to control this disease. Your individual meal plan, an exercise plan, and medication can help keep your blood sugar under control most of the time, Beebe adds.

Graze. Spread your calories, especially those that come from carbohydrates, throughout the day in order to keep your blood sugar levels at optimal levels, Beebe says. So instead of two large meals, you may want to eat five or six smaller meals like half a sandwich and an orange.

Don't forget fiber. Food high in water-soluble fiber like beans, oat bran, fruits, and nuts can help people with diabetes control their blood sugar, Beebe says. Soluble fiber slows the absorption of carbohydrates, so your blood sugar level may not rise as quickly. Try eating at least 20 grams of fiber a day. For example, start your day with a bowl of oatmeal for breakfast. Then have a peach for a midmorning snack, a bowl of chili for lunch, and lentil bean soup along with your dinner. You'll be well on your way to reaching your goal.

Treat yourself. In the past, people with diabetes were told that they could not eat certain foods, namely, refined carbohydrates like sugar, cookies, or sweets. But more than 30 research studies have shown that all carbohydrates have similar effects on blood sugar. That means a cookie elevates blood sugar about as much as a slice of bread or piece of fruit, Beebe says.

"For the most part, there is no reason why a person with diabetes can't include a cookie or other dessert item in a healthy meal plan," Beebe says. "It's simply unrealistic to expect that somebody is never going to eat sugar. It's the total amount of carbohydrates you eat each day that is really important."

Moderation is the key, she adds. Try to keep your simple-sugar intake down to 10 percent of your total calories each day. If you eat 2,000 calories a day, for example, you can allocate about 200 calories—that's about one scoop of ice cream or one or two brownies—to your sweet tooth.

Pay heed to your feet. Inspect your feet and between your toes every day, Dr. Krasner says. Diabetes can damage nerve endings in your feet and toes, making it difficult for you to feel sores, blisters, and other injuries. Look for cuts, breaks in the skin, or swollen, red areas. Consult your doctor or podiatrist about any infections, puncture wounds, or open sores on your feet.

Keep your feet clean and dry. Bathe your feet with warm water and mild soap every day. Dry them carefully, especially between the toes. Apply a thin coat of moisturizing lotion if the skin on your feet feels unusually dry. Wear clean socks and comfortable, well-fitting shoes. Never go barefoot. You're more likely to injure your feet if you do, Dr. Krasner warns.

Get a green light to drive. If you use insulin or diabetes pills and have a history of low blood sugar (hypoglycemia), test your blood sugar level before you begin driving, Dr. Krasner says. If your blood sugar is below 100 milligrams, don't get behind the wheel until you've stabilized your blood sugar to over 100 milligrams. Hypoglycemia can cause loss of conscious while driving, he says. If you are driving and feel symptoms of hypoglycemia, such as extreme confusion, fatigue, or irritability, pull to a stop by the side of the road and treat yourself for it immediately.

DIARRHEA

That aching in your gut and sudden need to get to the nearest toilet is, granted, not one of life's more elegant moments. But try to appreciate the episode for what it is: an overly protective measure by your body to get rid of something it sees as a threat to you. In simple terms, your digestive system identifies a problem—a food ingredient it can't digest or is allergic to, a spice or flavoring that irritates it, an invading bacterium bent on real harm—and moves to expel the offending pest.

Fortunately, most diarrheal episodes don't persist indefinitely. "Most cases of diarrhea are self-limited and resolve within 7 to 14 days," says Jorge Herrera, M.D., professor of medicine in the division of gastroenterology at the University of South Alabama College of Medicine in Mobile. See your doctor if it persists longer than that or if you have any of the other warning signs in "When to See a Doctor" on page 156. Diarrhea can be very harmful to you. But you can minimize its effects. Here's how.

Try This First

'Lyte up the town. You've heard that you should drink more water when you have diarrhea, but you might be better off drinking a sports beverage instead. During a diarrhea attack, you rapidly lose important body fluids and minerals called electrolytes. Electrolytes include glucose, sodium, potassium, chloride, magnesium, and phosphorous, all things your body needs to function properly, says Roger L. Gebhard, M.D., gastroenterologist at the Veterans Affairs Medical Center and professor of medicine in the division of gastroenterology at the University of Minnesota, both in Minneapolis. Just drinking water, he says, dilutes the remaining electrolytes in your body.

Instead, Dr. Gebhard suggests quaffing sports drinks such as

Gatorade or an electrolyte solution such as Pedialyte. Try to replace the approximate volume lost in diarrhea by drinking about eight ounces after every visit to the bathroom, plus two to four cups per day. If the volume is clearly larger, compensate by drinking even more. If that isn't handy, help yourself to some fruit juice or flavored drinks to help restore the balance.

Other Wise Ways

Keep it plain. What you eat during a bout of diarrhea is just as important as what you drink. This is not the time to eat any new

MANAGING YOUR MEDS

Many medicines can trigger a bout of diarrhea. Often, it can be an unexpected reaction or sensitivity to a medication, so be sure to ask your doctor about a possible substitute, says Jorge Herrera, M.D., professor of medicine in the division of gastroenterology at the University of South Alabama College of Medicine in Mobile. Some of the most common diarrhea causers include:

- Antibiotics such as amoxicillin (Amoxil) or azithromycin (Zithromax)
- Over-the-counter antacids (particularly those containing magnesium, like Maalox or Mylanta)
- Some anti-inflammatory medications prescribed for arthritis, such as naproxen (Naprosyn) or indomethacin (Indocin)
- Some medications used to lower blood pressure, like enalapril (Vasotec)
- Medications to treat constipation, especially stimulant laxatives containing bisacodyl or senna, such as Senokot, Ex-Lax, and Correctol, or laxatives such as mineral oil and castor oil

In fact, Dr. Herrera asserts that seniors are more susceptible to medicinal conflicts than other population groups. "As we grow older," he says, "the gut works a little bit less actively, so people get constipated and try to move their bowels every day." As a result, they rely on laxatives to get the desired effect. "An otherwise healthy person who's normally active should try not to supplement his normal diet with laxatives."

WHEN TO SEE A DOCTOR

Whenever diarrhea is accompanied by fever, blood in the stool, constant pain (instead of just cramps before or during a bowel movement), vomiting (for more than 24 hours), or dizziness when standing, consult a physician right away, says Jorge Herrera, M.D., professor of medicine in the division of gastroenterology at the University of South Alabama College of Medicine in Mobile. Such symptoms aren't run-of-the-mill and may signal a more serious ailment. Unless you are losing weight or the diarrhea is so severe that it interferes with your lifestyle, you can safely try to treat it at home for 7 to 14 days, advises Dr. Herrera. See your doctor if diarrhea doesn't make a run for it after two weeks.

and unusual foods that you've wanted to try, says Shobita Rajagopalan, M.D., assistant professor of medicine in the department of internal medicine at the Charles R. Drew University of Medicine and Science in Los Angeles.

Instead, Dr. Rajagopalan recommends a bland carbohydrate diet with foods such as rice, bread, or mashed potatoes. Foods that are sweet, sour, or spicy may stimulate peristalsis, the rhythmic, wavelike intestinal contractions that aid digestion and hasten diarrhea.

Mix it up. Dr. Gebhard offers a simple way to remember what to eat: Try the BRAT—bananas, rice, applesauce, and toast—diet, he notes, amending the formula to include a second T, which stands for tea.

K.O. with Kaopectate. Have some Kaopectate, says Dr. Gebhard. The remedy works simply by absorbing and binding irritating material in the gut, he adds. Follow the dosage instructions on the label.

Be antiantacid. Dr. Rajagopalan warns against antacids such as Maalox or Mylanta to treat diarrhea. "People often mistake bloating and gas with diarrhea symptoms," she explains, "so they take antacids. Unfortunately, these compounds contain magnesium, which can cause bowel movements."

Take a powder. For diarrhea, "a good natural remedy is carob powder, available at health food stores," says Andrew T. Weil, M.D., director of the program in integrative medicine and clinical professor of internal medicine at the University of Arizona College of Medicine in Tuscon. He recommends mixing one tablespoon of powder with applesauce and honey to make it palatable. Use this remedy no more than three times a day for no more than three days, until the symptoms subside, says Dr. Weil. Take it on an empty stomach with acidophilus, dried or liquid bacteria cultures that are considered friendly to the intestinal tract. When taking acidophilus, follow the instructions on the label. You'll find these ingredients in health food stores.

Know your body. Certain underlying medical conditions make some individuals more prone to diarrhea throughout their lives, say experts. If you have, for instance, food allergies, irritable bowel syndrome, lactose intolerance (LI), diabetes, or ulcers, you simply have to watch your diet more closely than other people do.

One of these conditions, LI, affects some 30 million Americans. People with LI lack an enzyme that digests lactose (a sugar found in dairy products). If they eat or drink dairy, they are likely to feel bloated, gassy, or diarrheal.

Dr. Gebhard notes that you can ask your doctor to administer a painless breath test to check for lactose intolerance. A confirmation of the condition could save you needless episodes of diarrhea.

Travel cautiously. Diarrhea sometimes is brought on when you take a trip outside the United States, especially to underdeveloped nations. This condition, known as traveler's diarrhea, is caused by bacteria that secrete toxins into the intestine. The microbes find their way into your system by way of food and water. Since you're just visiting, you haven't had time to build up the proper bacterial immunity.

Dr. Rajagopalan recommends several potential defenses against traveler's diarrhea.

- Drink bottled water.
- Peel all fruit that you intend to eat (the skin may have been washed with tainted water).
- Avoid raw and uncooked food.

Stick with the bottle. That country stream you noticed on your nature walk may look inviting, but don't drink from it. Dr. Herrera points out that many natural waterways can contain intestinal parasites that cause diarrhea. Carry bottled water with you and sip from that instead. If you're camping overnight and can't take along enough water, visit a camping-goods store to find out about water purifiers and water-purifying tablets.

DIVERTICULOSIS

Diverticulosis is a classic good-news–bad-news condition. On the one hand, it's a disease with virtually no symptoms, and it may never cause problems. On the other, diverticulosis can progress and become a related, though more serious, problem known as diverticulitis. Together, the two ailments are known as diverticular disease.

No question, you're at greater risk of getting diverticular disease as you get older. Diverticulosis, especially, is a common problem in America, reports Peter McNally, D.O, chief of gastroenterology at Evans Army Hospital in Colorado Springs, Colorado, and spokesperson for the American College of Gasteroenterology.

After you cross the treacherous waters of middle age, there's a very good chance that you'll get diverticulosis. According to the National Digestive Disorders Clearinghouse, about half of all Americans between 60 and 80 have diverticulosis, and almost everyone over 80 does.

Some definitions: A diverticulum is a grape-size pouch or sac that protrudes from the wall of the colon (large intestine). Sacs occur in other places along the gastrointestinal tract as well, but rarely. The pouches are thought to arise from excess pressure buildup in the colon, usually due to a lack of fiber in the diet. Doctors often compare the condition to an inner tube poking through weak spots on a tire.

Typically with diverticulosis, diverticuli (small multiple pouches) appear. Once established on the colon, they're permanent. Most people never know they have the condition, says Michael Epstein, M.D., founder of Digestive Disorders Associates in Annapolis, Maryland.

Diverticulitis occurs, though, when the diverticuli trap bits of stool or undigested food and become inflamed. This inflammation causes abdominal pain, usually around the left side of the lower abdomen. If the diverticuli become infected, the pain is accompanied by fever, nausea, vomiting, chills, and cramping. At this point, people often see their doctor, who diagnoses the disease. Because diverticulosis usually "flies below radar," people can miss opportunities to stop its transformation, says Dr. Epstein.

Fortunately, that transition from diverticulosis to diverticulitis may not occur—the statistical likelihood is 10 to 25 percent—and you can do things to improve your odds of never developing either affliction.

Try This First

Viva variety. In countries where dietary fiber is high, such as Africa and China, diverticular disease is virtually nonexistent. Although there's no conclusive evidence, that's a strong case for increasing your intake of fiber as part of a regular healthy diet, says Dr. McNally. "Try to get from 25 to 40 grams of fiber in your diet a day," he says. That's combined soluble and insoluble fiber because both can help. Soluble fiber, which dissolves easily in water, takes on a soft texture in the intestines that helps prevent dry, hard stools. Insoluble fiber passes almost unchanged through the intestines and adds bulk to the stool. Dr. McNally recommends incorporating high-fiber foods such as beans, whole grains like buckwheat, bran cereals such as Kellogg's All-Bran, fresh fruits like avocados, and vegetables such as artichokes into a daily regimen. Add fiber to your diet slowly. Too much, too soon may lead to gassiness, bloating, and diarrhea. Each week, increase your daily intake by no more than five grams, the amount of fiber in one cup of cooked carrots, says Dr. McNally.

Other Wise Ways

Raise your glass. Dr. Epstein says that increasing water and fiber at the same time is a good idea. Lacking sufficient fiber, the bowel has to work harder to push the stool out. He advises drinking plenty of fluids, six to eight glasses daily, which just means a tall glass every couple of hours. Not sure you're getting enough water? Test

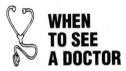

WHEN TO SEE A DOCTOR

Most people never know they have diverticuli (small multiple pouches that generally develop on the colon) until one of the sacs becomes inflamed. By then, the disease may have progressed into diverticulitis, a more serious complication.

Talk to your doctor if you feel unexplained pain in the lower left part of your abdomen, says Peter McNally, D.O, chief of gastroenterology at Evans Army Hospital in Colorado Springs, Colorado, and spokesperson for the American College of Gastroenterology. The pain may be accompanied by a fever and sweating, especially during bowel movements. If you have these symptoms or if you notice bloody stool, "see your doctor that day," says Dr. McNally.

yourself by examining your urine. "It should look light, not dark," says Dr. Epstein.

Build a base at breakfast. Another good idea: Mix a tablespoon of powdered fiber with a glass of orange juice in the morning. "It's a real simple, healthy way to start the day," says Dr. McNally. Check your pharmacy shelves for powdered fiber that comes in different flavors, consistencies, and sizes, like Metamucil and Citrucel.

Investigate veggies. "In the best of all possible worlds," says Joanne Curran-Celentano, Ph.D., R.D., associate professor of nutritional sciences at the University of New Hampshire in Durham, "you want to get a lot of fiber from vegetables" and not only because of their fiber content. Vegetables contain other desirable nutrients that are good for the body, such as cancer-fighting beta-carotene. Her favorites include kale and squash.

Subtract seeds. Doctors are currently debating the effects of seeds on diverticulosis. Some experts say that seeds of all types can aggravate the condition and lead to diverticulitis. Dr. Epstein, for instance, tells people to at least cut back on seeds as well as corn, nuts, and popcorn.

Stay active. As you age, physical activity falls off, notes Bryant Stamford, Ph.D., director of the Health Promotion and Wellness Center at the University of Louisville in Kentucky. Without the benefits of exercise, the gastrointestinal tract slows down, which can make diverticular disease worse. So try to get a little bit of exercise—even if it's just a walk around the block—every day, he suggests.

MANAGING YOUR MEDS

Sometimes, taking medicine is a catch-22. That's especially true if you have diverticulitis, because taking a pain medication may make your situation worse. Sure, the pain may go away for a time, but the pain medication may make your already sluggish colon move even slower and make your diverticulitis worse, says W. Steven Pray, Ph.D., R.Ph., professor of nonprescription drug products at Southwestern Oklahoma State University in Weatherford. Beware of constipation-causing pain medications, especially narcotics like codeine, which is found in products such as Tylenol with codeine, and morphine (Duramorph).

For more information on medications that can cause constipation, see "Managing Your Meds" on page 119.

Before taking corticosteroids, for example, fludrocortisone (Florinef), cortisone (Cortone Acetate), and dexamethasone (Decadron), be sure to tell your doctor that you have diverticulitis. These drugs can mask symptoms of diverticulitis and ulcers, says Dr. Pray.

Several drugs may even cause diverticulitis, warns Dr. Pray. Before taking donepezil (Aricept), which is used to treat Alzheimer's disease; risperidone (Risperdal), which is prescribed for psychotic disorders like schizophrenia; or sertraline (Zoloft), which is used to treat depression, alert your doctor if you have diverticulosis or are at risk for it.

If you already have diverticulitis, your doctor may have prescribed an antispasmodic such as hyoscyamine (Gastrosed). This powerful medication may interact with certain other medications. Be sure to tell your doctor if you are also taking any of the following:

- Over-the-counter diarrhea medicine containing kaolin and pectin (Kapectolin) or attapulgite (Kaopectate)
- Antifungals such as ketoconazole (Nizoral) that are used to treat serious fungus infections
- Tricyclic antidepressants such as amitriptyline (Elavil)
- Over-the-counter and prescription potassium supplements, which may be used to treat high blood pressure, such as potassium chloride (Kay Ciel)

DIZZINESS

Scientists are discovering that the topsy-turvy sensations astronauts endure following prolonged space flights are similar to the dizzy feelings that many Americans experience as they age, says William H. Paloski, Ph.D., director of NASA's life sciences research laboratories at the Johnson Space Center in Houston.

For astronauts, the answer is simple—the body's balance system needs gravity to work properly. So in the weightless environment of space, the balance system essentially shuts down, and astronauts must adapt to living in a world where up and down are meaningless. Once astronauts land, it takes time to get used to relying on their balance mechanisms again. As a result, they may feel dizzy and disoriented for a few days, Dr. Paloski says.

On Earth, particularly for older adults, dizziness also is a sign that the body's balance mechanisms are out of whack. Fatigue, stress, anemia, anxiety, inner-ear infections, and other common ailments can cause dizziness at any age. But many chronic conditions associated with aging, such as diabetes, heart disease, high blood pressure, and arteriosclerosis (hardening of the arteries), also can affect your balance, says Brian W. Blakley, M.D., chief of otolaryngology at the University of Manitoba Faculty of Medicine in Winnipeg and author of *Feeling Dizzy*. Here are a few ways to stop this topsy-turvy sensation.

Try This First

Get down. For mild dizziness, the best thing you can do is lie down, relax, and wait for the dizziness to go away, Dr. Blakley suggests. Often, the sensation will disappear within a few minutes. Even if you're at some social occasion, excuse yourself, take a break, and lie down on a couch or stretch out in a lounge chair with your feet as high as possible, at least higher than your heart. You want to elevate your legs to stimulate blood flow to your brain. If there's no place to lie down, just retire for a minute—even go to the john if you have to—sit down, and lower your head between your legs until the dizziness subsides, he suggests.

Other Wise Ways

Eat three squares a day. Skipping meals can result in low blood sugar, a common cause of dizziness, Dr. Blakley explains. Similarly, eating unusual fare like an all-liquid diet can create a mineral imbalance in your body that could cause wooziness. Eat at least three well-balanced meals a day consisting of 3 to 5 servings of fruits and

MANAGING YOUR MEDS

Almost any drug can cause dizziness, particularly when taken in conjunction with another medication made with the same active ingredient, says W. Steven Pray, Ph.D., R.Ph., a professor of nonprescription drug products at Southwestern Oklahoma State University in Weatherford. Sleeping pills like Nytol and allergy medications like Benadryl, for instance, both contain the antihistamine diphenhydramine. If you take these two over-the-counter (OTC) products together, it may cause an overdose of antihistamines and greatly increase your risk of developing dizziness and other side effects. Always ask your doctor or pharmacist about drug interactions before taking any combination of medications, he suggests. In addition, be aware that the following drugs also can turn your world upside down.

- High blood pressure medications including terazosin (Hytrin) and prazosin (Minipress)
- Anticonvulsants that contain phenytoin (Dilantin)
- Antibiotics such as cephalosporins (cephalexin)
- OTC and prescription pain medications including aspirin, ibuprofen, and codeine as found in many pain medications, such as Tylenol with codeine

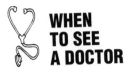

WHEN TO SEE A DOCTOR

Seek immediate medical attention if:

• Your dizziness is unexplained, severe, recurrent, or persistent.

• You also have difficulty speaking or swallowing.

• You also develop sudden weakness, numbness, or tingling on one side of your body.

• You also have a severe headache.

• Your vision suddenly gets worse or you develop double vision.

• You also have ringing in your ears or sudden loss of hearing in one ear.

• You feel dizzy after a fall or after a head injury.

vegetables; 6 to 11 servings of breads, cereal, and other foods made with grains; 2 to 3 servings of dairy products like milk and cheese; and 2 to 3 servings of meat and fish.

Shake the salt habit. Too much salt in the diet causes the body to retain fluid, which can disrupt the workings of the inner ear, according to Dr. Blakley. Avoid cheese, bacon, and salty snacks like potato chips, popcorn, and French fries. Read package labels carefully, and reach for foods that are advertised as having no salt added or being low in sodium or reduced sodium. Use herbs, spices, and fruit juices to season foods, he says. And be sure to rinse canned foods like tuna to remove salty juices.

Move like a snail. Rapid changes in head positions, particularly when you shift from lying down to standing up, can cause dizziness, Dr. Blakley explains. Move in stages. If you're getting out of bed, for instance, sit on the edge of the mattress for at least 30 seconds before standing.

Jump into the deep end. Practicing the very movements that cause dizziness can help your brain learn to compensate for the problem. As a starting point, Dr. Blakley suggests doing three repetitions of the following exercises, three or four times a day. These exercises are designed to stimulate the balance sensors in your inner ear. They are supposed to make you dizzy and should be done while sitting in a chair or other safe place so that you will not fall if you become dizzy. Keep your eyes open.

First, try some horizontal head rotations.

1. Start in a sitting position looking straight ahead.

2. Turn your head all the way to the right, keeping your chin parallel to the floor and moving it toward your right shoulder. Then turn all the way to the left, going back and forth, slowly increasing the speed of rotation of your head as much as you can in 20 seconds.

3. Rest a few seconds.

You can also try some vertical head rotations.

1. Start in the sitting position with your head turned a little, as if you are looking at an object to your right, and your chin parallel to the floor.

2. Move your head so that your left ear moves toward your left knee. Your ear will not touch your knee in this exercise. You will have to bend your neck. Move in this direction until your head is horizontal, usually about a foot above your knee.

3. Alternate between these two positions as quickly as you can for 20 seconds.

4. Rest a few seconds.

5. Do steps 1 and 2 in the opposite direction, turning your head to the left and then moving your right ear toward your right knee. Alternate between these positions as quickly as you can for 20 seconds.

Dry Eyes

L ike your car's windshield, your eyes have a built-in cleaning system designed to ensure better vision. To clean your windshield, you squirt fluid onto the glass and your wiper blades spread it around. To lubricate and clean your eyes, glands secrete tiny tears that get spread around by your eyelids when you blink. "Your eyes must constantly produce this tear fluid for you to feel comfortable and have clear vision," says Robert Cykiert, M.D., assistant professor of ophthalmology at New York University Medical Center in New York City. "Otherwise, they get dry and uncomfortable."

If you have dry eyes, you'll often feel like you have an eyelash stuck in your eye. Your eyes may burn, redden, and itch. Sometimes, your vision will blur.

Dry eyes become more noticeable as you age because your tear glands naturally stop producing as much fluid. In fact, the average person produces 60 percent fewer tears at age 65 than at age 18. The condition, however, is most common in postmenopausal women and may be related to hormonal changes. Rheumatoid arthritis and lupus can also cause dry eyes by inflaming those same glands.

Whatever has dried your eyes out, there are ways to combat the problem that will have you weeping with joy.

Try This First

Buy tears. Sold over-the-counter, artificial tears can provide the lubricant you need. You have your choice of dozens of products. All have their merits. But not all may be right for you, says Larry R. Taub, M.D., assistant professor of ophthalmology and director of comprehensive ophthalmology at Emory University School of Medicine in Atlanta. So choose those that are most comfortable to you.

Artificial tears have the following differences.

Thick versus watery. Thicker tears and ointments will stay on your eyes longer, but they can temporarily make your vision blurry. Ointments work best at night when it's impractical to keep getting up and applying tears. Dr. Taub suggests that you use thicker tears during the day when thinner tears stop working their magic. You can tell if tears are thick or thin by checking the active ingredients. Thicker tears contain methylcellulose.

Preservatives versus no preservatives. "Preservative" isn't necessarily a bad word. It makes your bottle of tears last longer. Tears without a preservative can only be used right after opening and then must be thrown away, which makes them more expensive. Some people, however, find tears containing preservatives to be irritating, says Dr. Taub. Use the kind with preservatives if you only need to apply tears four or five times a day. If you need more frequent applications, switch to a brand that is labeled preservative-free. It may cost a little more, but your eyes will thank you.

Once you choose a type of ointment or drops, try different brands in that class. Some may work better for you than others.

MANAGING YOUR MEDS

Any type of antihistamine—whether prescription or over-the-counter—can dry out your eyes, says Larry R. Taub, M.D., assistant professor of ophthalmology and director of comprehensive ophthalmology at Emory University School of Medicine in Atlanta. If you take antihistamines like diphenhydramine (Benadryl) for allergies, consider cutting back your dosage. Motion sickness medications like dimenhydrinate (Dramamine) also contain antihistamines. Or up your use of artificial tears, he says.

Other medications that may dry out your eyes include:

- Some heart medications such as propranolol (Inderal) that are used to treat high blood pressure
- Some antidepressants like amitriptyline (Elavil)
- Over-the-counter decongestants used for nasal stuffiness, such as pseudoephedrine (Sudafed) or phenylpropanolamine (Tavist-D)
- Anticholinergics like dicyclomine (Bentyl) and scopolamine (Transderm Scōp), used to treat intestinal or urinary problems

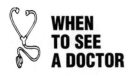

WHEN TO SEE A DOCTOR

If you can get by on three or four drops of artificial tears a day and your eyes aren't bothering you too much, you don't need to get help. But if you need to apply drops more often, consider seeing your eye doctor, advises Robert Cykiert, M.D., assistant professor of ophthalmology at New York University Medical Center in New York City.

An ophthalmologist can insert plugs into the tiny hole in the corner of your eyelid. The plugs will prevent tears from draining into the back of your nose. This is a quick, reversible office procedure that takes just a few minutes.

If you wear contact lenses, ask your doctor about getting refitted with a type that doesn't need as much moisture.

Other Wise Ways

Get rid of anti-redness drops. Stay away from eyedrops that are designed to ease red, bloodshot eyes, such as Visine or Murine. They may make your eyes look better, but the ingredients in these drops can actually dry you out more than they help, says Paula Newsome, O.D., optometrist and spokesperson for the Better Vision Institute in Charlotte, North Carolina.

Stay away from irritants. Pollen, pollution, smoke, and other airborne particles won't necessarily dry out your eyes. But they can make already dry eyes feel uncomfortable and red, explains Dr. Taub. So sit in the nonsmoking section at restaurants, run a filtered air conditioner during the summer, and wear the kind of sunglasses that wrap around your eyes in windy, dusty areas. Sunglasses will also keep the bright light from the sun from irritating your sensitive eyes.

Preserve your natural tears. Dry winter heat, a hair dryer in your face, or your car's air-conditioning vent all can suck the moisture from your eyes. So keep that blast of air pointed in a different direction. And use a humidifier during winter months, says Dr. Taub. Such methods will keep you from robbing your eyes of their own moisture.

Apply a warm compress. Heat will stimulate your glands to produce more oil, which will keep your tears from evaporating as quickly, says James Gigantelli, M.D., director of ophthalmic plastic and reconstructive surgery at the University of Missouri in Columbia. Fill a washbasin with hot tap water and immerse a washcloth. Apply the washcloth to your eyes for about 10 minutes twice a day.

Drink plenty of water. Guzzling down glass after glass of water won't solve your problems entirely. But it can aid you in your quest to keep your eyes moist, says Dr. Newsome. Aim for eight eight-ounce glasses per day.

Take reading breaks. When you read or work at a computer, you often forget to blink, which keeps the fluid that you do have from getting spread out over your eyes, warns Dr. Cykiert. You can't consciously remember to blink. You'll drive yourself nuts. But you can take a break every 10 minutes or so. That way you'll naturally resort to your normal blink rate.

Dry Hair

Bad hair isn't intentionally trying to ruin your evening, it's trying to tell you something. "Your hair is kind of smart, if you listen to it," says Barbara Bealer, assistant education director of the Allentown School of Cosmetology in Pennsylvania. "It tells you what it needs."

So what is your hair trying to tell you when its ends look like the bristles on a broom? "It's telling you to stop doing whatever is causing it to dry out and find a conditioner that will help replace some of the natural oils that are being stripped out," says Clay Cockerell, M.D., clinical associate professor of dermatology and pathology at the University of Texas Southwestern Medical Center in Dallas.

Whatever is causing the dryness, you can minimize the damage with these simple strategies.

Try This First

Condition the condition. After each washing of your hair, Dr. Cockerell suggests applying a conditioner specifically designed for dry hair. Look for a conditioner that says "for dry hair" on the label. Conditioners replace or lock in the natural oils that often get stripped out. Conditioning your hair after each washing should help you lubricate your once-dry hair, he says.

For best results, leave the conditioner in your hair for three to five minutes before rinsing, says Bealer. Deeper conditioners require longer timing, so check the directions before application.

Other Wise Ways

Oil it up. For both dry hair and a dry scalp, good old-fashioned castor oil provides an effective solution, says Kenneth Battelle,

170

owner and master stylist at Kenneth's Salon in New York City's Waldorf-Astoria Hotel. If you have a dry scalp, warm up some castor oil by putting a small amount into a pot and heating it on a very low setting until it is warm to the touch. Then massage it into your scalp. Wrap your head in a hot, steamy towel for 15 minutes and then wash, he says. (To get this effect, you can run towels through the washing machine using hot water but no detergent.) Or you can wrap your oiled-up head in a dry towel and sit under a hair dryer set on low for 10 minutes, he says.

If the ends of your hair are dry, but not your scalp, Battelle recommends applying the heated oil only to the ends of your hair. Leave it on for 10 to 15 minutes and then wash with a shampoo designed specifically for dry hair. Battelle notes that castor oil is very hard to get out of your hair, so you'll need to wash your hair with hot (not scalding) water and plenty of suds. If you don't have castor oil on hand, olive, mineral, avocado, or even vegetable oil should work just as well.

Wash every other day. If you have a problem with dry hair, your hair needs a day off between washings. "Somewhere along the way, it became vogue to wash your hair every day. But there's no rule that says you have to," notes Dr. Cockerell. "Constant hair washing with a harsh shampoo strips the natural oils," he says. By washing every other day, you're still getting your hair clean enough, and the alternating schedule helps save your hair from drying out.

Take a walk on the mild side. When you do wash your hair, use a gentle shampoo such as a baby shampoo, suggests Fredric S. Brandt, M.D., clinical associate professor of dermatology at the University of Miami School of Medicine. "Using a mild shampoo is a good idea because it won't strip away too many of your hair's protective oils," he says.

Turn to the rinse cycle. After swimming in the ocean or a pool, rinse your hair immediately to get rid of the salt or chlorine. "People of all ages who swim often should be sure to wash the chlorine or salt out of their hair as soon as possible, because it can do some damage to your hair over time," says Dr. Brandt.

Don't give your hair a knockdown blow. Folks with dry hair should avoid excessive blow-drying. When your hair is wet, just let it dry naturally. "That's better for the overall health of your hair," he

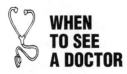

WHEN TO SEE A DOCTOR

says. If you must use a blow-dryer, use a spray-in conditioner while drying your hair to protect it from excess damage, he adds.

Spoon-feed it. People on low-fat diets might not be getting enough oils in their bodies—and if that's so, then their scalps and hair might be deprived. But of course, you don't want to add a lot of heart-hurting, fat-producing oils to your diet just to improve your hair.

The solution? Supplement a low-fat diet with some heart-healthy olive oil. "I suggest taking a teaspoon of olive oil per day," says Dr. Brandt. "You should see a difference in the dryness of your skin and hair in a week or two," he says. Try incorporating the oil into a salad dressing, or drizzle it over bread.

Dry Hands

They hurt, burn, and are often as dry as the Mojave Desert. Most folks refer to them as dishpan hands, but you don't even have to wash dishes to suffer from them.

Several factors can cause your hands to dry up. Living in an extremely dry climate, like Phoenix, can be a beautiful but dehydrating experience. The dry air absorbs the natural moisture throughout the body, including in your hands. And of course, several everyday chores can be hazardous to your hands' health, including dish washing, laundry, housecleaning, and bathing of grandchildren. These chores often involve the use of chemical agents such as household cleansers and solvents that damage and dry out your hands. Just the act of washing your hands also robs them of moisture.

Even if you don't expose them to hot water and chemicals, your hands tend to get drier with age. That's because your body loses some of its moisture with each passing year, says Dee Anna Glaser, M.D., assistant professor of dermatology at the St. Louis University School of Medicine. "Skin loses some of its thickness and water-retaining ability over time, even without aggravating factors like a really dry climate or constant contact with cleaning solutions," says Dr. Glaser.

Unless they get so dry that they crack and bleed, dry hands are more nuisance than nightmare. And there are ways you can bring moisture back into those dehydrated digits.

Try This First

Make lotion your favorite potion. Every time you wash your hands, put on a little moisturizer afterward, says Dr. Glaser. With every washing, you're removing moisture-encasing oils

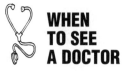

WHEN TO SEE A DOCTOR

from your hands as well as dirt and grime. By applying a hand lotion, you replenish those lost oils and keep your skin from drying out. "Find a hand lotion that you like and keep it near your sink and in your purse or desk, so that you can apply it to your hands after each time you wash them," says Dr. Glaser.

Over-the-counter lotions do just fine, says Stephen Schleicher, M.D., co-director of the Dermatology Center in Philadelphia. He recommends any of the following for his patients: Alpha Keri, Aquaderm, Aquaphor, Complex 15, Curel, Cutemol, Dermasil, Derma Centre, Eucerin, Keri, Lubriderm, Oil of Olay, Pen-Kera, and UltraDerm.

Other Wise Ways

Soften your soaps. The harsher the soap, the more oils and moisture you'll strip from your hands. Dr. Glaser suggests that you wash your hands with a gentle hand cleanser such as Dove or Oil of Olay. These soaps contain emollients, which are agents that soften or smooth the skin.

Oil 'em up. To buy a simple hand cream at the cosmetics department of your local department store, you might have to pay a small fortune. But just stroll down the vegetable oil aisle in the supermarket to find a hand moisturizer that's just as good and a lot less expensive. Regular vegetable shortening like Crisco soothes cracked, dry hands, Dr. Glaser says. To get the most out of the oil, rub it over your hands at night before you go to bed. Then put on a pair of old gloves. Not only will the gloves save you from ruining your linens but also they will force the oil to penetrate your skin, she says.

Wear washup gloves, too. You often put your hands into terrible conditions: hot water, bathroom cleaners, ammonia, bleach. Protect them from the ravages of such harsh substances by wearing a pair of vinyl gloves with cotton liners. The vinyl outside keeps the water off your hands, while the cotton liner absorbs sweat so that your hands won't get wet inside. Wear them whenever you wash dishes or use any other possible irritants such as chemicals and cleaning products.

Tap into water. Drink at least eight glasses of water per day, says Dr. Glaser. Dry hands are the result of a lack of moisture in the skin, so not drinking enough water may aggravate dryness in the hands.

DRY MOUTH

Call it what you will—slobber, drool, or spittle—saliva is a wondrous substance. It's your first line of defense against predatory fungi, viruses, and bacteria that are lurking in every crevice of your jowls. It's loaded with protective minerals like calcium that help keep your teeth strong. It helps you swallow soothing teas, colas, and wines. It allows you to savor the taste of flavorful foods. Its lubricating moisture even helps you pronounce words clearly. In short, saliva keeps your mouth a flourishing utopia.

Without enough of it, your mouth can quickly become something akin to Death Valley—a harsh, arid environment vulnerable to ravages of tooth decay and gum erosion.

"Dry mouth is very serious in terms of the health of the mouth," says Philip C. Fox, D.D.S., clinical director of the National Institute of Dental Research in Bethesda, Maryland. "Dry mouth can play a tremendous role in the development of cavities, fungal infections, and tooth loss."

Often, dry mouth is triggered by autoimmune disorders like rheumatoid arthritis, lupus, or Sjögren's syndrome. Other chronic ailments that are common among seniors, like diabetes and Parkinson's disease, also can dry out your mouth. In addition, anemia, anxiety, stress, and depression can slow saliva production to a trickle. More than 400 drugs, including many used to treat high blood pressure and some heart conditions also can cause your mouth to feel as arid as the Sahara. Radiation therapy and other cancer treatments can also trigger dry mouth.

"We can't always cure dry mouth, particularly if it is caused by a disease," says Gretchen Gibson, D.D.S., director of the geriatric dentistry program at the Veterans Administration Medical Center in Dallas. "That doesn't mean you can't do something to relieve it."

Try This First

Take H₂O wherever you go. Keep a water bottle handy and take frequent sips, Dr. Fox suggests. Sipping will help keep your mouth better lubricated than gulping down a glass of water all at once. Take small swigs. Ultimately, you want to be quaffing about a cup of water every hour, he suggests.

Other Wise Ways

Hold your grounds. Overindulging in caffeine will make a dry mouth worse. Limit yourself to no more than one cup of coffee or tea a day, Dr. Gibson suggests.

Skip the sodas. Dry mouth and carbonated beverages don't mix, Dr. Ettinger says. Without sufficient saliva to break it down, the acid in sodas and other carbonated drinks will further dry out your mouth and can severely damage your teeth and gums.

MANAGING YOUR MEDS

More than 400 prescription and over-the-counter medications can contribute to dry mouth, says Ronald Ettinger, D.D.Sc., director of geriatric dental programs at the University of Iowa College of Dentistry in Iowa City. If you suspect that one of your medications is causing mouth dryness, ask your doctor or pharmacist if another drug might be less dehydrating. Among the common drugs taken by seniors that can cause mouth dryness are:

- Calcium channel blockers like verapamil (Calan, Isoptin), used to control irregular heartbeats
- Antidepressants like amitriptyline (Elavil)
- High blood pressure medications like prazosin (Minipress) or propranolol (Inderal)
- Diuretics such as furosemide (Lasix) or chlorothiazide (Diuril)
- Antihistamines found in over-the-counter products such as chlorpheniramine (Chlor-Trimeton), brompheniramine (Dimetapp), and diphenhydramine (Benadryl)

WHEN TO SEE A DOCTOR

Any persistent dry mouth lasting more than a day or two should be brought to the attention of your dentist, says Ronald Ettinger, D.D.Sc., director of geriatric dental programs at the University of Iowa College of Dentistry in Iowa City. In particular, seek dental care if:

• You have to drink fluids frequently to alleviate thirst and the dry feeling in your mouth.

• Dryness interferes with your ability to eat or speak.

If your dentist can't find the source of the problem, ask for a second opinion, Dr. Ettinger urges.

Lose the brew, too. Alcohol is another favorite beverage that dries the mouth, Dr. Gibson says. So cork your alcohol consumption but also be wary of hidden alcohol in medicines and mouthwashes, which can be as high as 26 percent alcohol. As an alternative, look for alcohol-free mouth rinses.

Snuff the smokes. Reason 3,577 to quit: Tobacco smoke burns the moisture right out of your mouth, says Robert Henry, D.M.D., dentist in Lexington, Kentucky, and past president of the American Society for Geriatric Dentistry.

Moisten the air. Put a cool-air vaporizer in your bedroom. This can add much needed humidity to the air and prevent you from waking up with dry mouth, says Ronald Ettinger, D.D.Sc., director of geriatric dental programs at the University of Iowa College of Dentistry in Iowa City. You'll find vaporizers in most pharmacies or variety stores.

Brush up on oral hygiene. If you have dry mouth, your teeth and gums are more susceptible to infection, which not only can lead to tooth loss but also can make your mouth feel even drier. So it's particularly important to brush after every meal and floss at least once a day, Dr. Ettinger says.

Get a squirt of instant wetness. Saliva substitutes like Optimoist and moisturizing gels and toothpastes like Oralbalance and Bioténe can provide temporary relief from dry mouth, Dr. Gibson says. These over-the-counter products, which can be used as needed, help coat and protect your gums and mouth, particularly at night. They also can be used under dentures to provide moisture and reduce friction.

"The Oralbalance and Biotène products work because they contain many of the proteins and enzymes you find in real saliva," Dr. Gibson says. "But they're only an interim solution because they will not make you produce more saliva."

Gnaw on a sugarless delight. Chew on a piece of sugarless gum, or suck on a piece of sugarless hard candy for 5 to 10 minutes every two hours. This can help stimulate your salivary glands so you'll have a more sustained flow of fluid in your mouth, Dr. Gibson says.

Blaze a homeopathic trail. If you have dry mouth accompanied by cracks in the corners of your mouth, loss of taste, and dehydration, try a 30X daily dose of Natrum muriaticum, a homeopathic remedy available at most health food stores, suggests Flora Parsa Stay, D.D.S., dentist in Oxnard, California, and author of *The Complete Book of Dental Remedies*. Or you can take a 6X dose of Bryonia, another homeopathic remedy, three times a day to help relieve a parched mouth.

Dissolve the tablets under your tongue. Do not eat or drink for 15 minutes before or after taking one of these remedies, Dr. Stay says. If you don't see improvement within 10 days, try another remedy.

Homeopathic remedies are extremely dilute doses of substances that would otherwise cause the symptoms that you're suffering. According to homeopathic practice, the correct remedy depends on your particular symptoms. The notations 30X and 6X (as well as C measurements) are standard measurements in homeopathy and refer to a remedy's potency, which is listed on the label.

Dry Skin

L ife can be hard on your skin. So many showers, baths, and swimming pools. So many hours in the sun, wind, and rain. Like the natural forces that can erode mountains, these everyday experiences have the unfortunate power to erode the skin's protective layer of lipids, or oils.

By the time you've seen the passage of 22,000 days or so, your skin has been through a lot. Whatever it shows on the surface, just underneath it's wearing a bit thin—and where skin cells are skimpy, your body has a harder time holding moisture. The diminished lipid layer no longer holds moisture very well, says Norman Levine, M.D, professor and chief of dermatology at the University of Arizona Health Sciences Center in Tucson. And when you have only a skinny layer for moisture storage, you tend to get dry, sensitive skin.

But you don't have to give in to the forces of nature. You can even counteract the wear-away work of the elements that are against you. As it happens, there are a number of ways you can re-capture your lost moisture. Here's how you can literally save your skin.

Try This First

Rebuild your barriers. The best answer to dry skin, say Dr. Levine and other experts, is to rebuild your skin's protective barrier with a good moisturizer. Apply it all over at least twice a day. The moisturizer can replace some of the missing elements that used to allow your skin to retain fluids and keep itself moist.

Almost any moisturizer is fine, says Guy F. Webster, M.D., Ph.D., associate professor of dermatology at Thomas Jefferson University in Philadelphia. "Even petroleum jelly is a good moisturizer be-cause it seals the skin and prevents moisture from being exposed to air and then evaporating." Dr. Webster also notes that when purchasing a moisturizer, you should look for the ingredient urea acid or lactic acid. The better moisturizers will contain one of those.

Other Wise Ways

Go for a lipid cleanser. Most soaps contain detergents that break down and wash away the skin's natural oils, which is precisely what you don't want to happen. When you wash, use a gentle soap substitute that is designed to cleanse your skin without removing the oil. Look for body washes that contain lipids. (Lipid cleansers will have an oil such as mineral, linseed, castor, or soybean oil listed as part of the ingredients.) These products are gentle on the skin and are excellent moisturizers, says Mary Ruth Buchness, M.D., chief of dermatology at St. Vincent's Hospital and Medical Center in New York City and associate professor of dermatology and medicine at New York Medical College in Valhalla. Cleansers that contain lipids include Nivea Visage Gentle Cleansing Lotion, Noxema Plus Cleansing Cream, and Ponds Cold Cream Deep Cleanser.

Lather up with moisturizing soaps. There are many moisturizing soaps available. Among the most widely recommended by dermatologists are Basis for Dry Skin or Neutrogena Dry Skin.

MANAGING YOUR MEDS

Many medications can dry out your skin, says W. Steven Pray, Ph.D., R.Ph., professor of nonprescription drug products at Southwestern Oklahoma State University in Weatherford. Drugs prescribed for edema (water retention) are meant to dry out the body. These include loop diuretics such as furosemide (Lasix), and potassium-sparing ones, for example, triamterene (Dyrenium). And many high blood pressure medications, for example, chlorothiazide (Diuril), have a similar diuretic effect. If you are currently taking medication and are concerned about dry skin, ask your doctor about the side effects of your medications. But be sure you don't drop any medication, especially for high blood pressure, unless your doctor is informed and gives consent.

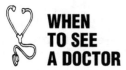

WHEN TO SEE A DOCTOR

If your dry skin is so severe that you're constantly scratching it raw or if it actually cracks and bleeds when you're just doing everyday things like walking or flexing your hand or arm, you may have a skin problem that can be treated. Your first line of defense may be an over-the-counter 1-percent hydrocorti-sone cream, says Norman Levine, M.D, professor and chief of dermatology at the University of Arizona Health Sciences Center in Tucson. Just follow the package di-rections. If you don't get any relief, consult your doctor, suggests Dr. Levine.

Other good soap substitutes include Cetaphil or Phisoderm.

Or go the water route. The fact is, you don't have to use a soap or soap substitute all over your body. Just wash your face, hands, and odor-producing areas of your body such as your armpits and groin. Just rinse off the rest, suggests Dr. Levine.

Ration your bathing. It seems ironic, but one of the greatest threats to a skin's ability to stay moist is water itself, especially when it's piping hot. Hot water is especially de-structive to the skin's natural oils, says Dr. Levine. Bathe as infrequently as possible, he advises, especially in winter when the air is dry. Once every two, three, or even four days might be enough for you. And when you do take a bath or shower, use lukewarm water and avoid lingering too long.

Leave a little water behind. After your shower or bathe, pat yourself dry, leaving a little moisture on your skin, advises Dr. Buchness. Then apply your moisturizer. By applying your moisturizer on top of your slightly wet skin, you are sealing in the moisture and thus preventing it from es-caping.

Hydrate with alpha hydroxy. Doctors may argue over the value of alpha hydroxy acids (AHAs) for eliminating wrinkles. But AHAs can remove dry, dead, and scaly skin and then moisturize the new tissue below. AHA moisturizers, which are made from milk, fruit, and sugarcane, trap water and hold it within your skin. By eliminating dead cells and plumping up the new ones, these mois-turizers help keep your skin moist and youthful, says Dr. Buchness.

Give your skin a vacation. Before you go on your next vacation, consider what the climate will be like. "Very often, people who suffer from dry skin don't think about where they go on vacation and then find that their skin is even drier and more irritated when they go," explains Dr. Buchness. If you're in a humid place like New Orleans, your dry skin condition may ease a little. But what if you head for Arizona, where the temperatures are high and the humidity is down in the single-digit figures? That's just the kind of place where your skin could be most miserable. Instead, plan a trip to a place where your skin will get relief, too.

EARACHES

Sometimes, an earache isn't really coming from the ear. Often, ear pain is referred pain, meaning that it is really coming from somewhere else nearby. It could be a throat problem or pain from a nearby joint (the jaw, for example). Ear pain could even signal a toothache, says Charles P. Kimmelman, M.D., professor of otolaryngology at Cornell University Medical College and attending physician at Manhattan Eye, Ear, and Throat Hospital, both in New York City.

Ear pain, of course, may also mean that your ear just hurts. Sometimes, this is the result of an ear infection. To be sure of what's causing the discomfort, you should see your doctor any time you have an earache that lasts more than a day or two.

But until you get to the doctor's office, you can soothe earache pain in a number of ways.

Try This First

Crank up the heat. You can use heat to treat earaches, says Michael Wynne, Ph.D., associate professor in the department of otolaryngology at the Indiana University School of Medicine in Indianapolis. Lay a warm, damp washcloth, heating pad, or hot-water bottle wrapped in a towel over the outside of your ear. You can apply the heat steadily for as long as the pain lasts. The heat over your ear will help stimulate circulation and relieve the pressure that causes the pain of earaches, Dr. Wynne says.

Other Wise Ways

Drop in some oil. Put a couple of drops of warm baby or mineral oil in your ear canal (as long as you're certain that you've never had a ruptured eardrum), says Jennifer Derebery, M.D., otologist at the House Ear Clinic and Institute and assistant clinical professor of otolaryngology at the University of Southern California School of Medicine in Los Angeles. Once again, the warmth should soothe your pain. You can warm the oil by holding the bottle under hot water for a minute or two. Before you put the oil in your ear, put a dab on the back of your hand. If it's too hot for your hand, you can bet that it's too hot for your ear canal. After inserting the drops, wipe any excess oil off the outside of your ear.

Massage a little. Earache pain can be very sharp, so people tend to tense up, Dr. Wynne says. Relax that tension with a little light massage. Using your fingertips, apply gentle pressure and rub your jaw and neck with circular strokes for 5 to 10 minutes. Massaging the large muscle groups in the jaw and the back of the neck helps reduce tension and improves overall relaxation, thereby decreasing some of the discomfort, he says.

Quit abusing cotton swabs. Cotton-tipped swabs are fine for cleaning your outer ears, but when you start using them to clean out wax from inside your ear canal, you may as well be sending out an engraved invitation to an ear infection. So don't. Not only can swabs break the inner ear's delicate skin and make way for infection, Dr. Wynne says, but they can cause problems when they accidentally get shoved in too far or break off and damage an eardrum. And earwax, believe it or not, is a first line of defense against infection and, therefore, ear pain. Too much aggressive earwax removal clears the way for bacteria to proceed unhindered to your inner ear.

Swim smart. Getting lots of water in your ear can happen when you do a lot of swimming. That can also have an effect on your earwax, softening it, lowering its acidity, and causing the general irritation known as swimmer's ear. To combat this problem, you can use earplugs while swimming. Of course, some people are prone to swimmer's ear and can even get it from showering. Putting a few drops of the product Swim Ear or rubbing alcohol in your ear canal can dry up the moisture that leads to swimmer's ear. Better yet, mix a solution that is 50 percent alcohol and 50 percent white vinegar. Use an eyedropper to put a couple of drops of the solution in your ear after swimming, Dr. Wynne suggests. The alcohol helps

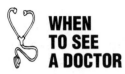

WHEN TO SEE A DOCTOR

If you have ear pain after any kind of blow to the ear, see your doctor immediately because you may have damaged your eardrum. If your ear pain is accompanied by dizziness, loss of hearing on one side, headaches, and facial paralysis, absolutely get it checked out by your doctor. Such symptoms indicate a potentially serious problem, such as a benign growth on the nerve to your ear.

evaporate the water that can lead to irritation, and the vinegar helps keep the acidic value of the ear canal high.

Clear your tubes. If you have a cold or flu and have to be flying, think about taking a decongestant a half-hour before you board (and before you land, if your flight will last longer than the effect of the medication) to help keep the eustachian tubes in your ears clear, explains Dr. Wynne. It is the blockage in these tubes, which lead from your ear to your nose, that make it difficult for your ears to adjust to altitude changes. That allows pressure to build up behind your eardrums, causing pain.

Keep your jaw flapping. Any time you face a change in altitude and pressure, do things that keep you swallowing, says Dr. Wynne. That opens the eustachian tubes and thus can prevent ear pain. Chew gum, yawn, sip a drink—it all helps equalize the pressure that builds in your ears when the plane is ascending or descending.

EAR HAIR

It's God's little practical joke, says John F. Romano, M.D., clinical associate professor of dermatology at New York Hospital–Cornell Medical Center in New York City. "He takes the hair from your head and puts it on your ears and nose."

The humor may be lost on you if you're the one who suddenly finds that he has fuzz growing out of his ears. This new growth of hair is unfortunately a normal part of male aging. No one is entirely sure what makes it happen, but one theory is that as you age, the hair follicles in and around your ears and nose may become more sensitive to the male hormone testosterone, which stimulates the unwanted hair growth.

Science has not successfully tackled the problem of permanently removing hair, but there are some things you can do on a regular basis to keep the hair in check.

Try This First

Get a close shave. Shaving around the outer ear and the lobe is an effective, albeit temporary, method for getting rid of external hair, Dr. Romano says. You can make it easier by lathering up but then removing the lather just prior to shaving to improve visibility. Some of the softening effects of the cream will remain. Or you can use your electric shaver to gently shave the hairs off your lobe and outer ear.

For the peskier hair that seems to congregate just at the edge of your inner ear, your best and safest bet is to invest in a personal grooming shaver. These reasonably priced shavers differ from a standard electric razor in that they are much smaller in width and are designed for smaller surfaces, making it easy to mow down hair found growing just outside the ear.

187

Other Wise Ways

Melt it away. Using chemical depilatories on the outside of your ear is another way to remove the hair. Just remember that under no circumstance should you stick the depilatory into your ear canal, Dr. Romano says. Be sure to limit the product to only the lobe and rim and go nowhere near the opening, he says. Brands such as Neet and Nair can be purchased in any store. If using a chemical depilatory is a new thing to you, be sure to follow the instructions on the back of the package. It's always advisable to test a small amount of depilatory on your skin first in case you might be sensitive to it.

Snip what's sticking out. A small pair of scissors can be used to cut away ear hair on the inner ear, especially if the hair is sticking out of the ear and you can see it with a mirror. If it's bothering you and you can't see it, don't use a scissors on your own, Dr. Romano says. One slip, and you could do serious damage to your eardrum or ear canal. Ask your doctor to help you.

Keep your ears clean. Excess ear hair can have an effect on your hearing in a roundabout way. Earwax can get all tangled in your ear hair and pile up, causing temporary hearing loss, Dr. Romano explains. To avoid this problem, wipe your outer ear with a warm, damp washcloth daily. You can also purchase wax removal kits.

Earwax

Formed by glands near the outer ends of the ear canals, earwax is there to trap dirt and dust particles and lubricate the skin in the ear canals, thus protecting your sensitive inner ears. It also has antifungal and antibacterial properties, which protect you from infection. Normally, it is formed in a thin translucent layer that gently migrates toward your outer ear, where it dries up and flakes away.

Sometimes, the wax can build up and block your ear canals. And the older you are, the more wax problems you may have, says Michael Wynne, Ph.D., associate professor in the department of otolaryngology at the Indiana University School of Medicine in Indianapolis. "Older adults tend to have more problems with wax, and that's just simply because the rate of skin growth in the ear canal doesn't occur as rapidly," Dr. Wynne says. That can cause the natural migration of the earwax to slow down.

Seniors, however, can also have the opposite problem, says Ernest Mhoon, M.D., professor of otolaryngology at the University of Chicago. Wax glands can atrophy, causing an underproduction of wax and, consequently, itchy ears.

Wax is not simply a cosmetic problem. Wax can become so impacted that it can block the ear canal and cause hearing loss. That needn't happen if you use these strategies.

Try This First

Follow your mom's advice. To take care of earwax, all you may need is a warm, wet washcloth. Use it to clean out the bowls of your ears every time you bathe or shower. This can help ensure that you don't have wax pileups in your ear canals, explains Dr. Mhoon.

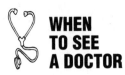

WHEN TO SEE A DOCTOR

If you experience pain, bleeding, or pus coming from your ears, be sure to see a doctor before you try to clean out your ears. Any of these symptoms might indicate an infection, says Michael Wynne, Ph.D., associate professor in the department of otolaryngology at the Indiana University School of Medicine in Indianapolis.

Also, if you have trouble hearing, earwax may only be part of the problem, says Dr. Wynne. Be sure to see your doctor to determine whether you have some persistent hearing loss for other reasons.

Other Wise Ways

Soften it up. The worst thing about wax accumulation is that it can also harden, becoming like a rock in your ear canal. To avoid that, use an eyedropper and put one or two drops of warm oil into your ear a couple of times a week. You can use mineral, baby, or vegetable oil. The warm oil keeps the wax soft and lets it continue to migrate out of your ear, says Dr. Wynne.

Put in some peroxide. Some hydrogen peroxide that is diluted by 50 percent with distilled water can soften up the earwax, helping it on its natural journey out of your ear, says Dr. Wynne. Using an eyedropper, tilt your head to one side—the problem ear should be facing the ceiling—and squeeze two or three drops of the hydrogen peroxide/distilled water mixture in your ear. You can place cotton in your ear to keep the hydrogen peroxide from leaking out of your ear canal. After a couple of minutes, remove the cotton and allow everything to drain out.

Watch the wax kits. Earwax kits that you buy in the pharmacy can be effective, but you have to use them correctly, says Jennifer Derebery, M.D., otologist at the House Ear Clinic and Institute and assistant clinical professor of otolaryngology at the University of Southern California School of Medicine in Los Angeles. The kit comes with a rubber bulb that you fill with water, then squirt it into the ear.

But if you use one of these kits, you have to follow the instructions carefully. Before you use the bulb, you have to tilt your head and pull your ear up and back to straighten out your ear canal. If it's not lined up just right, you might end up pushing the wax deeper into your eardrum.

Your best tactic is to enlist the aid of a family member, advises Dr. Derebery. And be sure you don't use this method if you know or suspect that you have a hole in your eardrum, she warns. The water can get into the hole and cause an infection.

Trim that hair. In older men, ear hair can get tangled with the earwax, preventing it from migrating out of the ear, says Dr. Wynne. Keep the hair in and around the opening to your ear canal trimmed if this is a problem.

Give your hearing aid a rest. Like ear hair, hearing aids can block the natural path of earwax and trigger a buildup, says Solomon Greer, M.D., ear, nose, and throat doctor in private practice in Chicago. "People with hearing aids can have high accumulations of wax because the wax doesn't come out as easily as it should." The best thing to do is make sure you clean your hearing aid nightly. Wiping it off with a tissue should do.

ECZEMA

Eczema is a term doctors use to describe all kinds of red, blistering, oozing, scaly, brownish, thickened, and itchy skin conditions. Outbreaks can occur on the face and neck, in the folds of elbows and knees, on the hands, or, in extreme cases, over the entire body. While no one knows the cause, doctors say that allergies, sensitivity to environmental conditions like dry furnace air and scratchy clothes, and possibly stress can trigger eczema flare-ups.

Although many people outgrow eczema when they reach adulthood, others have outbreaks their whole lives. Eczema can be especially irritating for seniors because their oil-producing glands are not as active as they used to be, says John F. Romano, M.D., clinical assistant professor of dermatology at New York Hospital–Cornell Medical Center in New York City. This can lead to dry skin, and thus, greater irritation. And sometimes older skin heals more slowly, especially in the lower legs, because of reduced circulation, Dr. Romano adds.

There are several types of eczema, and some of them require very different treatments. Since many types appear alike, it might be tricky to get a correct diagnosis. But that's what you need, says Dr. Romano.

Once you know what you're dealing with, you can manage eczema a number of ways, all of which begin with an effective skin-care routine.

Try This First

Maintain moisture. To prevent the dry skin that is at the root of eczema, you need to trap some moisture. Apply a soothing skin cream right after you finish bathing, says K. William Kitzmiller,

M.D., dermatologist in private practice in Cincinnati. The best of the heavy creams or lotions, called emollients, are oily but unscented. Nivea cream, petroleum jelly, or even solid vegetable shortening are excellent for people with eczema, says Dr. Kitzmiller.

Emollients are safe to use as often as needed. "When you step out of the bath or shower, liberally apply your emollient and then blot your skin dry," suggests Dr. Kitzmiller. Since water gets into your skin when you bathe, the emollient helps trap the moisture and hold it there, he says.

Other Wise Ways

Have some hydrocortisone cream. Most eczema flare-ups can be relieved by nonprescription 1-percent hydrocortisone cream such as Cortaid, according to Dr. Romano. Don't apply it every day, however, because it can cause spider veins and stretch marks. Intermittent use, no more than three times a week, should keep irritation in check, he says.

Time your baths. Doctors used to tell people with eczema to take quick baths—no longer than 10 minutes—to avoid having their skin dry out. Ignore that old thinking, says Kristin Leiferman, M.D., professor of dermatology at the Mayo Medical School in Rochester, Minnesota. Instead, take a leisurely bath for 10 to 20 minutes per day. Your skin cells will absorb water through their membranes and become hydrated. "You'll know that you've been in long enough when your skin starts to pucker and crinkle," notes Dr. Leiferman.

Turn down the temp. When you take that bath, though, use lukewarm water. Hot bath water *can* dry out the skin. And hot water can also irritate skin that's already tender, explains Dr. Kitzmiller.

Eliminate scented products. Added fragrances are a chief cause of skin allergies and irritant reactions, according to Dr. Kitzmiller. If you have eczema, try to avoid any skin-care products that have fragrances.

Dr. Leiferman recommends nonirritating soaps and cleansers, like Dove or Aveeno, that don't have a lot of fragrance, color, or additives.

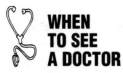

WHEN TO SEE A DOCTOR

Eczema can have many different causes, so if you develop an outbreak, it's smart to see a doctor to determine what's causing the itching, says John F. Romano, M.D., clinical assistant professor of dermatology at New York Hospital–Cornell Medical Center in New York City. Definitely get checked out if you have patches of skin that are:

- Painful
- Hot to the touch
- Oozing a puslike discharge

Milk it for all it's worth. Whole milk compresses are a low-cost way to soothe eczema flare-ups and reduce itchiness, says Dr. Kitzmiller. Saturate a gauze pad or cotton cloth with equal parts cold milk and ice water and apply it to the skin for about three minutes, he says. Resoak the cloth and reapply it at least two more times for three-minute soaks. You can repeat this treatment several times a day, he suggests, but be sure to rinse your skin with cool water after each application. Otherwise, you'll start to smell like sour milk.

Ice the itch. Another way to control the itch of eczema is to hold a plastic bag of ice on the affected area, says Dr. Kitzmiller. Wrap the ice pack in a towel and hold it on the inflamed zone as long as necessary.

Choose nonitchy clothing. Anything you can do to reduce itchiness is going to minimize damage to your skin caused by scratching, says Karen K. Deasey, M.D., chief of dermatology at Bryn Mawr Hospital in Pennsylvania. Choose cotton clothing and cotton bedding whenever possible. When your body is in contact with cotton, your skin stays cool and can breathe. Synthetic fabrics can be irritating, and so can wool.

Turn to mild detergents. You can further reduce the itchiness of clothes by using mild laundry detergents such as Tide and Ivory and by rinsing garments twice to clear away all traces of detergent, says Dr. Deasey.

Shun the softeners. Avoid fabric softeners, advises Dr. Deasey, because they contain fragrances that can make your skin itch. She also suggests staying away from the newer blue liquid detergents because they leave residues on clothes, and if your skin reacts to those residues, you'll itch.

Humidify your surroundings. Anything you do to add moisture to the air is going to help relieve the dry skin and itch of eczema, says Dr. Kitzmiller. Ideal humidification, he says, is about 50 percent, "just short of making the windows sweat." You can add moisture to the air in your home with a cold-air humidifier or by placing shallow pans of water near radiators, Dr. Kitzmiller says.

Protect your hands. Hand rashes are an extremely common form of eczema. Many household items could be causing these rashes, including soaps and detergents, solvents, cleaning agents, chemicals, and the ingredients in skin and personal care products.

MANAGING YOUR MEDS

If your eczema is normally under control but you have a flare-up, your doctor may prescribe a topical steroid cream such as fluocinonide (Lidex). Although many people express concerns about the side effects of topical steroids, side effects are rare as long as the medication is used appropriately, says John F. Romano, M.D., clinical assistant professor of dermatology at New York Hospital–Cornell Medical Center in New York City. Just be sure to use topical steroids as directed by your doctor.

Also, be on the alert for prescription drugs that can dry out skin and aggravate an eczema condition, says Dr. Romano. Among the medications that are known to cause problems are:

• Diuretics used to treat heart disease and high blood pressure, such as hydrochlorothiazide (Esidrix), that reduce fluid levels in the body and can dry the skin
• Some neurological and psychiatric medications, such as lithium (Eskalith), can also irritate sensitive skin

Be careful with niacin, advises Dr. Romano. Too much can cause flushing, a trigger for at least one kind of dermatitis. If you are taking a prescription for niacin, be sure to take your recommended daily dose and no more. And alert your doctor if you have dermatitis symptoms accompanied by oily skin or seeping in the itchy area.

And once your hands become dry and chapped, they're even more vulnerable to household agents that could make them itch. Even innocuous-looking substances like water and baby products can make an outbreak worse when your hands are super-dry.

If you have eczema on your hands, doctors recommend wearing a pair of vinyl gloves with cotton liners to protect you from irritants whenever you do dishes or housework. Have four or five pairs and keep them in the kitchen, bathroom, and laundry areas. Be sure to dry out your gloves between cleaning jobs, he says. And always replace gloves that develop holes.

Relax for your rash. "Stress is a definite contributing factor in eczema as well as in other skin conditions," notes Dr. Kitzmiller. "Skin disorders have multiple causes and a person's emotional state can play a large part. If you are feeling stressed out or are particularly worried about something, it will only aggravate your condition."

Stress causes your body to release histamines, which make you itch, Dr. Kitzmiller explains. When you start to feel stressed, take 10 deep breaths, meditate, or go for a walk, he says. "Do whatever it takes to calm down and relax."

Reduce dust mites. Many doctors think that people with certain types of eczema may be affected by allergens produced by dust mites in the house. Take measures to ban the mites from contact, and your skin condition might improve, says Dr. Kitzmiller.

Bedding, mattresses, curtains, and carpets are all prime real estate for these mites. Regular vacuuming, damp dusting, and routine washing and airing of bedding are the most effective ways to reduce their population, he says.

EMPHYSEMA

If you seriously injured your back, you'd most likely go to rehabilitation therapy to get it into shape. You might not be able to do the things you did with your back before, but you'd learn how to use it effectively and work with your limitations.

Well, the same goes for your lungs. If they've been damaged by a disease like emphysema, you have to learn how to use your lungs so you get the most from them. It's called pulmonary rehabilitation, and it's a way for people with emphysema to lead as active lives as they possibly can.

"It's the major thing we have to offer. It does not improve the way the lungs function, but it offers the prospect of improving your general condition. It teaches you how to function better with what you have," says Mark J. Rosen, M.D., chief of the division of pulmonary and critical-care medicine at the Beth Israel Medical Center in New York City.

Over time, emphysema destroys a system of saclike structures in your lungs, called alveoli, that moves oxygen into your bloodstream and takes carbon dioxide out. These sacs are thin, fragile, and easily damaged.

When the alveoli are destroyed, holes form in the lungs. The lungs transfer less oxygen to your bloodstream, causing shortness of breath during exercise and then eventually at rest. The lungs also lose elasticity, making it harder for them to expand and contract, which in turn causes you to have a hard time exhaling.

Although there is a genetic form of emphysema, "it is mostly a smokers' disease," says Barry Make, M.D., director of pulmonary rehabilitation at the National Jewish Center for Immunology and Respiratory Medicine in Denver.

Currently, there is no cure, but you can learn to manage the problem. The following tips offer some rehabilitation exercises as

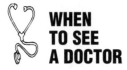

WHEN TO SEE A DOCTOR

If you have emphysema, it won't take long for your regular family doctor to identify the symptoms of shortness of breath and cough. After that, you should see your regular doctor or a pulmonary specialist on a regular basis, says Barry Make, M.D., director of pulmonary rehabilitation at the National Jewish Center for Immunology and Respiratory Medicine in Denver. Without proper care, the disease can progress and eventually damage your heart as well as your lungs. Also see your doctor if:

• Your symptoms get worse.

• You have congestion in your lungs.

• You have swelling in your legs.

well as lifestyle changes that will make your life easier with emphysema. "Even with severe emphysema, there are certain things that can be done," Dr. Rosen says.

Try This Now

Put your lips together and blow. An exercise called pursed-lips breathing is taught to people with emphysema to help their lungs work better, Dr. Make says. Inhale fully through your nose. Purse your lips lightly as though you are going to blow out a candle and exhale slowly and fully. Practice the exercise daily and use it when you feel short of breath during exertion. You can also use it when you feel anxious.

Other Wise Ways

Quit smoking. Don't assume that because you already have emphysema it is too late to stop smoking. "No matter what stage you are, if you stop smoking, you will stop further damage and prevent decline from emphysema," Dr. Make says.

Maintain a smoke-free environment. Keep away from other people who smoke and places where you're likely to encounter secondhand smoke, says Henry Gong Jr., M.D., professor of medicine in the division of pulmonary and critical-care medicine and environmental health service at the University of Southern California School of Medicine in Downey. Smoke or pollutants can make it harder for you to breathe, he says.

Breathe the right way. Proper, more efficient breathing means filling your lungs with air from the bottom up. To do this, you need to learn how to breathe from your diaphragm, the group of muscles between your chest and your stomach, Dr. Make says. It is often easier to learn how to do this when you are lying down. Place your hand on your belly. While relaxing your stomach, inhale slowly through your nose. Keep your abdomen relaxed so that your diaphragm drops down and your stomach expands. The hand on your stomach should move up if you are breathing with your diaphragm. Slowly breathe out of pursed lips.

Take a walk. Whether it be down the street or down your hallway, take a stroll every day, Dr. Make says. While exercise won't get rid of emphysema, it builds endurance, meaning you will be able to do more without getting tired and winded as quickly. Dr. Make recommends walking because it is the easiest and cheapest activity, although you could also use a treadmill. Walk as far as you can each day, trying to go farther over time.

If the pollution is bad, it doesn't mean you can't exercise, Dr. Make says. You just have to find an indoor place to walk. Go to a mall with air conditioning and walk around there.

MANAGING YOUR MEDS

People with emphysema may be put on bronchodilators such as ipratropium (Atrovent) and albuterol (Proventil), medicines that open up the air passages and make it easier to breathe, says Mark J. Rosen, M.D., chief of the division of pulmonary and critical-care medicine at the Beth Israel Medical Center in New York City. Typically, these inhalers are conveniently packaged so you can carry them around in your purse or pocket and use them when you need them.

Whether or not you're taking bronchodilators, you should be aware of other medications that might make it harder for you to breathe. Be sure any doctor who's prescribing medications knows about your emphysema condition before you take the following:

- Heart disease medications such as beta-blockers like acebutolol (Sectral) or propranolol (Inderal)
- Beta-blockers such as betaxolol (Betopic) and carteolol (Ocupress), used to treat glaucoma

Search for quality air. Air pollution can make life harder on people with emphysema. Watch for or listen to local air-quality reports on the television or radio news, Dr. Make says. If the pollution is high, take it easy that day, he advises. Also, trust your own judgment. Many people with emphysema can feel when the pollution is up even without air-quality reports. If you have some trouble breathing, lighten your load for the day.

Find shortcuts. It's the little things that can save you energy and effort when you have emphysema. Buy slip-on shoes instead of sneakers and shoes that need to be tied, says Michael S. Stulbarg, M.D., professor of clinical medicine and director of the clinical pulmonary center at the University of California, San Francisco. Take showers instead of baths. Put things that you use regularly in easy-to-reach places. These steps, though small, can help conserve your energy to do things you really want or need to do.

Go belt-free. Tight clothes, especially around the stomach and waist, restrict your breathing, so dress in loose, comfortable clothing. While you are overhauling your wardrobe, get rid of girdles or tight belts, Dr. Make says. They also pinch your waist and make it difficult to breathe.

Make the temperature just right. "Temperatures too hot or too cold put more stress on your lungs," Dr. Make says. So when the heat is on, retreat to a nice air-conditioned house or shopping mall. When Jack Frost is about, try to stay inside a warm house if you can. If you must venture out, bundle up and wrap a scarf around your nose and mouth to help warm the air before you inhale.

EYESTRAIN

At some point in your life, someone probably told you that reading in a dark room would ruin your eyes. The same wisdom applied to sitting too close to the TV or reading a book two inches from your face.

The thing is, it's not true. Yes, reading in poor lighting may make your eyes hurt. But it won't ruin your vision. In fact, your vision changes over time all by itself, dim light or not. You will notice, however, that your eyes hurt when trying to perform such feats as you age. That's because you'll have more trouble focusing up close, a condition called presbyopia. It's a natural part of aging, says Robert Cykiert, M.D., assistant professor of ophthalmology at New York University Medical Center in New York City.

You see, you were born with perfect eyes. "Children have very soft, pliable lenses and strong eye muscles. They are able to tolerate focusing much easier. That's why children can read books with their chins resting on the page and sit close to the TV. As we age, our ability to focus decreases," says Joseph Kubacki, M.D., professor and chairman of the ophthalmology department and assistant dean for medical affairs at Temple University School of Medicine in Philadelphia. "The lens becomes less and less pliable and the muscles that control the focusing become less robust. Since it's harder to focus, you feel eyestrain more easily."

Eyestrain isn't as serious as some eye problems, but it can certainly make the niceties of life—reading a favorite book, focusing on hobbies like needlepoint, enjoying a candlelit dinner—more problematic. Here are some strategies for taking the strain out of your eyes.

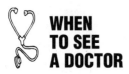

WHEN TO SEE A DOCTOR

Try This First

Take a break. Your eyes get a workout when you try to focus on something close. But they get a chance to relax when you stare off into the distance. Take a short rest break, or as many breaks as you need, to relieve the strain and help prevent eyestrain in the future. When you read, work at a computer, or sew, periodically stop what you're doing and look at least 10 feet away or farther for about 30 seconds every 20 minutes or so, says Larry R. Taub, M.D., assistant professor of ophthalmology and director of comprehensive ophthalmology at Emory University School of Medicine in Atlanta.

"If you are focusing at a given distance, it's like lifting your arm up and holding it there—the muscle goes into a spasm. It's much more fatiguing to do that than to move around and relax," says Dr. Kubacki.

Other Wise Ways

Bat your eyes. Try to remember to blink, says Dr. Kubacki. Your eyes start to hurt after a lot of reading or computer work because you tend to stare without blinking and your eyes get dried out. If you find that you're doing a lot of staring and not much blinking, remind yourself to shut your eyes every now and then.

Make sure your glasses still work. Because your ability to focus continues to decrease with age, the glasses you wore 5 or 10 years ago may not be strong enough for you today. Most likely, you need glasses with a higher magnification.

You can try finding reading glasses at your local drugstore. But first you should see an ophthalmologist or optometrist for an exam to rule out eye disease. If your prescription is equal in both eyes and you don't have an astigmatism (an unequal curvature of the surfaces of the eye), you can try a pair of reading glasses sold in stores. Otherwise, your doctor can order prescription lenses for you to use at the distances prescribed. If your glasses are made for you to read at a computer's distance, for instance, and you wear those same glasses to read a book, you'll strain your eyes. People typically read a book at 14 inches but use a computer at 20 inches, says Dr. Cykiert.

Read in bright light. Though reading in a dark room will not ruin your eyes, it can poop them out, says Dr. Kubacki. The same with reading with just a reading lamp and no other lights on. "If there's too big a gradient between the light in the background and your reading light, your pupil doesn't know what to adjust to, so it constricts and dilates," says Dr. Kubacki. Use a reading light with a 75- to 100-watt bulb and also keep other 60-watt room lights on.

MANAGING YOUR MEDS

A few medications may make it harder to focus your vision, which can cause eyestrain if you don't do something about it, says W. Steven Pray, Ph.D., R.Ph., professor of nonprescription drug products at Southwestern Oklahoma State University in Weatherford.

Common medications that may blur vision include:

- The glaucoma medication acetazolamide (Diamox)
- Antiarthritic and anti-inflammatory medications such as fenoprofen (Nalfon), ibuprofen, ketoprofen (Orudis KT), or naproxen (Aleve)
- Antidepressants such as amitriptyline (Elavil) and imipramine (Tofranil)
- The antihypertension medication chlorthalidone (one of the ingredients of Combipres)
- The psoriasis drug etretinate (Tegison)
- Antibacterial and antibiotic agents such as sulfonamides (ingredients in Bactrim DS) and tetracyclines (Doxycycline)

FATIGUE

Feeling tired is a given at certain times—when you've walked more than usual, worked long hours in the garden, or taken a long-distance flight. But fatigue can come from unexpected sources, too. In the hustle, bustle, and travel of a Christmas visit to see your children and grandchildren in another state, you can end up pretty exhausted by the time Christmas morning dawns.

On a smaller scale, if your coffeemaker breaks down and you don't get your morning cup, fatigue can come along about midmorning. Even the glare of a computer screen—forcing you to squint—can be fatiguing.

One of the things older people have a difficult time recognizing about fatigue is its relationship to stress, says Maria Simonson, Sc.D., Ph.D., director of the health, weight, and stress clinic and professor emeritus at Johns Hopkins Medical Institutions in Baltimore. "They try to find physical causes. If they have something go wrong with them, it must be with their bodies. They forget the psychological aspects of their minds."

True, your body is changing and there are physical developments during aging that contribute to fatigue. The older you are, the more sleep problems you have and the more sedentary you might be. And maybe you're less likely to eat balanced, healthful meals. These and other factors can leave you feeling sluggish during the day.

But fatigue is not an inevitable part of aging. You have the power to change many of the factors that cause that rundown feeling, says Stephen Langer, M.D., specialist in thyroid problems and chronic fatigue in Berkeley, California, and author of *Solved: The Riddle of Illness*.

Perk yourself up with these tips.

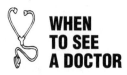

WHEN TO SEE A DOCTOR

Fatigue can be a symptom of many other medical problems from anemia to cancer, so see your doctor if your fatigue has gone on longer than a month and doesn't seem to have a cause. If you find yourself falling asleep at inappropriate times—during work, a conversation, or a bridge game—you need to see a sleep specialist, advises Sonia Ancoli-Israel, Ph.D., director of the sleep disorders clinic at the Veteran's Affairs Health Care System in San Diego, professor of psychiatry at the University of California, San Diego, and author of *All I Want Is a Good Night's Sleep.*

Try This First

Get moving. Exercise and physical movement are sure ways of beating back fatigue. For four to six hours after you exercise, your body's metabolism and temperature remain up, leaving you feeling more alert and awake. And it doesn't take a lot to keep your body rhythms on course and give you a charge of energy. "If you can walk 20 to 40 minutes three or four times a week, it's perfect," Dr. Langer says. Remember to concentrate on doing what you like to do. And do the exercise when it is convenient. That way you will be more likely to stick to it.

Other Wise Ways

Socialize. No one knows exactly why, but increased social interaction seems to help people feel less fatigued. "One theory holds that increasing mental activity—just like increasing physical activity—increases blood flow to the brain," says Phyllis Zee, M.D., Ph.D., director of the sleep disorders center and associate professor of neurology at Northwestern University Medical School in Chicago. "And we find that not only does it improve deep sleep in older people but also their mental ability increases during the day."

Find something useful to do. Loneliness and boredom contribute to fatigue, Dr. Simonson says. Doing some volunteer work or joining a hobby group might seem like a small thing to do. But once you start doing it, you may find that participation puts a whole new incentive in your daily life. "Make yourself valuable to people," advises Dr. Simonson.

Eat right. A diet that is 60 percent carbohydrates, 20 percent protein, and 20 percent fat is the optimum to maintain energy, Dr. Langer says. Most of us rely on refined foods such as pasta, white rice, white bread, and packaged food products, which are less nutrient-dense than their whole-food counterparts. If you can shift your diet to include more whole grains, fruits, and vegetables, you'll probably see a bit of change. All these foods are sources of energy that are also packed with nutrients.

Treat constipation with C. Constipation can interfere with the body's ability to absorb key nutrients, leading to potential deficiencies in vitamins and minerals, says Dr. Langer. (For more information, see Constipation on page 118.) Start taking a vitamin C supplement, which helps loosen the stool as well as provide antioxidants, he advises. He recommends a powdered form of C that will be less irritating to the stomach. Dr. Langer suggests beginning with 1,000 milligrams (usually one-quarter teaspoon) three to four times a day and slowly increasing your intake to your own personal level of bowel tolerance. Powdered vitamin C is available at health food stores.

Go for some ginseng. The herbal remedy ginseng has been used by people for centuries to put a little spring in their steps. When you're picking a ginseng product, examine the label to make sure it has at least 4 percent ginsenosides, suggests Varro Tyler, Ph.D., distinguished professor emeritus at Purdue University in West Lafayette, Indiana, and author of *The Honest Herbal*. Dr. Tyler recommends taking two 100-milligram capsules a day. Make sure to

MANAGING YOUR MEDS

Sedatives such as Valium (diazepam) and over-the-counter sleeping pills can lead to daytime symptoms including fatigue. If a drug that you are taking causes daytime drowsiness or fatigue, ask your doctor or pharmacist if you can take the medication before you go to bed rather than during the day when you want to be awake and alert, says Margaret Moline, Ph.D., director of the sleep-wake disorders center at New York Presbyterian Hospital–Cornell Medical Center in White Plains, New York.

get American ginseng or Asian ginseng, which tend to be more effective, says Dr. Tyler, who cautions that Siberian ginseng is not as well-tested. (Ginseng may cause irritability if taken with caffeine or other stimulants, and it should not be taken by people with high blood pressure.)

Pick up some ginkgo biloba. You may want to try ginkgo biloba if you feel that you're in a mental fog. This herb helps fend off mental fatigue by improving circulation to your extremities and your brain, Dr. Langer says. Try taking 120 milligrams of it a day.

Do not use this herb with antidepressant MAO inhibitor drugs such as phenelzine sulfate (Nardil) or tranylcypromine (Parnate), aspirin or other nonsteroidal anti-inflammatory drugs (NSAIDs), or blood-thinning medications such as warfarin (Coumadin).

Write it down. Stress and worry can add to fatigue, especially if you let your problems plague you in the night, says Lauren Broch, Ph.D., director of education and training at the sleep-wake disorders center at New York Hospital–Cornell Medical Center in White Plains, New York. You can't make worries vanish, of course, but there's an organizing trick that can outfox the worrywart part of your brain.

Make a list of all the things that are bothering you, suggests Dr. Broch. Do it sometime late in the day or early in the evening to help you feel more in control of your problems so you can stop worrying before you try to rest. For every item on the list, think of a potential resolution. Then put the list away and use the rest of your time leading up to bedtime to relax.

Get enough quality sleep. Are you able to sleep soundly each night? Even though you may be spending enough time in bed, it's quality that really counts, says Margaret Moline, Ph.D., director of the sleep-wake disorders center at New York Presbyterian Hospital–Cornell Medical Center in White Plains, New York. When older patients complain about fatigue, she finds, the real problem can often be a sleep disorder that impacts the quality of their sleep. "If you spend eight hours in bed every night and still don't feel refreshed in the morning, talk with your doctor," advises Dr. Moline.

Rise and shine the same time each day. Varying sleep patterns can often leave people with a jet-lag feeling even if they've never left home. Go to bed at the same time each night, and try to rise at the same hour each morning. The regular sleep time ensures that your body will sleep efficiently, says Dr. Zee.

Monitor sleeping pill use. If you take an over-the-counter sleeping pill right before bedtime every night, you may still experience its lingering effects when you try to wake up the next morning, says Melanie Cupp, Pharm.D., clinical assistant professor of pharmacy and a drug information specialist at the West Virginia University School of Pharmacy in Morgantown. Dr. Cupp says that sleeping pills can have a carry-over, almost hangover, effect the next day, causing drowsiness that can be so bad that it impairs driving.

Brighten your world. Colors can have an amazing effect on how people feel, says Dr. Simonson. The colors on the warm end of the spectrum—yellows, oranges, and reds—are the higher energy, stimulating colors. But don't go repainting your whole house in magenta yet. She suggests that you use these colors strategically in every room of your house, in objets d'art, rugs, and other accessories. Place these colors where the eye will linger. In the bedroom, carefully limit the use of energizing colors, but make sure to have one particular object that will help rouse you in the morning. "This has an instant, energizing effect," Dr. Simonson says.

Power nap. If you take a nap, for how long do you nap? If you nap for more than a half-hour, your body goes into its deep-sleep phases and you feel very groggy when you are wakened. As long as you nap in the early part of the afternoon and limit the nap to a half-hour, you probably will feel more refreshed for the rest of the day, says Sonia Ancoli-Israel, Ph.D., director of the sleep disorders clinic at the Veteran's Affairs Health Care System in San Diego, professor of psychiatry at the University of California, San Diego, and author of *All I Want Is a Good Night's Sleep*.

Treat your blues. Feeling depressed affects your sleep and your energy levels. "Depression will affect sleep. It might make you sleep more, it might make you sleep less, but it will generally make you feel more fatigued," Dr. Broch says. If you suspect that the blues are making you feel blah, consult with your doctor.

Caffeinate or decaffeinate your life. The stimulant caffeine and fatigue have an intimate and conflicting relationship, says Roland Griffiths, Ph.D., professor in the departments of psychiatry and neuroscience at Johns Hopkins School of Medicine in Baltimore.

On a short-term basis, caffeine can work. If you don't have it regularly and you need something to keep yourself awake during an important meeting or event, drinking a caffeinated beverage will help boost your feelings of wakefulness and well-being. That dose of caffeine can also increase your ability to concentrate. So caffeinated coffee, tea, soda, or even chocolate may help you get by in the short term.

But the watchwords here are "short term." If you start using caffeine habitually, you'll start to feel fatigued whenever you don't get enough. So to maximize the benefits of your caffeine intake, use it either intermittently (about every third day) or minimally (less than 75 milligrams a day), says Dr. Griffith. That's about a half-cup of coffee or two six-ounce cups of tea.

Take care of your eyes. If you have an eyeglass prescription that's not up-to-date or you're doing a lot of close-up work such as reading, the strain on your eye muscles will make you feel tired, says Stephen Miller, O.D., executive director of the College of Optometrists in Vision Development in St. Louis.

In addition to your eye muscles tiring, if you can't see something well, you may move closer or hunch over so you can see. That's certainly true if you're doing anything that requires viewing at a close distance all day long, such as reading, sewing, or other detail-oriented hobbies, says Dr. Miller. All that hunching over can lead to muscle fatigue and strain in your back, neck, and shoulders.

So take a break every 15 minutes or so, look away, or perform another task. Do anything that allows your eyes to relax and helps you avoid fatigue.

If you're experiencing eyestrain regularly, be sure to call your eye doctor for an appointment. Your prescription may need adjusting or you may have to start wearing some type of corrective lenses. Dr. Miller recommends an annual eye exam for older adults.

Halt the hunching. Be sure that hunching over doesn't become a habit, says Dr. Miller. If you're using a computer, adjust your seat position so you can sit erect about 20 to 26 inches away from the screen. You should be looking down slightly at about a 15- to 20-degree angle when viewing the screen. Keep your feet flat on the floor and your arms bent at about a 90-degree angle when using the keyboard. And if you do a lot of reading, position the book so you don't strain your shoulders. Sit upright and hold your reading material about 14 to 18 inches from your eyes. Use good lighting that doesn't glare or cast shadows. Frequent breaks from work—taking time to walk or stretch—can help keep your neck-area muscles loosened up.

Do like birds of a feather. Some people get up at the crack of dawn. Others don't get going until the afternoon and are most productive in the wee hours of the morning. Sleep specialists call people with these predilections larks and owls. If you're an owl trying to fit into a lark's schedule, you're going to end up tired. If possible, consider changing your routine, maybe even your job, to fit your pattern. "For people who are constitutionally one way or another, it helps to find a lifestyle that matches their constitutions," says Patricia Prinz, Ph.D., professor of behavioral nursing and adjunct professor of psychiatry and behavior sciences at the University of Washington in Seattle.

FEARS AND ANXIETY

Some fears are tougher to lick than others. And certainly, people over 60 have plenty to be anxious about, like crime, loss of loved ones, chronic illness, disability, and loneliness. But just as certainly, the vast majority of these fears (unpleasant responses to a real external threat or danger) and anxieties (responses to unreal or imagined danger) can easily be conquered, even at age 60, 70, or 80, experts say.

"It's important for older people who feel anxious to know that they're not going crazy and they're not alone. There are other people who are having these problems. Anxiety can be treated. You don't have to suffer," says Shirley Babior, licensed clinical social worker in San Diego and co-author of *Overcoming Panic, Anxiety, and Phobias*.

Although some people are naturally jittery throughout their lives, aging seems to magnify many fears, says Bernard Vittone, M.D., psychiatrist and director of the National Center for the Treatment of Phobias, Anxiety, and Depression in Washington, D.C. As a person ages, some areas of the brain that regulate anxiety become more sensitive. These changes in the brain combined with life experiences such as accidents, injuries, and the deaths of loved ones make people over 60 prone to an array of frights.

If everything isn't fine, try these anxiety-relieving tips.

Try This First

Breathe through one nostril. When you feel fearful or anxious, block off one side of your nose with a finger and take 8 to 10 slow, deep breaths through your open nostril, Dr. Vittone suggests. Deep breathing helps you tame your fears. Blocking one nostril forces you to take in air much more slowly so the deep breathing will be more effective. "My patients tell me over and over again that breathing through a single nostril works wonders for decreasing feelings of anxiety," Dr. Vittone says.

Other Wise Ways

Double-check that threat. Many worries have no basis in reality, notes Dr. Vittone. So before you work yourself up into a panic, ask yourself four questions.

1. What is the worst thing that can happen?
2. How bad is that really?
3. What is the likelihood of it happening to me?
4. How many times has this happened to me or my friends in the past?

MANAGING YOUR MEDS

Anxiety is a common side effect of more than 150 prescribed and over-the-counter medications. Ironically, among the prime offenders are a class of antianxiety drugs known as benzodiazepines, says George T. Grossberg, M.D., director of geriatric psychiatry at St. Louis University School of Medicine. These drugs, including alprazolam (Xanax), can cause a paradoxical effect in some people that actually worsens anxiety instead of relieving it. If this happens to you, consult your physician. Other medications that may trigger anxiety include:

- Diphenhydramine (Benadryl) and over-the-counter cold, flu, and allergy preparations containing dextromethorphan, for example, Comtrex Nighttime
- Virtually all decongestants, including those available over-the-counter, like pseudoephedrine (Actifed, Sudafed)
- Bronchodilators containing theophylline, such as Slo-bid and Theo-Dur
- Steroids, including those used to treat rheumatoid arthritis
- Beverages and over-the-counter and prescription medications that contain caffeine, like coffee, stimulants such as Vivarin and No-Doz, diet pills, and pain relievers such as Anacin or Excedrin (Check the labels on these over-the-counter products before buying)

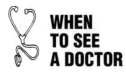

WHEN TO SEE A DOCTOR

Consult your physician if:

• You find yourself avoiding situations, places, or people in order to avoid feeling anxious.

• You worry excessively and have difficulty putting it out of your mind.

• You have panic attacks (short, unexplained periods of intense fear or discomfort).

• You have difficulty concentrating on tasks.

• You have frequent bursts of anger or irritation.

• You have insomnia or frequently feel unusually tired during waking hours.

"Frequently, older people who ask these questions of themselves discover that they're worried about something that would simply cause mild embarrassment or something that they've never known to happen to anyone," Dr. Vittone says.

Even if there is a threat, these reality checks can motivate you to take action to reduce the risk. If you're worried, for instance, about a household fire, you can ask your local fire department for a safety inspection and for advice about how to get out of your home quickly, suggests Dr. Vittone.

Take in the sights and sounds. Whenever you feel anxious, take a moment to focus on your senses. What are you smelling? Hearing? Seeing? Tasting? Touching? If you see a leaf on the sidewalk, for instance, pick it up and exam it carefully. Zeroing in on your senses will keep you in the present moment and prevent you from dwelling on catastrophic thoughts about the future, Dr. Vittone says.

Fill the gaps. Retirement and other events in later life often leave gaps in our lives. Fear will fill those holes unless you find other ways to fill them. So stay active and involved with friends, family, and your community, recommends Dr. Vittone. Be adventurous. Take an exotic trip. Take a ride on a roller coaster with your grandchildren. Take dance lessons. Do and be as much as you can, and there won't be holes in your life where fear can seep in.

Do the hustle. Daily exercise such as a 15-minute walk around the block, washing the dishes, or just stretching in a chair several times a day can relieve tension, anxiety, and fear, Dr. Vittone says.

Exercise stimulates the production of endorphins, your brain's own morphinelike chemicals, explains Una McCann, M.D., chief of the unit on anxiety disorders at the National Institute of Mental Health in Bethesda, Maryland. "Endorphins fill your entire body with a sense of calm and well-being."

Dump the second cup. After age 60, as little as one cup of coffee can trigger severe anxiety in some people, Dr. Vittone says. That's because the brain becomes more caffeine-sensitive as it ages. In fact, caffeine—the active ingredient in coffee, teas, and some sodas—may be the single worst substance that an anxious older person can consume, according to Dr. Vittone. Limit yourself to no more than one eight-ounce cup of caffeinated coffee, tea, or soda a day. If even one cup seems to spark anxiety, make a complete switch to decaffeinated beverages, he says.

Cork the champagne. Alcohol may feel relaxing, but that feeling is deceptive. As you sip it, alcohol numbs your brain's anxiety centers, so you feel more at ease and less fretful. But as it wears off, alcohol can trigger a rebound effect in your brain, causing you to feel more fearful and anxious than you did before you took your first drink, explains Dr. Vittone. If you imbibe, one or two drinks a day probably won't aggravate your anxiety, he says. But drinking more than that will. (A drink is defined as one 12-ounce beer, 5-ounce glass of wine, or 1½-ounce shot of liquor.)

FEVER

When you're older and you get sick, you may not feel as hot as you used to. Literally.

"Older people usually don't get as high fevers as young people do in the presence of infection. A person in her twenties or thirties might have a temperature of 104°F, but an older person might have 101°F or maybe only 99°F," says Peter V. Lee, M.D., professor emeritus of family medicine at the University of Southern California School of Medicine in Los Angeles.

Why that's the case is a bit of a mystery. Certain medications, such as sedatives or antitremor drugs for Parkinson's disease, can inhibit your body's ability to generate a fever, says Thomas C. Rosenthal, M.D., professor and chairman of the department of family medicine at the State University of New York in Buffalo. Mostly, though, it's just natural for older people to run lower fevers when they're sick.

Even a low fever is one you have to watch, however. For someone over 60, a temperature reading that hovers around 100°F for more than 24 hours could be a sign of a high-grade illness or infection and warrants a visit to the doctor, says Dr. Lee. "A fever is the same thing as rapid heart rate or elevation of blood pressure. It's a signal that something is wrong," he says.

If you do have a mild fever caused by a cold or flu, here are some suggestions to make you more comfortable.

Try This First

Keep up with the fluids. A fever can cause you to lose almost an extra quart of fluid a day, Dr. Rosenthal says. So make sure you drink eight or more eight-ounce glasses of fluid per day. Plain old water is the best, but juices and clear sodas can also help you keep hydrated. Avoid liquids that have caffeine or a lot of sugar in them. They can actually cause you to lose more water in the long run.

Other Wise Ways

Take two and . . . you know. Take two regular or extra-strength acetaminophen or aspirin. These medications can bring the fever down and make you more comfortable, Dr. Rosenthal says. Nonsteroidal anti-inflammatory drugs (NSAIDs) such as ibuprofen can also help and may hold the fever down longer.

Don't overdo exercise. If you already exercise, you can continue to do so even while you have a low fever. But don't overdo it. You can't sweat out a fever. If you normally run or jog, switch to a walking pace when you're sick. "Go ahead and move, but don't push yourself," advises Dr. Rosenthal.

Take a quick dip. If you're feeling uncomfortable and want to cool off, give yourself a sponge bath or a good soak in the tub but keep the water lukewarm. You don't want to plunge into a very cold or very hot shower, because that could make you feel dizzy and affect your balance, says Susan Black, M.D., doctor in private practice in Tewksbury, Massachusetts. If you have a fever, the lukewarm water will actually feel cool and soothing.

MANAGING YOUR MEDS

If you're allergic to a medication, one of the ways your body will tell you is through fever. But it won't always happen right away, says Peter V. Lee, professor emeritus of family medicine at the University of Southern California School of Medicine in Los Angeles. If you develop an unexplained fever, sometimes accompanied by a rash or joint pain, within 7 to 10 days after taking a new drug regularly, you might be allergic to it. Talk to your doctor immediately about a substitute.

If you're taking aspirin for your fever, it's important to remember that many medications may interact with it, warns W. Steven Pray, Ph.D., R.Ph., professor of nonprescription drug products at Southwestern Oklahoma State University in Weatherford.

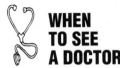

WHEN TO SEE A DOCTOR

Children can get a little fever from just cutting teeth. But once you're an adult over age 60, a fever of over 100°F is cause for concern, says Susan Black, M.D., doctor in private practice in Tewksbury, Massachusetts. So please see your doctor:

• If a fever over 100°F lasts for more than 24 hours, it could be a sign of serious infection.

• If you have fever and chest pain, it could be a sign that you have or are developing pneumonia.

• If you have fever and a stiff neck, it could be a sign you have meningitis.

• If you have fever and abdominal pain, it could be any one of a number of infections, from kidney infection to bowel infection.

Don't starve a fever. Starving yourself while you have a fever won't really affect the fever, but it can make you feel weaker and sicker. Although you may not have very much appetite when you're sick, do try to eat a little something, even if it's only a cup of broth and some crackers. "If the food doesn't upset your stomach, it's fine to eat," Dr. Black says.

Figure out what your base temperature is. Because people over 60 can run temperatures that are cooler than younger adults, it pays to learn what your normal temperature is when you're not sick. Dr. Black suggests that you take your temperature when you are well for a week, every morning and again after 4:00 P.M. each day to get a sense of what's normal for you. A problematic fever is two points or more above your normal temperature.

FLATULENCE

When we were kids, flatulence was one of the funniest subjects imaginable. But when you reach a certain age, it's no longer a laughing matter. As we age, our gastrointestinal tracts frequently become more finicky, which in turn can lead to increased trouble with flatulence.

It's embarrassing, to be sure, but don't necessarily view it as a health problem, says Roger L. Gebhard, M.D., gastroenterologist at the Veterans Affairs Medical Center and professor of medicine in the division of gastroenterology at the University of Minnesota, both in Minneapolis. Most of us produce roughly one to three pints of gas daily, and the only way to relieve that pressure is through burping or flatulence. "The average person passes gas 14 to 20 times a day," Dr. Gebhard says, "which may seem like a lot, but it's actually perfectly normal."

Still, you'd probably prefer to decrease the likelihood of embarrassing episodes. There are a number of simple things you can do to ward off rumblings from down under, says Dr. Gebhard. If flatulence keeps you grumbling, here's how to keep it under control.

Try This First

Ration the gas supply. "Most flatulence originates in the carbohydrates of foods we eat," says Dr. Gebhard. "If there are certain foods that you suspect are causing the flatulence, cut those foods out of your diet for three days to see if it reduces the problem. By that time, you'll know, and you can quickly use trial and error to discover the worst offenders."

Here's what's going on. Remember that one to three pints of gas we mentioned? Most of it is produced by harmless bacteria living in your large intestine, Dr. Gebhard says. Whenever you eat a carbohydrate, your digestive system can't fully break it down. The bacteria living there will do it for you, but this produces gas as a by-product.

Depending on which particular carbohydrates you eat or enzymes you may lack (most often the lactase that breaks down dairy products), a number of different foods could cause problems with flatulence. Beans, vegetables high in cellulose (like broccoli and cauliflower), dairy products, and foods or supplements high in fiber are the most common problems, says Dr. Gebhard. Of course, all these contribute to a healthy diet, he points out, so you don't want to eliminate them completely. But cutting back on the one causing the most problems may make a big difference.

Other Wise Ways

Stop milking it for all it's worth. You may have discovered that milk as well as milk products like cheese and ice cream seem to trigger a lot of gas. That's understandable. As we grow older, our bodies produce less of an enzyme called lactase that breaks down the natural sugar in milk called lactose. Lack of that enzyme also causes gas.

If you still like milk for a good dose of bone-strengthening calcium, take it with an over-the-counter lactose digestion aid such as Lactaid, says Harris Clearfield, M.D., professor of medicine and director of the division of gastroenterology at Hahnemann University Hospital in Philadelphia. They help your body digest the lactose before any bacteria can get to it. Also, most supermarkets offer reduced-lactose milk or cheese.

Break down the beans. You can turn down the volume of the musical fruit and certain hard-to-digest beans by adding a few drops of a product called Beano to your food, says Dr. Gebhard. Beano works to break down the complex sugar found in those foods, making life simpler for your digestive system.

Give them a good soak. Another way to stifle those problematic beans is to soak them in a pot of water overnight, then pour out the water and refill the pot before cooking, says James Duke, Ph.D., botanical consultant, author of *The Green Pharmacy*, and a former ethnobotanist with the U.S. Department of Agriculture who specializes in medicinal plants. This helps to remove the offending carbohydrates. Better yet, add a small whole carrot to the pot of beans after soaking them, he suggests. Carrots can help soothe the digestive tract.

Swallow smartly. The amount of air that you swallow can have a big impact on how much gas you pass, although most of it will come out as belches, says Dr. Gebhard. When you eat and drink rapidly, you tend to swallow air without realizing it, he says. You also gulp down too much air when you chew gum, suck on hard candy, or smoke. And some people gulp air just because they're nervous, so that's another thing to watch out for. Also, ill-fitting dentures can lead to higher amounts of air-swallowing. So if you wear dentures, it might be worth checking with a dentist to make sure they fit properly.

Meanwhile, slow down when you're having dinner, sip rather than gulp, and try to be aware of times when you tend to swallow air, Dr. Gebhard suggests. As a last resort, become one of those people who constantly chews on a pen. The pen will keep your teeth separated, making it virtually impossible to swallow large amounts of air.

Say goodbye to soda. The carbonation in soft drinks, seltzer water, beer, and other carbonated beverages can cause gas problems, says Dr. Clearfield. It's gas that keeps the beverages bubbly, and when that gas goes to your inner gut, it still has the fizz in it. Stay away from these beverages for a few days to see if your symptoms improve, he suggests.

Stick with it. Any new addition to your diet like a high-fiber supplement or eight-bean chili recipe may cause flatulence in the short term. But if you continue to get your fill of fiber, your body may adjust, says Dr. Gebhard. So if a food or supplement is important to your health, don't give it up because of a one-time gas attack. Start small and gradually increase the amount you're taking in, he recommends. You might try adding about five grams of fiber more than you're used to each day for one week, then an additional five the next week, and so on until you are consuming 25 to 35 grams of fiber per day. Over time, your body might produce less gas in response.

Stamp out sorbitol. Sorbitol, another sugar that our bodies have trouble digesting, is used as an artificial sweetener in sugar-free gums, candies, and many dietetic foods, reports Dr. Gebhard. It's also found naturally in certain fruits such as apples, pears, prunes, and peaches, but only the concentrated form packed into food products causes flatulence problems. If you consume a lot of these products, try cutting back, he suggests.

Spice things up. Herbs known as carminatives may help the problem by soothing the digestive tract, says Dr. Duke. Among these are anise seed, basil, bergamot, coriander, dill, fennel, lemon balm, marjoram, oregano, peppermint, rosemary, sage, and thyme. Adding a touch of one or more of these herbs to your food or tea can be a flavorful way to solve the problem.

Choose charcoal. Activated charcoal tablets are an over-the-counter solution that may absorb gas and provide some relief, says Dr. Clearfield. While the medical evidence for charcoal's effectiveness is still somewhat murky, there's no harm in giving it a try, he says. Follow the package directions for dosage. Just don't be alarmed if your stools turn black. It's a common result of taking the tablets.

FOOD POISONING

Not all of the old ways are the best ways. Earlier this century, when iceboxes and Depression-era frugality were the norm, untold numbers of people put themselves at risk for contracting food-borne illnesses, says Nancy Cohen, R.D., Ph.D., professor of nutrition at the University of Massachusetts at Amherst.

Even if you can't quite remember those days, you may follow habits that were started back then. "If you grew up in a time when you were used to being thrifty, saving energy, and saving food and if you grew up with an icebox, you didn't want to put something warm or hot in the icebox. You cooled it to room temperature first, or the ice would melt," explains Dr. Cohen. Despite the fact that almost everyone now uses electric refrigerators, the practice of letting food cool still survives, says Dr. Cohen, and it's dangerous because it allows bacteria in food to be at temperatures in which they thrive.

These bacteria include *E. coli*, which is found in unpasteurized milk and undercooked ground beef, and salmonella, which is found in raw chicken, raw meat, and eggs. Other foods that come in contact with the bacteria can also become contaminated. But along with these freeloaders are viruses and parasites that give rise to food-borne illnesses, or what's more commonly called food poisoning. Learning how to prevent food poisoning is critical for seniors, says Margy J. Woodburn, Ph.D., professor emeritus of nutrition and food management at Oregon State University in Corvallis.

"When you do have a food-borne illness, the consequences are more apt to persist or to lead to secondary types of illness," Dr. Woodburn says. "Your immune system does not respond as quickly or as well as a younger person's. In fact, if food poisoning is very severe, it can even be life-threatening."

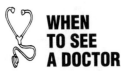

WHEN TO SEE A DOCTOR

Diarrhea and vomiting are your body's way of getting rid of things that are bad for it. So they may not be pleasant symptoms, but they're okay up to a point. If your vomiting and diarrhea last more than 24 hours or if you become dizzy and disoriented and start hallucinating, you need to see your doctor right away, says Clarita E. Herrera, M.D., clinical instructor in primary care at the New York Medical College in Valhalla, New York. You may have something other than food poisoning or you may have a case of it that needs medical attention.

Also, some illnesses such as a bleeding ulcer masquerade as food poisoning. "If you ever see any blood in your vomit or stool, you want to call right away," says Dr. Herrera.

Other changes in aging bodies can put seniors at risk for contracting food poisoning. For example, one line of defense against salmonella is the acidity of the stomach, but as people age, their stomachs become less acidic, says Sonja Olsen, Ph.D., medical epidemiologist with the Centers for Disease Control and Prevention. "So one of the main natural barriers declines," she says.

The tricky part of food poisoning can be knowing if you have it at all. Symptoms such as cramps, diarrhea, vomiting, and fever range from mild to severe. Those symptoms might show up within hours of eating the bad food, but sometimes the onset doesn't begin for days and it can be mistaken for a stomach flu. The Centers for Disease Control and Prevention can only give an estimated number of food poisoning cases—as many as 33 million every year—because so many cases go unreported.

Because of the terrible consequences of these illnesses—*E. coli* can cause kidney failure and brain damage—you should check with your doctor immediately if you have frequent or bloody diarrhea or if diarrhea or vomiting lasts more than 24 hours. And if you can, Dr. Woodburn suggests, save a little bit of the food that you suspect made you sick. Your doctor may use it for further testing to determine what type of foodborne illness you've contracted.

Try This First

Practice proper preparation. The best way to ensure that you don't come down with food poisoning is to practice safe food preparation and sanitation to prevent cross-contamination, which occurs when the bacteria in raw meat juices are transferred from a surface to a food that's eaten without further cooking. If you truss a chicken on the counter, for example, and later make a sandwich on that counter without cleaning it, you risk that kind of contamination.

To stop cross-contamination, stick to the following habits, advises Dr. Woodburn.

• Wash every kitchen surface and utensil with hot soapy water after food has been prepared on it or with it.

• Use disposable paper towels instead of dishcloths to clean and dry utensils or kitchen counters. If you do use dishcloths, get a fresh one every day, Dr. Woodburn says. Otherwise, they can become breeding grounds for bacteria.

• Sponges can also harbor bacteria, so replace them regularly, throw them in the dishwasher, or boil them, Dr. Woodburn suggests.

• When cleaning the sink, use scouring powders with a chlorine base to kill bacteria, Dr. Woodburn warns.

• Wash your hands well with soap and water after handling raw meat, poultry, seafood, and eggs.

Other Wise Ways

Think cold and shallow. When storing cooked foods, you want the food to cool fast. That means not leaving a cooked dish or perishable foods out at room temperature for more than two hours. "What you want to do is keep foods out of the danger zone, which is 40°F to 140°F," Dr. Cohen says. Between those two temperatures, bacteria multiply rapidly and cause illness.

While it may be easier to stick an entire pot of something in the fridge, the depth of the food in the pot may not allow it to cool down fast enough. Instead, divide up the food and store it in shallow containers so it's no more than two inches deep. That will expose the food to the cold air inside the refrigerator and allow it to cool more rapidly.

Coddle with cooling. To avoid spoilage, delicate fruits and vegetables—raspberries and lettuce, for instance—should always be stored in a cool refrigerator. They'll not only stay fresher but also they'll be less likely to get bacteria or mold.

Keep the fridge frigid. Sure, you might want to save on electricity bills, but not at the risk of your health. Refrigerators should be kept at 40°F or lower to slow the growth of bacteria, and freezers should be kept at 0°F or lower, Dr. Cohen says. Check the accuracy of the internal temperature setting in your refrigerator with a store-bought refrigerator thermometer.

Make sure your goose is cooked. You want the inside of a chicken or hamburger to be so hot that you kill off harmful bacteria and viruses, so investing in a meat thermometer is a wise precaution. Ground or cubed meat may have bacteria throughout, so cook to a temperature of 160°F (which is medium) or even better to 170°F (which is well-done). Poultry should be cooked to 180°F for optimal taste and safety. When preparing poultry, don't wash it first, because that gives bacteria a chance to spread.

Sorry, Charlie, no sushi. Eat fish and shellfish that have been cooked. Shellfish, especially oysters, are particularly dangerous when eaten raw, because they often carry viruses and bacteria that cause serious illness, says Dr. Woodburn.

Use a cutting-edge solution. Wash every cutting board with hot soapy water and rinse it. To further sanitize it, you can use a bleach solution. In a small washtub, mix one tablespoon of bleach with one gallon of water. Dip the cutting board in the solution, then let it air dry, says Dr. Cohen.

Ditch the nicked ones. Don't use a cutting board with lots of deep nicks in it, regardless of whether it is wooden or plastic, Dr. Cohen advises. No matter how well you think you've dried it, there can still be moisture in those nicks, where bacteria survive.

Let water run over. Fruits and vegetables should be washed under running water or washed twice, Dr. Woodburn says. Leafy vegetables such as lettuce should be separated and washed as leaves, not as a whole head. If you're peeling a fruit or vegetable, it's still best to wash it first. The action of the knife cutting into the skin can spread germs.

Clean your hands. An excellent strategy for washing your hands is using soap and water as hot as you can stand for 20 seconds or as long as it takes to sing "Happy Birthday," recommends Dr. Woodburn. When you are washing, use a lot of friction. Scrub between fingers, under nails, and under jewelry. Dry your hands with disposable paper towels, not dishtowels, which are often breeding grounds for bacteria and could recontaminate your hands after washing.

Follow the law of thaw. Frozen foods should be thawed in the refrigerator, not at room temperature. Foods may be thawed in the microwave but must be immediately cooked, not left out or returned to the refrigerator, says Dr. Cohen.

Throw it out. It may seem like common sense, but if a food doesn't look right or smell right, don't take a chance by eating it. Don't think that if you cut or scrape off a moldy part, the rest will be okay to eat. "There are microscopic edges to that mold," explains Dr. Cohen. You may be able to see where the mold is growing, "but what else is growing that you can't see?" Most leftovers don't last more than a few days stored in the fridge, she notes.

If it bulges, throw it out. Bacteria that cause botulism like to hide out in canned foods, in a low-acid and airless environment. While modern methods of preparing canned goods have reduced the risk of botulism, approximately 100 cases of the disease still occur in the United States every year, a quarter of which are transmitted through food, says Dr. Olsen. If you have a can that is swollen or leaking—typical signs of botulism—throw it out. You don't even want to taste it. Botulism causes blurred vision, difficulty swallowing and speaking, paralysis, and sometimes death.

Look for a clean, well-lit place. When you're eating out, certain strategies can help you avoid food poisoning. Avoid dishes that are made with raw or undercooked eggs, such as hollandaise sauce, Caesar salad, fresh mayonnaise, and chiffon pie. Ask your server to ask the cook whether these dishes have been made traditionally by using raw eggs, or with a pasteurized commercial egg product. If it's the pasteurized product, you won't have to worry about possible contamination from salmonella (the bacteria that can cause serious digestive problems), explains Dr. Cohen.

Scan the hand that feeds you. Check out your server. Are his hands clean? Is he handling your food in a sanitary manner? Does the whole restaurant seem to be tidy and well-run? If the answers are no, the restaurant may also have a problem following food safety standards, cautions Dr. Woodburn.

Monitor the warmth. If foods that are supposed to be served hot or cold are served to you lukewarm, send them back, says Dr. Woodburn. She also advises caution when eating salad mixtures such as pasta salad or chicken salad, which are handled after they are prepared and may not have been stored at the correct temperatures.

If It Gets You

If you do get food poisoning, it's often accompanied by diarrhea or vomiting. Your doctor may recommend an electrolyte drink such as Recharge to help restore lost fluids and minerals. In addition, here are some home remedies that can help you recover.

Brew a broth. A broth that's high in potassium might help since potassium is one of the electrolytes your body needs, advises Sherry Briskey, naturopathic physician and staff physician at Southwest Naturopathic Medical Center in Tempe, Arizona. To four cups of water add one cup each of diced celery, diced carrots, parsley, and spinach and bring to a boil. Drink three to four cups for two to three days during and after diarrhea or vomiting has stopped. If diarrhea or vomiting continue, contact a doctor. Not only will drinking the broth contribute to your liquid intake but also the mineral-rich vegetables in it will help you restore electrolytes.

Try charcoal. Some naturopathic doctors recommend activated charcoal. Capsules are available in drugstores and health food stores. Or you can eat a piece of burnt toast for the same effect, says Thomas Kruzel, naturopathic physician in private practice in Portland, Oregon. "That will do in a pinch," he says. The one thing to remember is not to be alarmed when the charcoal turns your stool black.

Go on a BRAT diet. One way to lessen the effects of diarrhea is to focus on a BRAT diet for two to three days or until symptoms stop, Dr. Briskey says. Those letters stand for bananas, rice, applesauce, and toast. "Those kinds of foods help to firm up the stool a little bit," she says.

FOOT ODOR

R ight now, as you read this, millions of microscopic creatures are living on your feet. It might give you the heebie-jeebies to think about it, but these little guys, called bacteria, are perfectly normal inhabitants for feet to have. In fact, they know something that never occurred to you. Your feet are a great feasting ground. But if you overfeed them, they can really start to stink up the place.

"With sweating and high temperatures, your skin will flake. Bacteria will feed on these flakes," says Walter J. Pedowitz, M.D., associate clinical professor of orthopedic surgery at Columbia University in New York City. That would be fine if they cleaned up after themselves. But instead, the feasting bacteria produce organic substances called fatty acids, and those are the leftovers that start to reek on your feet.

In other words, if you stick your foot into a leather shoe and go cut the grass during a warm day, you're creating a land of plenty for these microscopic creatures. It's kind of like feeding a bunch of cowboys an endless supply of beans while they lounge around in a room with little air circulation.

Thankfully, the aging process gives you some natural protection against foot odor. You have 3,000 sweat glands per square inch of skin on your feet. Over the years, these sweat glands release less and less sweat. Less sweat means less food for bacteria. So teenagers and young adults usually have more problems with foot odor than people who are 60-plus.

This doesn't mean, however, that you are totally immune. If you don't practice good hygiene, even an older foot can start to smell.

Foot odor may also signal an infection. People with diabetes often have dry, cracked skin on their feet. These cracks provide footholds for yeast, bacteria, and fungi to set up camp. Left uncontrolled, these cases of athlete's foot and other skin infections can smell. At

229

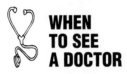

WHEN TO SEE A DOCTOR

If home remedies aren't helping, you probably have either a low-grade infection or overactive sweat glands. To halt a low-grade infection, your doctor may prescribe topical or oral antibiotics or antifungal medication, says Walter J. Pedowitz, M.D., associate clinical professor of orthopedic surgery at Columbia University in New York City.

that point, you may need to see your doctor, who can prescribe an antifungal ointment.

But for everyday smell protection, there are ways to keep those little inhabitants in check and keep your feet smelling fresh.

Try This First

Throw out those stinking shoes. No matter what you do to make your feet smell better, if you shove them back inside a pair of smelly shoes, they'll stink all over again. If you have smelly shoes, get rid of them and treat yourself to a new pair, says Dr. Pedowitz.

Other Wise Ways

Change shoes and socks often. Aim to change your shoes and socks at least once a day. But gauge your shoe and sock changes by how much your feet sweat. As soon as you notice that they are wet, it's time for a change. Wash each pair of socks after wearing them. Try to rotate your shoes so they have a day to dry out between wears, advises Dr. Pedowitz.

Buy absorbent socks. Thick, soft socks will soak up the sweat, keeping it away from your skin. Stay away from nylon, which doesn't breathe or absorb moisture but does pick up odor fast, says Dr. Pedowitz.

Add inserts. Sold over the counter, shoe inserts such as Odor-Eaters are widely available in stores and can help keep your feet odor-free, notes Dr. Pedowitz.

Apply some powder. Dust your feet with baby or foot powder. The powder will absorb some of the sweat, adds Dr. Pedowitz.

Buy breathable shoes. Although you always believed a good leather shoe was the best thing you could put on your foot, it's not. Once odor gets into leather shoes, it won't get out. They're ruined. Plus, leather makes your feet sweat. So opt for canvas or nylon shoes that have as little leather as possible, says Alan J. Liftin, M.D., dermatologist in private practice in Livingston, New Jersey.

Wash what you can. In addition to washing your socks, also remember to take out any inserts or pads in your shoes and wash those regularly too, Dr. Liftin says.

Take a tea bath. If your problem is excess sweating, soak your feet in a bucket of strongly brewed black tea, says Dr. Pedowitz. The tannic acid in the tea will kill the bacteria and close down your pores, keeping your feet dry longer. Use two tea bags per pint of water and boil for 15 minutes. Then remove the bags and add two quarts of water to the tea. Soak your feet for 30 minutes daily for about a week.

MANAGING YOUR MEDS

If your doctor prescribes oral antibiotics or antifungal medication, make sure to speak up about other medications you may be taking. This is a good general precaution and should be a routine part of the prescription process, says Walter J. Pedowitz, M.D., associate clinical professor of orthopedic surgery at Columbia University in New York City. Your doctor can then prescribe the right type of medication for you.

Before heading to the doctor's office, however, check your medicine chest. Some seemingly innocuous medications may contribute to foot odor simply because they can increase sweat production. Here are some possible culprits.

- Aspirin, which increases sweat production
- Thermoregulation medication, such as dantrolene (Dantrium), that can increase or decrease peripheral circulation, which could mean sweaty feet
- If you are taking hyperthyroid medication such as methimazole (Tapazole) or hyperadrenal medications like dexamethasone (Decadron), be aware that these conditions often cause additional sweating in the feet.

FOOT PAIN

When you really think about it, it's amazing that our feet last as long as they do. The 26 bones, 33 joints, 107 ligaments, and 19 muscles and tendons in your feet take 8,000 to 10,000 steps a day, covering more than four times the circumference of the globe in a lifetime. An average day of walking puts several hundred tons of pressure on your feet, which is partly why your feet are easier to injure than any other part of your body.

And when your feet have a problem, they'll let you know it. First, they send you signals like calluses, black toenails, and bunions. If you only deal with the signals or the symptoms but don't solve the underlying problem, your feet will eventually send you another message that's impossible to overlook—pain.

Usually, the problem in question is that your shoes don't fit right or that you were born with certain foot problems that need to be corrected by a doctor, says Neil Scheffler, D.P.M., podiatrist and president of health care and education for the Mid-Atlantic Region of the American Association of Diabetes in Baltimore. Other factors, however, also come into play. For instance, putting on extra weight as you age can add a tremendous amount of pressure to your feet. Here are some other age-related causes of foot pain.

Plantar fasciitis. The most common cause of heel pain, plantar fasciitis (pronounced fas-ee-eye-tis) becomes more prevalent as you get older. That's probably because your plantar fascia (a strong, elastic band of fibrous tissue that runs from your heel to your forefoot) gets less flexible over time. As the fascia inflames under the constant strain of walking or standing, it pulls at your heel, sometimes creating a bony prominence called a spur. Though the spur sounds painful, it's really the tight pull against your heel that causes the pain, says Tzvi Bar-David, D.P.M., podiatrist with Columbia-Presbyterian Medical Center in New York City.

"Think of the plantar fascia as a bowed string that creates the arch of your foot. When you step on this bow, you flatten it and tighten it," says Dr. Bar-David.

The telltale sign that you have plantar fasciitis is that you feel pain on the inner part of your heel. This usually occurs when you first get out of bed or stand up after sitting for some time.

Fat-pad loss. When you were born, you had nice cushy fat pads under your heels and your forefoot. But as you walked and walked over the years, these pads eventually got flattened out and slowly shrunk away. This is a natural process but can be a painful one since now you have little there to cushion your feet and absorb shock. You'll feel pain from fat-pad loss under your heel and the ball of your foot.

Arthritis. Use any joint often and rigorously enough, and eventually, you'll wear away the cartilage that cushions it. In most cases, an injury fails to heal correctly. Then inflammation causes your protective cartilage to rub away, and walking becomes painful. The feet tend to suffer mightily from arthritis because there are so many joints to damage. Arthritis manifests itself with pain, swelling, and lumps, most often in the top of your midfoot or in your toes.

Regardless of why your feet hurt, here are some strategies to nip pain in the bud.

Try This First

Stomp on pain. Nonsteroidal anti-inflammatory drugs (NSAIDs) such as ibuprofen can relieve the pain and swelling of most types of foot pain. Follow package directions. This is a temporary fix, however. You don't want to stay on over-the-counter painkillers for more than a few weeks, advises Dr. Bar-David. So make sure to try other strategies to relieve your specific foot problem.

Other Wise Ways

Bend some toes to stretch a tendon. Much of the pain from plantar fasciitis stems from a tight Achilles tendon (the band that runs down through your heel and connects with your plantar

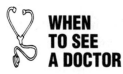

WHEN TO SEE A DOCTOR

Usually, simple reme-
dies are all you need to
banish pain. But if
home remedies don't
help, see your regular
doctor or podiatrist,
advises Tzvi Bar-David,
D.p.m., podiatrist with
Columbia-Presbyterian
Medical Center in New
York City.

Persistent heel or
other types of foot
pain may signal more
serious problems such
as a stress fracture or
adult flat-foot syn-
drome when the
tendon that holds
your arches up gets
torn. Such conditions
may require surgery or
immobilization. Also,
your heel pain may re-
sult from another
cause such as a disc
problem or arthritis in
your spine.

fascia). When it's tight, your plantar fascia gets less flexible. "Often, if you stretch the Achilles tendon, you'll end up relieving the plantar fasciitis," says Dr. Bar-David.

To stretch your Achilles tendon, get in a relaxed position—sitting or lying down—and bend your leg until your toes are within reach. Using both hands, pull your toes toward your shin and hold for 20 seconds.

Or lean in for tendon relief. Another Achilles tendon stretch can be done standing up in front of a wall. Place your hands against the wall and lean forward with your feet firmly planted flat on the ground behind you. Keep your back and feet flat and your knees locked. You will feel your calf stretching if you do this properly, notes Dr. Bar-David. Repeat this 10 times, holding each stretch for 30 seconds.

Vary your stretch times. The Achilles tendon stretches can help alleviate heel pain when it strikes, but you should also do them routinely. Be sure to stretch before and after exercising. Also, stretch before going to sleep and before getting out of bed in the morning. Though you might think your legs and feet are relaxed at night, most people sleep with their feet pointed, keeping the plantar fascia and the Achilles tight all night long, Dr. Bar-David says. So plantar fasciitis is often worst during the first few steps in the morning. By stretching before you rise, you can get your feet off to a good start.

Cushion that heel. Shop around for heel cups, or ask a podiatrist about some cushioning that will make your heel feel better. With extra cushioning, your heels aren't jarred so much by everyday walking or running. And with the slight heel lift, your Achilles tendon has a chance to relax, which eases the pull on your plantar fascia, explains Dr. Bar-David.

Switch to running or walking shoes. If your foot's natural padding has eroded over time, wear sneakers. They have extra cushioning in the heel, which helps make up for your somewhat reduced, natural fat pads, says James Michelson, M.D., associate professor of orthopedic surgery at Johns Hopkins School of Medicine in Baltimore. Lace-up shoes also will put less stress on the front of your foot if you have pain there.

Lose weight. If you've gained weight over the years, common sense tells you the extra pounds are putting extra pressure on your feet. This can create heel or forefoot pain, warns Dr. Bar-David. The lighter your body, the less your foot pain.

Get cushioned inserts. You can buy inserts to put in the sole of your shoe to absorb more shock. "Usually, it's all that's needed," adds Dr. Michelson.

Go for depth. If inserts and running shoes don't do the trick, go to a specialty orthopedic shoe store and ask for shoes that provide extra depth. These will allow you to stick even more cushioned in-

MANAGING YOUR MEDS

Over-the-counter nonsteroidal anti-inflammatory drugs (NSAIDs) such as ibuprofen and naproxen (Aleve) can zap pain but they may also cause side effects in some people. They include:

- Confusion
- Swelling of the face, feet, or lower legs
- Sudden decrease in urine output
- Stomach upset

If you suffer from any of these symptoms, talk with your doctor or pharmacist about a pain-relieving alternative that doesn't produce these kinds of side effects, advises W. Steven Pray, Ph.D., R.Ph., professor of nonprescription drug products at Southwestern Oklahoma State University in Weatherford.

serts into your shoe to absorb even more shock, according to Dr. Michelson.

Avoid high heels. If you're a woman, wearing high heels could contribute to arthritis and other foot pain. High heels also push all of the force of walking into the front of your foot, where things are tight and immovable. Switch to flats, says Dr. Michelson.

Get your feet measured. Shoes that are too tight will make your feet hurt even more. Most women wear their shoes two sizes too small, notes Dr. Michelson, and many haven't had their feet measured in at least five years. Since your feet grow as you age, the shoe that fit when you were 40 may be too small now. Have a clerk or a friend measure your feet for you while you are standing. And do this every time you buy a new pair of shoes, advises Dr. Michelson. Some other ways to make sure you get the right fit:

• Shop at the end of the day. Your feet swell over the course of the day and you'll want shoes that fit when your feet are at their largest.

• Keep in mind that one foot might be larger than the other. When you're shoe shopping, always fit shoes to your largest foot. (Use cushioning, if necessary, to fill in the gaps in the shoe for your smaller foot.)

• Make sure there's at least a half-inch between your longest toe and the end of the shoe.

Make ginger a habit. Fresh ginger is a great remedy for arthritis and other pain related to swelling, because it's a natural anti-inflammatory, says Neal Barnard, M.D., author of *Foods That Fight Pain* and president of the Physicians Committee for Responsible Medicine in Washington, D.C. Though you don't have to use a lot of it to get significant relief, you do have to take it regularly, he says.

Buy fresh ginger at the supermarket. Mince up one-half teaspoon to a teaspoon per day. Either put it in your food as a flavoring or mix it into some water and swallow it like a pill. Cloves, garlic, and turmeric, though less studied, have shown similar effects in some people, according to Dr. Barnard.

Rub hot peppers on them. Over-the-counter creams made from capsaicin, the active ingredient in hot peppers, can relieve arthritis and other foot pain, says Dr. Barnard. The lotion may at first cause a burning sensation, which goes away the more you use the stuff. Rub just enough to lightly cover the affected area on your feet whenever you feel pain. Wash your hands thoroughly after each application and keep the cream away from your eyes and other mucous membranes. It can really burn.

Modify your exercise. If your feet hurt because you give them a regular pounding every time you take a brisk walk, change your routine, says Donna Astion, M.D., associate chief of foot and ankle service for the Hospital for Joint Diseases, Orthopaedic Institute in New York City. For instance, try taking every other day off, alternating between weight-bearing activities such as running and non-weight-bearing activities such as cycling. If you run, alternate between hard tar roads and softer surfaces like trails.

Soak them. Treat your feet to a soak in Epsom salts and warm water. The soak can drain swollen tissues and help relieve pressure. Follow the directions on the package, which usually recommend one tablespoon of Epsom salts dissolved in each quart of water.

FRAGILE SKIN

Yes, you're familiar with the crow's-feet around your eyes and the subtle skin folds along your neck, but what are these cracks, these flakes, these spots and growths?

They're all signs that, like the rest of your physical body, your skin is getting a little more fragile as you age. In fact, your skin is likely to become more fragile in several ways. It becomes drier and more wrinkled and also tends to heal more slowly than it did when you were younger. The good news is, there are several things you can do to protect your skin. But first, here's a look at what causes fragile skin.

"One of the major reasons skin becomes fragile is because it becomes thinner the older you get," says Arthur K. Balin, M.D., medical director of the Sally Balin Medical Center for Dermatology and Cosmetic Surgery in Media, Pennsylvania, and co-author of *The Life of the Skin*. The top two layers of the skin, the epidermis and dermis, become thinner and contain fewer blood vessels, he says. With the decline in the number of blood vessels and overall quantity of blood flowing to cells, the tissues shrink.

A big contributor to this form of skin aging is the sun. "The sun breaks down capillaries, which reduces the amount of blood getting to tissues," says Frederic Haberman, M.D., assistant clinical professor of medicine (dermatology) at Albert Einstein College of Medicine in New York City and director of the Haberman Dermatology Institute in Ridgewood, New Jersey. "It also dries out the skin and breaks down the underlying layer. The result is that the sun makes the skin thinner, drier, and more fragile."

Doctors advise that your best line of defense for protecting and soothing fragile skin is to prevent overexposure to sunlight and, as much as possible, to keep your skin moisturized. It's also a good idea to support your skin with antioxidants, those immune-boosting and cancer-fighting nutrients in food that prevent the decay of cells and tissues, experts say.

Try This First

Go soak yourself. Once your outer layer of skin becomes thin, it can no longer hold moisture as well as it did during its youth, says Hillard Pearlstein, M.D., assistant clinical professor of dermatology at Mount Sinai School of Medicine in New York City. So you need to take steps to replenish the moisture. The best way, says Dr. Pearlstein, is to soak in a lukewarm bath for 15 minutes. But don't overdo it.

Many doctors recommend that people with fragile skin bathe only two or three times per week and use only the mildest soaps. Also, they say, you should avoid hot showers or baths because hot water is more drying than cool. And you should use soap only on odor-producing areas such as the armpits, genitals, and feet; rinse the rest of your body with cool water.

Other Wise Ways

Moisturize twice a day. You should moisturize your skin every morning and evening whether or not you've bathed that day. If you apply moisturizer after you've bathed, it will help hold the water in. "The moisturizer will not rebuild skin," Dr. Pearlstein says, "but it

MANAGING YOUR MEDS

If you find that your skin is becoming more fragile, it may be because of a prescription you're taking. The category of drugs known as adrenal corticosteroids, which includes such prescription medications as cortisone (Cortone), prednisone (Deltasone), and dexamethasone (Decadron), used to treat adrenal problems, arthritis, and skin diseases, may in some cases thin your skin and make it more susceptible to injury, says W. Steven Pray, Ph.D., R.Ph., professor of nonprescription products at Southwestern Oklahoma State University in Weatherford.

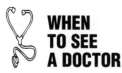

WHEN TO SEE A DOCTOR

Being thin-skinned is not enough, by itself, to call the doctor. But fragile skin can be the unwelcome result of a lifetime of sun exposure that carries other risks, too. You should report any changes in a skin growth or lesion to your doctor, recommends the American Academy of Dermatology.

will make the skin feel better and offer some protection against further moisture loss."

Use a moisturizer that contains petroleum jelly or lanolin, advises the American Academy of Dermatology. These are among the best and least irritating of moisturizing ingredients. If your moisturizer irritates your skin, consult a dermatologist for recommendations.

Try an antioxidant. Many people see an improvement in their skin after daily application of a skin lotion that contains the antioxidant vitamins C and E, says Dr. Haberman. (One brand containing both vitamins is Neutrogena New Hands.) Those who benefit from these topical lotions say the lotions make their skin feel stronger and that they appear to delay some of the damage done by overexposure to sunlight.

Create a daily shield. The sun's rays attack your skin like piercing arrows. "You have to stay out of harm's way to protect fragile skin," advises Dr. Pearlstein. "That protection starts with applying an adequate sunscreen each day, of at least a sun protection factor of 15."

Cover up, especially in summer. You should never deliberately sunbathe, but always wear a wide-brimmed hat to shade your face and neck, Dr. Pearlstein recommends. Also, wear long sleeves and light trousers. Finally, be sure to put on gloves when you're gardening, to protect the backs of your hands.

Walk on the shady side of the street. "I tell my patients to walk before 10:00 A.M. and after 4:00 P.M., when the sun's rays will do less damage to the skin," Dr. Pearlstein says. "I also tell them to walk on the shady side of the street to avoid the direct rays of the sun."

Try some acid on your skin. Alpha hydroxy acids (AHAs) are showing promising signs in the skin's fight against aging and sun damage, according to the American Academy of Dermatology. Some studies suggest that AHAs may reduce wrinkles and improve the skin's overall appearance. AHAs, which are found in milk, fruit, and sugarcane, are present in many moisturizing creams and lotions. You may see them listed as glycolic acid or lactic acid. You can safely use AHAs at home, notes Dr. Pearlstein. Look for over-the-counter skin preparations containing AHAs. Follow the package directions for usage.

GALLSTONES

Like a good friend, the gallbladder quietly serves us well until we mistreat it and it demands our attention. Located on the right side of the body under the liver, the gallbladder is a small pear-shaped organ that aids in digestion. Its main function is to store bile from the liver until the bile is needed to break down fats during digestion.

If too much cholesterol or calcium is in the bile, gallstones can form, but that in itself is not always a problem. Most people with gallstones never even know that they have these deposits, which can range in size from a grain of sand to a golf ball. Sometimes, when gallstones pass through a duct, they can get stuck, and that can cause a gallbladder attack. You'd know if you had one: You'd experience pain in your upper-middle or right abdomen, moving around to your back; nausea; and vomiting. These are all signs of gallstone problems, says Robert Charm, M.D., gastroenterologist in Walnut Creek, California, and professor of gastroenterology and internal medicine at the University of California, Davis. At that point, surgery is sometimes the best option.

If others in your family have had the problem or if you're overweight, you could be more prone to gallstones. Women who have had several children or who are on estrogen replacement therapy also tend to have a higher risk of developing gallstones, says Roger Gebhard, M.D., gastroenterologist at the Veterans Affairs Medical Center and professor of medicine in the division of gastroenterology at the University of Minnesota, both in Minneapolis. While many older people have gallstones, age doesn't put you at risk for them. But once you have gallstones, they don't go away on their own, explains Dr. Gebhard.

Even if sex and heredity are ganging up to raise your risk, that doesn't mean you're destined to get gallstones. Here are some things you can do to discourage the stones from getting started.

Try This First

Eat light. Since being overweight is a common risk factor for gallstones, do what you can to keep the weight off. Especially steer clear of large fatty meals, says Mike Cantwell, M.D., clinician and coordinator for clinical research at the Institute for Health and Healing at the California Pacific Medical Center in San Francisco. "Fat makes the gallbladder work harder, increasing the likelihood of gallstones."

Other Wise Ways

Lose a little at a time. While it's important to avoid being overweight, don't embark on a crash diet to get there. Losing weight fast can actually increase your risk of developing gallstones, explains Dr. Cantwell. Yo-yo dieting (a cycle of quick weight loss followed by weight gain) is especially hard on the gallbladder. It creates a situation where the gallbladder sits unused for a time, then suddenly gets overused. This stop-start activity only increases the likelihood of gallstone formation. A slow, steady weight-loss program that includes regular meals of low-fat foods and plenty of exercise is the way to go.

MANAGING YOUR MEDS

Thankfully, hardly any drugs can cause gallstones to develop or worsen. But gemfibrozil (Lopid), a drug prescribed to reduce triglyceride blood levels and raise high-density lipoprotein (HDL) cholesterol, has been linked to gallstone formation, says W. Steven Pray, Ph.D., R.Ph., a professor of nonprescription drug products at Southwestern Oklahoma State University in Weatherford. If you've been using this drug, talk to your doctor about this side effect. He may wish to prescribe an alternative.

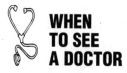

WHEN TO SEE A DOCTOR

In most cases, when you have gallstone pain, you'll need to see a doctor to confirm the diagnosis and determine the best way of dealing with the problem, says Martin Brotman, M.D., gastroenterologist at the California Pacific Medical Center in San Francisco. If your doctor decides to remove your gallbladder, your worries about gallstone pain are over. And don't fret; your digestive system will function just fine without that extra internal appendage.

But if your doctor doesn't operate, be alert to any recurrence of symptoms. If the pain returns, you'll need to return to your doctor.

Put on your walking shoes. If you don't exercise regularly, you could be risking gallstones. Regular exercise steps up metabolism (the pace of energy-burning), notes Dr. Charm. "When metabolism is slow, small gallstones can develop. Even simple activities like stretching or walking help gallbladder health."

Pump up the fiber. Yet another reason for eating meals high in fiber is that it'll reduce gallstone risk, says Dr. Charm. "Fiber helps lower cholesterol produced by the liver." And cholesterol, remember, is one of the building blocks of gallstones.

GLAUCOMA

Political opponents were fond of saying that President George Bush lacked "vision" for America's future. They were almost right.

In April 1990, White House doctors discovered that the 65-year-old president had a budding case of glaucoma in his left eye. Although he had not lost any vision, he immediately began using eyedrops twice a day to prevent future loss of sight.

"I haven't felt a thing," Bush told the press at the time.

Like Bush, many people afflicted with this insidious disease aren't aware that they have it. In fact, glaucoma is often called the silent thief of sight because it usually strikes slowly, painlessly, and without warning. Yet it afflicts more than three million Americans—most of them over age 60. Each year, it affects another 50,000 people worldwide and causes blindness in more than 1,000.

"You should never take your eyesight for granted, particularly because of diseases like glaucoma. Most people don't realize that they have had visual losses from glaucoma until the losses are very advanced. Your vision may be 20/20 right up to the end—and then it's snuffed out. And unfortunately, those losses are irreversible," says Anne Sumers, M.D., ophthalmologist in Ridgewood, New Jersey, and a spokeswoman for the American Academy of Ophthalmology.

But if glaucoma is detected and treated early, the progress of the disease can be halted and most of your vision can be saved with a regimen of eyedrops once or twice a day, Dr. Sumers says. Years after his diagnosis, for instance, Bush's vision was still in tip-top shape.

To understand how glaucoma robs vision, imagine that your eye is like a small sink, says Robert Ritch, M.D., medical director of the Glaucoma Foundation in New York City. The faucet is a gland behind the iris that constantly produces fluid that bathes the eye. The drain is a ¹⁄₅₀-inch-wide opening called the trabecular meshwork. As

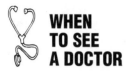

WHEN TO SEE A DOCTOR

Because it has no symptoms, glaucoma will sneak up on you. That's why it's important for everyone over age 60 to have an annual eye exam that includes a glaucoma check, says Anne Sumers, M.D., ophthalmologist in Ridgewood, New Jersey, and a spokeswoman for the American Academy of Ophthalmology.

In between exams, see an optometrist or ophthalmologist if you experience any of the following symptoms.

• Morning headaches
• Recurrent blurry vision
• Seeing rainbow-hued halos around lights at night
• Decreases in your peripheral (side) vision
• Pain around your eyes after watching television or leaving a dark theater

you age, this drain tends to clog and the fluid meets more resistance in flowing out of the eye. Since the eye is a closed compartment, fluid buildup results in raised pressure, or intraocular pressure (IOP), inside the eye, putting excessive pressure on the optic nerve. As the IOP increases, the nerve slowly begins to die and your peripheral (side) vision fades. Untreated, it eventually leads to almost total blindness. Once it is detected, the first line of treatment is to lower IOP. You'll need to regularly take medication to control it.

If you've been diagnosed with low-pressure glaucoma, in addition to taking medication, there are several things you can do to help keep it under control.

Try This First

Go for ginkgo. In addition to any prescription medications, ask your doctor about using ginkgo biloba, an over-the-counter herbal remedy that Dr. Ritch believes helps preserve vision. "Ginkgo appears to increase blood flow to the eye and prevent the death of cells in the optic nerve," he says.

Look for ginkgo extracts containing 6 to 7 percent terpenes, a component of the herb that Dr. Ritch suspects plays a key role in stopping optic nerve damage. He suggests taking 120 milligrams of the herbal remedy twice a day for two months, then cutting back to 60 milligrams twice a day. Doses of ginkgo biloba higher than 240 milligrams of concentrated extract can cause skin rash, diarrhea, and vomiting. Don't use ginkgo if you're taking monoamine oxidase (MAO) inhibitor drugs like phenelzine sulfate (Nardil) or tranylcypromine (Parnate), aspirin or nonsteroidal anti-inflammatory medications, or blood-thinning medications like warfarin (Coumadin).

Other Wise Ways

Set your sights on antioxidants. Studies strongly suggest that antioxidant vitamins C and E can relieve low eye pressure and slow the development of glaucoma, Dr. Ritch says. He recommends

MANAGING YOUR MEDS

The eyes are much more than the windows to the soul. They also are potent pathways for medications into your body.

"For some reason, a lot of people don't think of their eyedrops as medicine. They know that these drops affect the eyes, but they don't seem to realize that the drugs in these drops can get into the bloodstream and cause side effects in the entire body," says Anne Sumers, M.D., ophthalmologist in Ridgewood, New Jersey, and a spokeswoman for the American Academy of Ophthalmology. "So whenever you are being treated for glaucoma, it is extremely important to let all of your doctors know what medications you are taking."

Medications known as beta-blockers (Timoptic, Betoptic, Betagan) that are often used to treat glaucoma can cause asthma attacks, dizziness, impotence, fatigue, depression, memory loss, and other symptoms that your physician wouldn't necessarily associate with glaucoma unless he knew you were being treated with these drugs, Dr. Sumers says.

Ask your ophthalmologist or pharmacist about side effects before taking any glaucoma medications, including:

- Pilocarpine (Isopto Carpine, Pilocar) and other miotics (can cause headaches and blurred vision)
- Methazolamide (Neptazane, MZM) and other carbonic anhydrase inhibitors (can cause depression and kidney stones)
- Brimonidine tartrate (Alphagan) (can cause headaches and fatigue)
- Latanoprost (Xalatan) (can cause a pigmentation of the iris, which may turn the patient's blue eyes to brown)

taking 2,000 milligrams of vitamin C and 800 international units (IU) of vitamin E daily. (Vitamin C in amounts above 1,200 milligrams may cause diarrhea in some people. Also, although vitamin E is generally sold in doses of 400 IU, one small study showed a possible risk of stroke in dosages higher than 200 IU. Consult with your doctor if you are at high risk for stroke.)

Walk away from it. Regular aerobic exercise like walking can help lower pressure in the eye, increase blood flow to the optic nerve, and slow the progression of the disease, Dr. Ritch says.

In fact, research conducted at Oregon Health Sciences University in Portland on a group of sedentary people who began a program of brisk walking for 40 minutes three times a week found that those with glaucoma reduced their eye pressure by 20 percent. And those people who did not have glaucoma saw a 9 percent reduction in eye pressure.

Stick to your schedule. Timing is critical when using glaucoma medications, Dr. Sumers says. To get 24-hour coverage from your medication, you have to properly space out your doses.

"Some people think that three doses a day means at breakfast, lunch, and supper. That's not going to work, because the last dose of medication is going to wear off before you get another one the next day," she says. "So if you're supposed to use eyedrops three times a day, allow a full eight hours between treatments."

Don't skimp. If you don't think you got enough medication into your eye, try again, Dr. Sumers suggests. "You can't overdose on eyedrops. It's better to use an extra drop than to not get enough in."

Try the squeeze play. After you insert your eyedrops, press a finger against the tear duct in the inner corner of your eye for about one minute, Dr. Ritch says. It will help keep medication in your eye, where it is needed, rather than allowing it to run down your face. Keep your eyes shut while doing this, so the drug can be properly absorbed, he suggests. It is particularly important to leave about 10 minutes between medications if you're using two different eyedrop medications. If you don't wait long enough, the second drop will wash the first drop out of the eye before it has chance to do its job.

GOUT

D oes your toe hurt like the dickens today?

If the answer is yes, the cause may date all the way back to your adolescence. Somewhere in your teen years, the bad stuff called uric acid started to circulate in your blood in increased amounts. Basically a waste product, excess uric acid is a leftover. It enters your system after your body has absorbed all the energizing fuel it wants from meats and other foods. The excess is supposed to make a rapid migration to your kidneys, and they're supposed to siphon it off to the outside world the next time you get the urge to go.

People who develop gout, however, get in a nonproductive wrestling match with the flow-through of uric acid. Either their kidneys can't handle all the acid in their systems or their kidneys don't do a good job of flushing away normal amounts. Either way, uric acid builds up. Over time, it crystallizes and finds a resting place in your lower joints, says Jim O'Dell, M.D., professor and chief of rheumatology and vice chairman of the department of internal medicine at the University of Nebraska Medical Center in Omaha. These crystals are annoying. And your joints, very annoyed, rebel by swelling up, getting tender, and hurting like—well, just an awful lot.

In men, gout problems tend to surface in the midforties. But because of changes related to menopause, gout hits later for women, usually striking when they're in their midsixties, says Dr. O'Dell.

Some people get gout, some don't—but the selection process is more than random. Family history plays a role. If your grandpa had it and so did your mom, you're at greater risk than the gout-free family next door.

There are also dietary factors. Some foods such as meats, anchovies, mussels, and especially alcohol create a lot more uric acid than others. If your body can't shed the excess, you're being

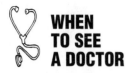

WHEN TO SEE A DOCTOR

If your gout attacks become more frequent, see your doctor. He can try to lower the levels of uric acid in your blood with a prescription for allopurinol (Zyloprim) or probenecid (Benemid), says Richard S. Panush, M.D., chairman of the department of medicine at Saint Barnabas Medical Center in Livingston, New Jersey.

set up for gout every time you eat these foods.

Your first gout attack may feel like a throbbing pain that suddenly flares up, usually just after you get out of bed or during the middle of the night. If you're lucky, you may never have another attack. Chances are, however, that you'll feel this pain again within six months to two years. And if you don't treat the problem, the attacks will grow longer and more frequent.

Half of people who have gout feel it in their big toes, though their ankles and knees also may be affected. Despite the pain it inflicts, gout itself is not a fatal disease, says Dr. O'Dell. The trouble is, it's strongly linked with certain more serious problems like high blood pressure, diabetes, kidney stones, and high cholesterol. So when you're seeing the doctor for pain relief, you may also be checked out for these other problems.

But once you have the doctor's diagnosis and advice, you're on your own. Here are some gout resisters that might help make the road smoother for you.

Try This First

Cool it down. When an attack flares up, reduce pain by packing your toe in ice, says Nancy Becker, M.D., rheumatologist in private practice in Kansas City, Kansas. Loosely fill a plastic bag with crushed ice and wrap a towel around the bag. With the towel between your toe and the bag of ice, apply this compress all around your toe. Use the ice pack up to three times daily, leaving it in place for 20 minutes during each treatment.

Other Wise Ways

Take an anti-inflammatory. Your pain is mostly a result of swelling. So over-the-counter anti-inflammatory medication such as ibuprofen may be helpful. Just make sure to let your rheumatologist know what you've been taking, says Dr. O'Dell. Anti-inflammatories can mask some of the symptoms of gout, making an accurate diagnosis more complicated.

Ban alcohol. Alcohol boosts your uric acid production. Stay away from the stuff, and you'll help manage gout, notes Dr. O'Dell.

Repudiate purine-rich foods. Foods rich in a substance called purine can elevate uric acid levels. Fortunately, the foods you usually have to reject are also bad for your heart health, so you have a twofold reason to shun them. Try to cut back on the following: organ meats, anchovies, consommé, gravies, herring, mussels, pork roast, poultry, roast beef, and sardines, suggests Dr. O'Dell.

Maintain a healthy weight. If you are over your ideal weight, you'll have higher levels of uric acid in your blood that may lead to

MANAGING YOUR MEDS

People with gout who also have a circulatory disease may have a problem because some of the medicine used to manage heart disease, such as diuretics like chlorothiazide (Diuril) or furosemide (Lasix), can raise uric acid levels, says Richard S. Panush, M.D., chairman of the department of medicine at Saint Barnabas Medical Center in Livingston, New Jersey. If you have a doctor for a heart condition and you see a rheumatologist for gout, be sure both of the doctors know what you are taking.

Side effects to the commonly taken gout medications include:

- Diarrhea
- Itching
- Nausea
- Rashes
- Stomach pain
- Vomiting

more frequent and intense gout attacks, says Richard S. Panush, M.D., chairman of the department of medicine at Saint Barnabas Medical Center in Livingston, New Jersey. Being overweight can also put you at higher risk for heart problems. Slowly but surely, lose those pounds, and you'll stack the deck in favor of fewer gout attacks.

Keep your toe in the water. Dehydration can trigger a gout attack. Whenever you drink plenty of fluids, especially water, you're activating the flush-out process that helps get the uric acid into your kidneys and then out of your system, says Dr. Panush. Make sure to get eight or more tall glasses of water every day. An easy method is to carry around a water bottle and take frequent sips.

GRIEF

The death of a loved one is never easy. And as we get older, each loss can seem that much more painful and close to the heart. Each year, for instance, about 800,000 Americans are widowed. According to data from the U.S. Bureau of the Census, 47 percent of women and 14 percent of men 65 and older will have lost their spouse. Add in the deaths of countless friends and relatives, and you could be lugging around a hefty load of grief.

But although it hurts, grief also heals.

"The death of a loved one, particularly a spouse, is one of life's most stressful events," says Laura Slap-Shelton, Ph.D., clinical psychologist with a specialty in neuropsychology at the Child Study Center in Bryn Mawr, Pennsylvania. "When you lose a spouse after many years of marriage, you not only have lost a person but also you've lost a lifetime of shared experiences and shared identity with someone you loved. Being able to weep over that loss and express anger and other uncomfortable feelings is part of the healing process. Grief will definitely help you heal your emotional wounds, but it will take some time."

How much time depends on the person. For some, grieving may end within a year. For others, it may take years to get over the period of mourning. Some sadness and a sense of missing your spouse may persist indefinitely for some. Grief counselors also know that bereavement is seldom tidy. It has no set course and can meander unpredictably through a vast array of emotions, including shock, denial, anger, despair, and acceptance.

"Most people feel numb or in shock immediately after the death of a loved one. It doesn't really sink in that the person is dead. This is actually healthy because the shock helps the survivor function in the first few days after the loss and do the necessary things like put together a funeral," says Daniel L. Segal, Ph.D., assistant pro-

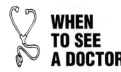

WHEN TO SEE A DOCTOR

Most people begin to shed their grief 6 to12 months after the death of a loved one. Seek counseling with a skilled psychologist or counselor if your bereavement persists more than a year and you have any of the following symptoms.

• You feel chronically depressed, anxious, or irritable.

• You have difficulty sleeping.

• You feel isolated, or your relationships with family and friends are deteriorating.

• Your use of alcohol or drugs has increased since the death of your loved one.

• You feel intensely guilty or unrealistically blame yourself for the death of your loved one.

• You are contemplating suicide or feel as if you want to die.

fessor of psychology at the University of Colorado at Colorado Springs.

In the weeks or months following the loss of a loved one, those in mourning commonly experience poor appetite, weight loss, insomnia, fatigue, forgetfulness, and concentration problems, says George T. Grossberg, M.D., director of geriatric psychiatry at St. Louis University School of Medicine.

But while grief isn't pleasant, repressing it is worse. In fact, people who bury their grief are more prone to lengthy bouts of clinical depression and other serious emotional problems than those who openly express their sorrow, Dr. Grossberg says.

So learning to cope with your feelings of loss and moving on with life is vital to your physical and emotional well-being. Remember, it is only natural to feel sad when a loved one dies. The best thing you can do is allow yourself to grieve and let the healing begin, Dr. Slap-Shelton says. Here are a few suggestions.

Try This First

Share your sorrow. Seek out friends and relatives who can understand your feelings of loss and are willing to listen. Talking will help you to accept and resolve the loss, says Harold G. Koenig, M.D., author of *Is Religion Good for Your Health?* and associate professor of psychiatry and behavioral sciences at Duke University Medical Center in Durham, North Carolina.

"It's very important to express and share those negative, painful emotions as soon as you can with someone you feel close to," Dr. Koenig says. "If you don't, those feelings are going to keep popping up and make it more difficult for you to function."

Other Wise Ways

Join a support group. Even more than family and friends, other people who have recently lost a loved one will understand the painful emotional roller coaster you are riding right now, Dr. Slap-Shelton says. "In a support group, you'll meet people who have been through similar experiences and have practical answers for many of the problems you're facing. You can cry and tell people exactly how you feel, without being judged," she says. Check the Internet, the classified ads in your local newspaper, or ask your clergy or doctor for information about bereavement support groups in your community.

Create a memorable memorial. Honor and remember your loved one in a way that has personal meaning for you, Dr. Segal suggests. Plant a tree, compile a photo album, volunteer your time at a favorite charity, or simply finish a project that your loved one started. Creating an ongoing legacy in memory of your loved one will help you heal, he says.

Let the words flow. Record in a journal your thoughts and feelings as you grieve, Dr. Slap-Shelton suggests. Think of your journal as a private and personal place where you can express your innermost emotions without being judged or criticized. It is often helpful to write a letter to your spouse as a means of expressing feelings directly to your lost loved one. Unloading your grief and safely storing it away in a journal also may help you feel less guilty about diving back into community life.

Speak the unspoken. Although it may be painful, picture the deceased person as you would like to remember him or her. Then take time to speak to the image of that loved one. Say all the things you wish you had said before the person died, says Dennis Gersten, M.D., psychiatrist in San Diego, imagery expert, and author of *Are You Getting Enlightened or Losing Your Mind?* If you're angry, sad, or feeling frightened, let the deceased person know that, too. This imaginary conversation can be remarkably healing, Dr. Gersten says.

Dive back in. Resume your daily routine as soon possible. Stay involved in religious activities, go back to work or your volunteer position, or get back into your exercise routine. Do many of the activities you enjoyed prior to the loss, Dr. Segal says.

"If you used to enjoy going to a movie once a week, it's important to keep doing that, even though your spouse isn't there. Find someone else to go with you. It will help prevent you from becoming isolated and dwelling on the loss," Dr. Segal says. "Doing that will be hard at first, but it will get easier and it will help you realize that life can and will go on. Survivors and others should realize that this is only the first stage of an ongoing process. Their loss may not have consciously registered yet."

Postpone major life changes. In the depths of grief, you may be more prone to make rash decisions that you'll quickly regret, Dr. Slap-Shelton says. So for at least a year after the death of your spouse, hold off on making important lifestyle decisions such as selling your home, moving, or remarrying.

Be patient with yourself. Don't try to rush yourself through your grief. Everyone recovers from a loss at his own pace. "The worst thing you can tell yourself is, 'It's been three months, I should be over this by now,' " Dr. Segal says. "You're just putting unrealistic pressure on yourself that will make you feel bad about yourself and make things worse."

Remember, some days will be better than others. You may feel absolutely great one evening but wake up the next morning filled with despair. That's a normal part of grieving that may persist for months. And that's okay, Dr. Segal says.

Get some good scents. The soothing fragrances of essential oils such as jasmine, rose, and lavender can help lift your spirits, relieve stress, and help you cope with grief, says John Steele, aromatic consultant in Los Angeles. The sparkling, lemony scent of melissa, also known as lemonbalm, is particularly effective for grief because it has antidepressant, euphoric qualities, Steele says. Apply a drop or two to a tissue or handkerchief and inhale whenever you're in need of some comfort, he suggests. Melissa, lavender, and other essential oils also can be mixed together to create a fragrance that is particularly uplifting for you. Essential oils are available at most health food stores.

Pray along the way. If you are religious, prayer can help you release your loved one to the care and protection of God, says Dr. Koenig. As you pray, imagine yourself in a beautiful place holding hands with your loved one. Now imagine that God walks up with his arms open, ready to receive the deceased. Give your loved one a deep embrace, put your loved one's hands into the hands of God, and let him or her go. Watch your loved one walk away with God (who has His arm around his or her shoulders) until they are completely out of sight.

This prayer ritual is so powerful that it has helped relieve grief-related depressions that have lasted for many years, Dr. Koenig says.

GUM PROBLEMS
AND TOOTH LOSS

A dreadful myth persists that tooth loss is an inevitable part of aging. Years ago, in Ireland and other European cultures, this belief was so pervasive that brides would have all their teeth removed and get dentures prior to marriage in order to spare their husbands the expense of it later in life, says Eric Z. Shapira, D.D.S., dentist in Half Moon Bay, California, and spokesperson for the Academy of General Dentistry in Chicago.

But these mass extractions were hardly warranted. Aging, dentists say, has little impact on the health of your teeth. "If you take proper care of your teeth and gums and get regular dental checkups, you should be able keep your teeth throughout your life," Dr. Shapira says. "In fact, I have a 98-year-old patient who still has all of her natural teeth. They're absolutely beautiful."

More people than ever before are preserving their natural teeth throughout adulthood, rapidly making toothlessness and full dentures relics of the past. In 1960, nearly half of all Americans 65 and older were toothless. By the mid 1980s, only about one in three seniors were wearing full dentures, says Stephen K. Shuman, D.D.S., associate professor of preventive sciences at the University of Minnesota School of Dentistry in Minneapolis. But while progress has been made, the typical American still only retains 16 to 19 natural teeth out of 32 after age 60.

The best way to ensure that you'll keep your full complement is by brushing and flossing at least twice a day to prevent cavities and receding gums (periodontal disease). These two tooth attackers are the top two causes of tooth loss in people over age 60, Dr. Shuman says.

Even if you've slacked off in your oral hygiene habits in recent years, perhaps because of a disabling ailment like arthritis or stroke, it still might not be too late to save your teeth, Dr. Shuman says. You just need to find ways to get back into the routine. Here are a few tips to help you take the bite out of tooth decay and gum disease.

Try This First

Plug in. Electric toothbrushes like Sonicare, Braun Oral-B, or Interplak will generally clean your teeth better than hand brushing, particularly if you have dexterity problems that make it difficult for you to brush and floss, says Jeffrey Astroth, D.D.S., chief of dentistry at the University of Colorado Center on Aging in Denver. "They have larger handles that make them easier to grip, and they clean between the teeth almost as well as dental floss. I wouldn't say they're better than flossing. But I've recommended these types of brushes to several of my patients," he says.

Other Wise Ways

Get a grip. If you have trouble holding on to a toothbrush, wrap the handle with aluminum foil or modeling putty, suggests Dr. Astroth. The foil or putty will enlarge the handle and make it easier to grasp. Or cut a small hole in opposing sides of a tennis ball or handball. Then stick the toothbrush handle through the holes. This, too, can make hanging on to the brush easier.

Brush up on your technique. Although you've been brushing for decades, here are a few reminders from Dr. Shapira.

• Use a soft-bristled brush unless directed otherwise by your dentist.

• Look in a mirror while you brush. If you can see what you're doing, it will help you clean your teeth more effectively.

• Place your toothbrush at a 45-degree angle against your gumline and massage in place in a circular motion.

• Move the brush back and forth gently in short (toothwide) strokes, four or five times on the outer, inner, and chewing surfaces of all teeth.

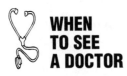

WHEN TO SEE A DOCTOR

Older Americans should have regular dental checkups at least twice a year. But, seek dental care as soon as possible if:

• You have loose or separating teeth.

• You have red, swollen, or tender gums.

• Your gums have pulled away from your teeth.

• Your gums bleed during tooth brushing and flossing, or they begin bleeding for no apparent reason.

• You have persistent bad breath.

• You notice pus between your teeth and gums.

• You notice a change in the way your teeth fit together when you bite.

• You notice a change in the fit of partial dentures.

• You have mouth sores that won't heal.

• For the inside surfaces of your front teeth, move up and down gently with the tip of the brush.

• Brush your tongue and gums to scrape away any odor-causing bacteria that accumulate.

• Replace your brush when the bristles become frayed, which is about every three to four months.

Be gentle. Don't clean your teeth the way you'd clean your kitchen sink, Dr. Shapira warns. Constant, forceful scrubbing can wear away tooth enamel and gums, making your teeth more sensitive and exposing the roots of your teeth to infection and other problems. To get an idea of how lightly you should be brushing, take your index finger and gently press it onto your palm until the skin on your palm underneath your finger blanches. It shouldn't take much pressure to do that, Dr. Shapira says.

Name that tune. Many people brush for less than 20 seconds. That's hardly enough time to adequately clean your teeth, says Nick Russo, D.D.S., vice president of the Academy of General Dentistry in Chicago. He recommends brushing for two to three minutes. If necessary, set an egg timer, or turn on a radio and brush for the duration of one song.

Some electric toothbrushes also have built-in timers, Dr. Shapira says.

Stick with gum. Chew sugarless gums, like Trident, or gum made with baking soda or hydrogen peroxide, like Arm and Hammer Dental Care or Biotène Gum, for 5 to 10 minutes three times a day. They can help control plaque buildup and prevent cavities, Dr. Shapira explains.

Be nutty about cheese. Eat a handful of peanuts or an ounce of aged Monterey Jack or Cheddar cheese after a meal or sugary snack to neutralize acids in the mouth that damage teeth and gums, Dr. Astroth suggests.

Follow the pyramid. The same nutritious foods that help build strong muscles and bones also strengthen your teeth and make them more resistant to cavities, Dr. Astroth says. Cavities are more common among seniors than you might suspect. Up to 68 percent of Americans 65 to 69 and more than 70 percent of those over age 70 may have root cavities at any given time, according to studies.

So eat a balanced diet daily that includes 6 to 11 servings of breads, cereals, and pastas; 3 to 5 servings of vegetables; 2 to 4 servings of fruits; 2 to 3 servings of yogurt, milk, and other dairy products; and 2 to 3 servings of fish, poultry, and nuts.

MANAGING YOUR MEDS

A long list of prescription and over-the-counter drugs can indirectly lead to tooth loss and gum disease, says Eric Z. Shapira, D.D.S., dentist in Half Moon Bay, California, and spokesperson for the Academy of General Dentistry in Chicago. In fact, more than 400 medications are known to sap saliva flow into the mouth. Without saliva to flush them out of the mouth, bacteria will flourish and damage both your teeth and gums. If you suspect that one of your medications is compounding your tooth or gum problems, consult with your doctor or pharmacist. Among the common drugs taken by seniors that can contribute to tooth loss are:

- Aspirin, acetaminophen, and other prescription and over-the-counter analgesics
- Nitroglycerin (Nitrostat) and other medications used to relieve angina
- Calcium channel blockers like verapamil (Calan), used to control irregular heartbeats
- Tricyclic antidepressants like amitriptyline (Elavil)
- High blood pressure medications like prazosin (Minipress) or propranolol (Inderal)
- Diuretics such as furosemide (Lasix) or chlorothiazide (Diuril)

Don't be too sweet. Limit your consumption of chocolate and other sweets, Dr. Shapira says. Remember that each time you eat sweets, harmful bacteria produce acids in your mouth for at least 20 minutes. It is this acid that causes tooth decay.

Snack on foods like nuts, popcorn, raw fruits, vegetables, and sugar-free drinks that don't promote decay. If you insist on eating sweets, do it just once a day, after you eat a well-balanced meal. And remember to brush immediately afterward to cleanse your mouth of bacteria and acids, Dr. Shapira urges.

Wash out your mouth. Gargle and rinse for 30 seconds just before bedtime with mouth rinses such as Viadent or Biotène. Or use a rinse like Fluorigard or ACT, which contain fluoride. They can help prevent cavities and flush harmful plaque and bacteria away from your gums, Dr. Shapira says. Avoid drinking any beverages for at least 30 minutes after using a fluoride mouth rinse, so that the fluoride can be properly absorbed by the teeth surfaces.

Tweak your gums. Flossing is fundamental at any age, Dr. Shuman says. If you can, at least once a day:

1. Break off about 18 inches of floss and wind most it around one of your middle fingers.
2. Wind the remaining floss around the same finger of the opposite hand. This finger will take up the floss as it becomes dirty.
3. Hold the floss tightly between your thumbs and forefingers. Guide the floss between your teeth using a gentle rubbing action. Never snap the floss into the gums.
4. When the floss reaches the gum line, curve it into a C shape against one tooth. Gently slide it into the space between the gum and the tooth.
5. Hold the floss tightly against the tooth. Gently rub the side of the tooth, moving the floss away from the gum with up-and-down motions.
6. Repeat this method on the rest of your teeth. Don't forget the back side of your last tooth. If you wear a bridge, be sure to floss the teeth around it.

If dexterity problems are making it difficult for you to use floss, consider using proxy brushes, Dr. Astroth suggests. These tiny, inexpensive brushes are easier for many older people to use, and they clean between the teeth almost as well as floss.

Get out and about. Without daily contact with others, the incentive to brush and floss your teeth can quickly fade. This is particularly true of seniors who have recently lost spouses or moved to new communities, Dr. Russo says. Join a jewelry-making, woodworking, or other hobby group. Get a part-time job. Volunteer at your church or synagogue. Dive into the outside world at least once a day, Dr. Russo urges. It will encourage you to maintain good oral hygiene.

Bar the drinks. Alcohol dries out your mouth and increases your likelihood of gum disease and tooth loss, says Dr. Shapira. If you drink, cut back to no more than one 12-ounce beer, 4-ounce glass of wine, or 1-ounce serving of liquor a day, Dr. Shapira urges.

Snub smoking. People over age 60 who continue to smoke are twice as prone to tooth loss as nonsmokers, says Elizabeth Krall, Ph.D., epidemiologist and associate professor at Boston University School of Dental Medicine.

Smoking causes bone loss that weakens a tooth's underlying support and promotes gum disease. In fact, smokers are five times more likely than nonsmokers to have gum disease, according to the National Institute of Dental Research.

In addition, smoking and chewing tobacco stain your teeth. These stains are a perfect place for plaque to hitch a ride on a tooth, causing cavities and aggravating periodontal disease.

Don't play dentist. Some drugstores sell over-the-counter devices that resemble scalers (instruments used by dentists and dental hygienists to remove tartar and other deposits from teeth). Although they may be tempting, leave them on the shelf, advises Heidi Hausauer, D.D.S., assistant clinical professor at the University of the Pacific School of Dentistry in San Francisco.

"I've had people come into the office who have used these over-the-counter dental instruments and chipped their front teeth with them. I've seen patients gouge roots and chip enamel off lower incisors," Dr. Hausauer says. "It's particularly unwise for an older person to use them, because he or she probably doesn't have the proper training or dexterity to use these products well. The person could take the device, inadvertently shove tartar farther down under the gum, and cause a severe infection." Instead of trying to do extensive cleanings yourself, get dental checkups twice a year, she urges.

Hair Loss

With each passing year, you've noticed more and more of your hair ending up in the sink or on your brush rather than on your head. It's not your mind playing tricks on you, says Dominic Brandy, M.D., clinical instructor in the department of dermatology at the University of Pittsburgh School of Medicine.

At maturity, the human scalp maintains an average of 100,000 hair follicles. At anytime, roughly 90 percent of the hairs on your head are in the growing phase, explains Dr. Brandy. The growing phase lasts from between two to seven years, depending on your age. At the same time, 10 percent of the follicles are in a three-month resting phase. During this resting phase, about 10 percent of the hair is shed from the follicle.

When you're young, your hair usually grows for six or seven years before falling. As the years pass, the growing stage gets shorter, lasting two to five years, says Dr. Brandy.

"As your hair grows for a shorter time, the hairs aren't as long or thick, and they fall out more regularly," says Judith Shank, M.D., clinical associate professor of dermatology at the University of Minnesota Medical School in Plymouth.

Hair loss is a mostly natural occurrence and may be hereditary. Some health conditions, however, may be causing you to shed more of it. Studies have linked hair loss to high cholesterol levels, and, therefore, it may indicate a risk of heart disease. Here are some ways to keep your hair in place or at least make the most of what you have.

Try This First

Pump some iron. In some cases, iron deficiency can also cause hair loss, says Fredric Brandt, M.D., clinical associate professor of dermatology at the University of Miami School of Medicine. "Senior citizens should make sure that they eat well-balanced diets with a daily serving of one or two iron-rich foods," says Dr. Brandt. Good sources of iron include lean red meat, cream of wheat, steamed clams, tofu, and broccoli.

Adding foods rich in iron is the best way to ensure that you get the recommended amount for people over age 50, which is 10 milligrams. Before turning to supplements, talk to your doctor, experts say, because high levels of iron can be toxic in adults.

MANAGING YOUR MEDS

If you're experiencing noticeable thinning at the top and back of your head, you may benefit from using over-the-counter minoxidil (Rogaine), says Dominic Brandy, M.D., clinical instructor in the department of dermatology at the University of Pittsburgh School of Medicine. For men, finasteride (Propecia) may be another option. Your doctor can provide more information, if you're interested.

Of course, there are items in your very own medicine chest that could be speeding up your hair loss. "But you have to be careful to sort out whether it's the medication that's causing your hair to fall out or the illness that these drugs are treating," says Judith Shank, M.D., clinical associate professor of dermatology at the University of Minnesota Medical School in Plymouth. The following may cause hair loss.

- Nonsteroidal anti-inflammatory drugs (NSAIDs) such as ibuprofen
- Anticoagulants such as heparin (Calciparine)
- DHEA, which is recommended by some doctors for natural hormone replacement therapy
- Beta-blockers like metoprolol tartrate (Lopressor) or other high blood pressure medicines such as penbutolol sulfate (Levatol)
- Antiseizure medications like phenytoin (Dilantin)
- Some gout medications such as sulfinpyrazone (Anturane)
- Some psoriasis medications like etretinate (Tegison)
- Some antituberculosis medicine like isoniazid (Rifamate)
- Excessive amounts of vitamin A and drugs related to vitamin A such as the acne medication isotretinoin (Accutane)

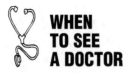

WHEN TO SEE A DOCTOR

The average person loses between 50 and 100 hairs every day, says Fredric Brandt, M.D., clinical associate professor of dermatology at the University of Miami School of Medicine. If you notice more than that on your brush or in your sink, it's time to see a doctor. You may have an underlying health problem like thyroid disease or iron-deficiency anemia that, once corrected, can end the follicle fallout.

Other Wise Ways

Get points for style. If your hair is thinning, get it styled in a manner that makes it appear thicker, says Barbara Bealer, assistant education director of the Allentown School of Cosmetology in Pennsylvania. Bealer suggests that women with thinning hair get an angled or blunt cut as opposed to a layered haircut. "When the hair is cut all one length, like a bob, it appears thicker than a layered cut," says Bealer. "An angled cut can create the illusion that your hair is thicker, which can mask the fact that your hair is thinning out a bit."

The same advice goes for men, Bealer adds. Don't make the mistake of trying to pull hair from one area to another; it will make the hair look thinner. Men may want to go with a slightly layered cut. A bit of layering can keep a man from looking like Prince Valiant while still getting the thicker appearance that comes from the hair being close to one length.

Keep it clean. Dirt and debris can sometimes choke off new hair growth, so keep your scalp clean by washing it daily, says Dr. Brandt.

Bealer recommends using Nioxin, a treatment for thinning hair available only through salons, or another hair treatment recommended by your styist. Nioxin is applied after each shampoo, to stimulate growth and cleanse the pores. This ensures that there is no debris such as excess oil blocking hair growth.

Add bounce with biotin. If your hair is starting to thin, take some biotin supplements, available at many health food stores. "Biotin is a B-complex vitamin that is necessary for your body to process dietary protein," says Dr. Brandt, who advises taking three milligrams (3,000 micrograms) of biotin once a day. Protein seals the moisture in your hair, keeping it thicker and fuller. If you want to get your biotin naturally, good food sources include corn, barley, milk, egg yolks, and fortified cereals.

Shampoo in thickness. If you suffer from thinning hair, try a hair-thickening shampoo such as Redken's Cat Protein Reconstructing Treatment, Bealer says. "These types of shampoos coat your hair with protein and can help seal in moisture, thus increasing the thickness of existing strands of hair within six months," Bealer says. Other hair-thickening shampoos on the market include Aussie Real Volume, Foltene Research, and Nexxus' Diametress Hair Thickening Shampoo.

Take time to de-stress. Try to keep your stress levels to a minimum, Dr. Brandt says. Older people often experience hair loss after a stressful event like the death of a loved one, he says. But left unchecked, everyday stress can build up and cause you to shed some hairs. For more information on managing stress, see Stress on page 504.

HAMMERTOES

D ay in, day out, you probably don't pay much attention to your toes. But then one day, you begin to notice that one of your toes looks odd. And by the time your 60th or 70th birthday rolls around, you may wonder why a number of your toes look as if they were cowering in fear.

Well, if you have a hammertoe—or a number of them—your poor piggies probably are cowering. Tucked inside stylish, ill-fitting shoes, they can take quite a beating, sight unseen. Not only that, a case or two of hammertoe can really hurt.

Usually, hammertoe starts with an imbalance created by two tendons, says Kathleen Stone, D.P.M., podiatrist in private practice in Glendale, Arizona. One tendon connects the muscles on the top of your foot to your toes, and an opposed tendon connects the muscles on the bottom of your foot to your toes. As the stronger top tendon starts to win the day-in, day-out tug-of-war, your toe's knuckle migrates up. Simultaneously, the end of your toe heads down. The result is a claw-shaped toe.

When shoes are too tight and too narrow, they scrunch your toes together into a tight space. Over the years, some toes may become permanently flexed. It can hurt just to walk, says Dr. Stone.

Even worse, each toe that's now sticking up in the most unnatural way will rub against your shoes and your other toes, creating painful corns and sometimes even ingrown toenails. The misaligned toe also encourages the fat pad that cushions the bottom of your foot to move away. Once that cushion is out of position, walking becomes even more painful, says Donna Astion, M.D., associate chief of foot and ankle service for the Hospital for Joint Diseases, Orthopaedic Institute in New York City.

Only a podiatric surgeon can set your toe straight. But you can keep matters from getting worse and prevent some pain with the following strategies, advises Dr. Stone.

Try This First

Get bigger shoes. You need shoes with wide toe boxes, says Dr. Stone. Look for shoes such as Easy Spirit and Nine West that come in different widths, he suggests.

Follow these fitting tips, advises Robert Schwartz, certified pedorthist (professional shoe fitter) and founder of Eneslow Pedorthic Institute in New York City.

• Shop for shoes near the end of the day, when your feet have swollen to their largest.

• Always have the salesperson measure your feet, and be sure you're standing when the foot measurement is taken.

• Look for shoes that are wide and long enough. There is no such thing as breaking in a shoe that is too narrow. You should be able to wiggle your toes while you are standing.

• When you're trying on shoes, make sure the ball of your foot feels comfortable.

• Get a shoe with extra depth to provide more room for your toe. If the shoes on display don't have enough depth, be sure to ask the store clerk for help.

Other Wise Ways

Move up a sock size, too. Too-tight socks or stockings will pull on your toe, encouraging it to pull up even more. So make sure your toes have plenty of wiggle room after you put socks or nylons on, recommends Dr. Stone.

Buy leather. Leather shoes are softer and provide more give than other types of shoes. This will give your toe slightly more mobility, says Schwartz.

WHEN TO SEE A DOCTOR

Usually, your hammertoe will be more of a nuisance than a serious issue. But if your toe suddenly becomes more painful, see a podiatrist as soon as possible, says Kathleen Stone, D.P.M., podiatrist in private practice in Glendale, Arizona.

Even if you don't require surgery, a podiatrist can fit you with custom-made orthotics and show you padding techniques, which will make your toe much more comfortable, says Dr. Stone.

HEADACHE

Some days, it seems like headaches are the price of modern life. We're bombarded with too much noise, too much stress, too much traffic, too much everything, and the result is a pounding headache.

Doctors estimate that over 45 million Americans have histories of getting chronic, recurring headaches. They figure that temporary tension-type headaches affect 70 percent of the population. Headache patterns begin in youth and middle age, say experts. And those patterns are likely to continue as you mature.

But all sorts of things can cause a headache at any age. Chocolate, cheese, red wine, cured meats, flickering fluorescent lights, stress, tension, or changes in sleep habits can trigger migraines. Chronic disease and neurological disorders can bring on headaches, as can something as mundane as coughing. According to one study, the most common cause of head pain is ice cream.

Each year, the vast majority of Americans who visit physicians for headaches suffer from what is known as primary headaches, says Alan Rapoport, M.D., director and co-founder of the New England Center for Headache in Stamford, Connecticut, and assistant clinical professor of neurology at Yale University Medical School. For these individuals, the headache itself is the primary problem and not just a symptom of some other disease. Primary headaches are divided into three general categories, says Dr. Rapoport: tension-type headache, migraine headache, and cluster headache.

Nine out of 10 people who get headaches have the tension-type. Also known as muscle-contraction headaches, some are caused by a tensing of muscles in the scalp and neck. With these, you'll feel a dull, achy pain, as if pressure were being applied to your head or neck. Tension-type headaches may be triggered by anxiety and stress, poor posture, muscle strain, or something out of kilter in your joints.

Migraines produce throbbing pain on one or both sides of the head. Other symptoms can include nausea, vomiting, light and noise sensitivity, fever, chills, flulike achiness, and sweating. Migraines may last from a few hours to days. You might get migraines several times a week or as infrequently as once every few years.

Cluster headaches are a relatively rare but very distinct type of headache that mainly affects men. The headaches come in series. They are sudden, excruciating one-sided headaches that can run from 45 minutes to two hours. Along with the headache comes nasal congestion. Typically, one eyelid droops, and the eye on the painful side gets irritated and watery. Dr. Rapoport says that cluster headaches occur chiefly in middle-age men. Fewer than one-tenth of 1 percent of the population gets this type of headache, and those in their senior years are even less likely to get them.

Then there are secondary headaches, which are probably most common to seniors. These are brought on by some other ailment like a sinus infection, temporomandibular joint disorder, shingles, glaucoma, brain hemorrhage, or meningitis, says Robert Kennedy, M.D., internist and director of geriatrics at Maimonides Medical Center in Brooklyn, New York. In older Americans, for example, dental and jaw problems caused by misaligned dentures often bring on headaches, says Dr. Kennedy. Cervical osteoarthritis can produce these headaches, too, by putting pressure on nerve roots in the neck and at the base of the skull. If you have chronic headaches, notes Dr. Kennedy, seek the advice of a headache specialist.

Although many tend to get fewer headaches as they age, says Dr. Kennedy, that fact won't be much comfort to you when headaches do strike. But the following remedies can come to the rescue.

Try This First

Take a break. Many times, headaches go away when you break your routine, explains Richard W. Besdine, M.D., professor of medicine and director of the center on aging at the University of Connecticut Health Center in Farmington. "Do some stretching exercises, take a walk in the fresh air, play a game on the computer. Do something you enjoy to get your mind off the pain."

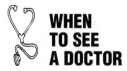

Often, relaxation and gentle exercise are all that's needed to relieve a mild tension-type headache, according to Dr. Rapoport.

Other Wise Ways

Keep a diary. The best way to beat a recurring headache is to keep a headache diary, says Robert Kunkel, M.D., migraine specialist at the Cleveland Clinic Foundation. In your diary, note when the headache begins, how long it lasts, and where it's located, like the base of the skull or left temple.

A diary should also chart what you were doing when the headache began, where you were, whether you were around any potential allergens, what you recently had to eat or drink, and whether you were feeling tense or emotionally upset. And include comments on any patterns you're noticing. For example, you might note that, "Headaches are more intense when I haven't had eight hours of sleep." This information will help you spot patterns that you may be able to alter, notes Dr. Kunkel. A diary can also help your doctor identify the best treatment, he says, while making you a better advocate for your own health.

Get physical. Regular exercise relieves headaches, says Dr. Kunkel, and reduces their frequency. Exercise causes the release of brain chemicals called endorphins, which are powerful natural painkillers, he says. Plus, people who exercise regularly tend to be in better health and have fewer headaches in general.

Try physical exercise like brisk walking,

jogging, swimming, bicycle riding, rowing, or aerobic dancing for 20 to 30 minutes a day. It can be very relaxing, calming, and therapeutic for someone with a headache, according to Dr. Kunkel. If the exercise makes a headache more intense, stop what you're doing and try something a little less jarring to your body. Check with your doctor before you begin an exercise program, says Dr. Kunkel.

Try the tried and true. You probably already knew this, but some over-the-counter pain medications, like Excedrin Migraine, Nuprin, and Orudis KT, provide very effective relief for most headaches, says Dr. Rapoport.

Mild headache pain can be treated with common painkillers like aspirin, acetaminophen, or ibuprofen tablets. "But take care not to use these too often," advises Dr. Rapoport, "because analgesics can cause rebound headaches." He suggests limiting use of these drugs to two or, at most, three days a week to avoid rebound headaches. Take no more per day than is recommended on the label.

MANAGING YOUR MEDS

Clinical research since the 1980s suggests that many people with daily headaches are suffering from a rebound effect that is due to overuse of some medications, says Alan Rapoport, M.D., director and co-founder of the New England Center for Headache in Stamford, Connecticut and assistant clinical professor of neurology at Yale University Medical School. When there's a rebound effect, you are actually getting increased and consistent pain from painkiller or tranquilizing medications that are supposed to make pain go away.

A rebound headache can be caused by both prescription and over-the-counter painkillers (Fioricet, aspirin, acetaminophen), sedative and tranquilizer drugs, and ergotamine tartrate (Cafergot), used for migraine. Fortunately, the headache often improves dramatically or goes away entirely when these medications are gradually stopped, says Dr. Rapoport. Daily prescription medications (such as antidepressants, beta-blockers, and calcium channel blockers) used to prevent headache then become more effective, he says.

Pinch yourself. Acupressure is a procedure based in a traditional Chinese medicine that may help relieve headaches by promoting the release of painkilling endorphins, says Dr. Kennedy.

Pinch the acupressure point on the same side that your head hurts. Using the thumb and index finger of one hand, lightly pinch the web of skin between the index finger and thumb of your other hand. Hold for three minutes, then release.

Cool it. An ice pack can relieve tension-type headaches, says Dr. Kennedy, by relieving muscle spasm and numbing the painful area.

To put the deep freeze on your headache, fill a plastic sandwich bag with ice cubes and wrap it in a damp towel, then hold it on the painful area for 10 minutes, suggests Dr. Kennedy. A bag of frozen vegetables or a specially made product called an ice pillow can be used in the same way, he says.

Give yourself a massage. Many tension-type headaches in older people are caused by arthritis in the neck, explains Dr. Kunkel. Gently massage your scalp and neck to help relieve the pain, he suggests. You can massage your scalp with your fingertips as if you were washing your hair.

Or softly knead the tight muscles of your neck and shoulders for as long as it feels comfortable. Or better yet, ask a loved one to massage your neck, head, and shoulders for 5 to 10 minutes, says Dr. Kunkel.

Roll out your neck. In addition to massaging tight muscles, Dr. Kunkel suggests doing neck rolls in the shower, where heat makes tight areas more pliable. Direct the spray to the back of your neck, let your chin hit your chest, and do big, slow rotations all the way around. Then switch directions, alternating after about five rotations per side, he says, and allowing the weight of your head to gently stretch stiff muscles. Stop if you feel any discomfort.

Boost vitamin B. Several studies have shown that vitamin B supplements can help prevent migraine, according to Dr. Rapoport.

In one Belgian study, people who took 400 milligrams daily of vitamin B_2, or riboflavin, reduced migraine intensity by 68 percent, he says. Other research found that patients improved when they started taking 50 milligrams of B_6.

B vitamins are generally safe because the body excretes any excess, Dr. Rapoport says. Nonetheless, check with your doctor before beginning vitamin therapy, he advises. Unstable gait and numb feet may occur, for example, in doses of B_6 at 50 milligrams to 2 grams daily over a prolonged time.

Magnify your magnesium intake. To prevent migraines, Dr. Rapoport recommends taking 250 to 400 milligrams of magnesium every day. Research suggests that magnesium deficiency is partially to blame for about 50 percent of migraines, he says. (People with heart or kidney problems should not take supplemental magnesium.) Supplemental magnesium may cause diarrhea in some people.

Keep regular hours. Migraines are commonly triggered by a change in sleep patterns, says Dr. Kunkel, who advises those prone to migraines to follow a routine as much as possible. It's best to go to bed and get up at about the same time each day, he adds, since this helps to regulate the brain's important biological clock.

While it's important to get enough rest, average six to eight hours. Avoid oversleeping, warns Dr. Kunkel, since this can also trigger a migraine.

Eliminate food triggers. Hammering headaches, especially migraines, can be brought on by different foods, says Dr. Rapoport.

One of the most common triggers is tyramine. Chocolate, red wine, and aged cheese all contain this chemical. It causes blood vessels to constrict only to rebound and dilate painfully later. Nitrites, found in cured or processed meats like turkey, ham, hot dogs, and bologna, can cause problems for some people. So can monosodium glutamate (MSG), which is found in meat tenderizers, canned and dry soups, and some Chinese food.

Eating salty snack food has been linked to headache attacks by some studies. Use of the artificial sweetener aspartame has been associated with headaches in some studies, but not in others.

Suspect foods don't cause problems for all people prone to migraine, says Dr. Rapoport. But if you might be susceptible, avoid many of these foods long enough to see if your headaches go away.

Turn down caffeine. If you consume caffeine every day then suddenly stop, you're setting yourself up for a major headache, explains Dr. Besdine. As with some other drugs, the lack of caffeine can cause a headache if your body has come to depend on it. This is why it's not a good idea to avoid caffeine altogether on the weekend if you're accustomed to having one or more cups per day, he adds.

To minimize caffeine's headache effect, Dr. Besdine recommends no more than two cups of caffeinated beverages a day. If you want to eliminate caffeine from your diet, it's best to do so very gradually, he says.

Don't skip meals. If you miss a meal, your blood sugar level drops, and that is one of the most common triggers mentioned by migraine patients, says Dr. Kunkel. Anyone prone to frequent headaches should avoid skipping meals, he says. Instead, have meals at regular intervals during the day, says Dr. Kunkel. And eat some protein, about three ounces at least three times each day.

Have a denture adjustment. If your bite isn't symmetrical because your dentures are out of alignment, it can cause headache pain by straining your jaw and facial muscles, Dr. Kunkel says. "Many older people hate to spend money updating or fixing their dentures, but it's really a small investment if it eliminates headaches and improves the quality of your life."

HEARING LOSS

Hearing loss is like having a juicy bit of gossip being told about you. No matter how vigilant you may be, you always seem to be the last one to know.

That's not entirely your fault, of course. As health problems go, hearing loss is a sneaky one, slipping up on you gradually. You may not notice the problem until you start telling your grandchildren to speak up. Or other people complain that your TV or radio is too loud. Or someone sends you on an errand and you come back with the wrong things.

When it starts to happen regularly, it can be annoying, frustrating, maybe even a little scary. But you don't have to accept it as a part of aging. As a first step, you should always see a doctor for an evaluation. Hearing loss can be caused by permanent nerve damage due to aging, says Ernest Mhoon, M.D., professor of otolaryngology at the University of Chicago. But the problem may also be something correctable, such as impacted ear wax. Only your doctor can help you determine which it is. If you are suffering hearing loss, here are some ways that you and your loved ones can make communication easier and more enjoyable.

Try This First

Get within eyeshot. Seeing a person can actually help you understand what he's saying. Try to look at people when they're talking to you, says Laurel Glass, M.D., former director of the University of California, San Francisco, Medical School Center on Deafness. You need to make sure you pick up all the visual cues and body language you can to help fill in the blanks of what you don't hear.

When you are talking with someone, make sure his face is not in

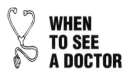

WHEN TO SEE A DOCTOR

shadows, or visual cues for speech reading will be lost, advises Michael Wynne, Ph.D., associate professor in the department of otolaryngology at the Indiana University School of Medicine in Indianapolis.

Other Wise Ways

Close the gap. Get within several feet of the person to whom you are talking. "The sound energy level is very important, and for every six feet you're away from the speaker, you lose half the energy volume of his voice," says Charles P. Kimmelman, M.D., professor of otolaryngology at Cornell University Medical College and attending physician at Manhattan Eye, Ear, and Throat Hospital, both in New York City.

Find a quiet spot. If you're going to do any kind of important communication, make sure you do it with the television off or in an environment that doesn't have a lot of distracting background noises, says Dr. Wynne. The radio, the dishwasher, and even the noise that a car makes while it's running can be loud enough to interfere with a conversation.

Ask people to speak slowly and clearly. It helps to have a couple of key phrases at your disposal, Dr. Glass says. This alerts the person with whom you are talking that you have a hearing loss. Simply asking "What?" or saying "I didn't hear you" may not be enough.

"You can say 'Could you slow down just a little and speak a little more firmly?'" Dr. Glass advises. Speaking firmly means putting a little more breath in the voice, not raising the voice, and talking louder.

Let friends and family help you. Communication is a two-way street, remember. If your hearing has been impaired, you can give people some helpful clues so they can communicate with you better, says Dr. Wynne. Let them know that if you don't understand something, they should repeat it again, the same way, without paraphrasing. If, after repeating it one time, you still don't understand them, then ask them to rephrase what they said.

Be a parrot. If someone is talking to you and you're not sure if you heard them correctly, you can double-check by repeating back to him what you think he just said, says Dr. Glass.

Keep your mouth free. Ask people to refrain from eating and chewing gum while talking, suggests Dr. Glass. That can obscure facial expressions. You want to take advantage of every auditory and visual cue you can when you are hearing impaired or if you're speaking to someone who is. And if you're a woman with a spouse who has a mustache or beard that covers his upper lip, you may want to ask him to keep it well-groomed so that it's easier for you to lip-read.

Show your good side. Usually, people with hearing loss have one ear that is better than the other. Be sure to sit with that ear closest to whatever it is you're trying to hear, says Dr. Mhoon. In social gatherings, focus on talking intimately with a small group of people, and sit so your good side is toward them.

Carry paper and pencil. If your hearing loss if very profound, the best thing to do is carry paper and a pencil with you so you can

MANAGING YOUR MEDS

Some diuretics, such as furosemide (Lasix), in high doses and some antihypertensive drugs, such as the combination bisoprolol and hydrochlorothiazide (Ziac), can cause hearing loss. Also, certain antibiotics, like gentamicin (Garamycin), can cause temporary or permanent hearing loss. Ask your doctor for advice if you are concerned about these side effects, says Laurel Glass, M.D, former director of the University of California, San Francisco, Medical School Center on Deafness.

at least communicate through writing, says Dr. Glass. If you don't understand what a person has just said, ask that person to write it out.

Clean out your ears. It may seem obvious, but we sometimes forget that wax buildup in our ears can muffle hearing. Make sure you're wiping your outer ear with a warm, wet washcloth every day, says Dr. Wynne.

Start protecting your ears. No matter how much hearing loss you have, you can always make it worse through exposure to loud noises. Some examples include running motors, power tools, and loud music. If you can't avoid prolonged exposure to loud noise, get some earplugs and wear them while you're exposed to the loud sounds, says Dr. Mhoon.

HEARTBURN

If there ever was an ailment that sounds just like it feels, it's heartburn. Coming hard on the heels of hearty meals, it's a searing pain in the middle of the chest. Its fiery flames, at their worst, seem to blaze all the way up from belly to throat. As the final insult, the burning is often accompanied by an acidic taste, as if the stomach was making mockery of whatever flavorful foods you've just enjoyed.

About the only good thing you can say about heartburn is that at least it has nothing to do with the heart, says Martin Brotman, M.D., gastroenterologist at the California Pacific Medical Center in San Francisco.

Instead, the trouble starts lower. Heartburn develops during an episode of acid reflux. That's when stomach acid works its way back up into the esophagus (the tube that carries food from the mouth to the stomach). While the stomach has a lining to protect its tender tissues from digestive acids, the esophagus wasn't meant to handle that hotbed of reflux irritation. As soon as the stomach acids touch unprotected esophagus, the result is heartburn, says Chesley Hines, M.D., gastroenterologist at the Center for Digestive Diseases in New Orleans.

After the age of 50, nearly half of us have a condition called hiatal hernias, which may be a setup for heartburn. To get a picture of a hiatal hernia, envision a small water balloon—that's your stomach—inside a big airbag, your abdomen. Tear a little hole in the top of your diaphragm in your abdomen, and your stomach will protrude. As it pokes up, that protrusion presses against the muscle that connects your esophagus to your stomach. The muscle allows acid to move into your esophagus, and you end up with the burning sensation of heartburn.

Having a hiatal hernia doesn't automatically mean you'll develop

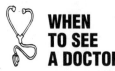

WHEN TO SEE A DOCTOR

Heartburn is usually nothing more serious than a penalty for overindulging at dinner, and everyone pays that price now and again. But if you have heartburn pain behind your breastbone during physical activities—while climbing the stairs, for example—see your doctor right away. Heartburnlike sensations during physical activity can sometimes be a sign of a hidden heart problem, says Martin Brotman, M.D., gastroenterologist at the California Pacific Medical Center in San Francisco.

heartburn. You're just at a greater risk for it. And fortunately, since so many of us are destined to have it, the hiatal hernia doesn't cause any other problems, according to Dr. Hines. Unlike other hernias, a hiatal one doesn't necessarily need to be repaired. All you have to worry about is taking care of the heartburn, if it strikes.

But whether the heartburn is caused by the hernia or originates from some other cause, prevention and treatment are the same. Here's what experts have to say.

Try This First

Neutralize acid now. The quickest way to get relief is to chew a couple of antacid tablets like Tums, Rolaids, or Maalox. These over-the-counter medications can quickly relieve heartburn once it starts, because they contain components that neutralize existing acid. "I like Tums because it has calcium," says Robert Charm, M.D., gastroenterologist and internist in Walnut Creek, California, and professor of gastroenterology and internal medicine at the University of California, Davis. Just be sure to take that Tums with your next meal, rather than on an empty stomach. Some people over 60 have trouble absorbing calcium carbonate on an empty stomach.

Other Wise Ways

Cut it off at the pass. Prevention is the best treatment for heartburn, says Roger L. Gebhard, M.D., gastroenterologist at the Veterans Affairs Medical Center and professor of medicine in the division of gastroenterology at the University of Minnesota, both in Minneapolis. "Pay attention to what foods seem to cause your heartburn, and avoid them in the future."

There are a number of foods that tend to relax the tight ring of muscle (the esophageal sphincter) that separates the vulnerable esophagus from the acid-producing stomach. These include fatty foods, peppermint, coffee with or without caffeine, alcohol, and chocolate.

Meanwhile, citrus juices, tomato-based foods and sauces, and spicy foods can irritate the esophagus. Very hot or very cold beverages can cause trouble and so can super-hot or icy food. In addi-

MANAGING YOUR MEDS

Both prescription and over-the-counter medications can cause heartburn, says W. Steven Pray, Ph.D., R.Ph., professor of nonprescription drug products at Southwestern Oklahoma State University in Weatherford. Here are just a few of them.

- Caffeine in any form, whether as a caffeinated beverage, as a stimulant (Vivarin), or to boost the potency of internal analgesics, as in the nonprescription product Excedrin
- Albuterol (Proventil) and metaproterenol (Alupent), which are prescribed to relieve some respiratory problems
- Blood sugar regulators such as glyburide (Micronase)
- Angina-relievers including nifedipine (Procardia)
- The osteoporosis drug alendronate (Fosamax)
- Aspirin and nonprescription and prescription nonsteroidal anti-inflammatory drugs (NSAIDs) such as ibuprofen, and oxaprozin (Daypro), which are used to treat inflammation, swelling, joint pain, and stiffness
- Tension-headache combination medicine with butalbital, aspirin, and caffeine (Fiorinal)
- Cholesterol-reducing drugs such as pravastatin (Pravachol) and fluvastatin (Lescol)
- Drugs for Parkinson's disease, such as selegiline (Eldepryl)

tion, beverages such as beer, cola drinks, and milk can stimulate the overproduction of stomach acids.

Don't dine and recline. Lying down too soon after eating often aggravates heartburn, says Dr. Charm. So allow yourself a three-hour break between eating and lying down. "You can sip a cup of decaffeinated green tea if you want a bedtime snack," he adds.

Rest the right way. When you do recline, try sleeping on your left side. "Some of my patients find that they are less likely to have reflux while lying on their left sides," says Dr. Gebhard.

Take a stroll. Instead of sitting or reclining after a meal, take a leisurely walk. If you stay upright for a while after a meal, gravity helps keep acid down in your stomach where it belongs. Too cold or too late to walk around the block? "Stroll around the house," suggests Dr. Gebhard. "Check out each room or look at the pictures on the walls."

Make gravity a friend, not a foe. If you have heartburn at night, elevate the head of your bed six to eight inches with blocks. "More pillows under your head won't work, because that will fold your body in half and cause acid to reflux up into the esophagus," explains Dr. Gebhard.

Lunch like a king. Then dine like a pauper. "Try eating a bit more for lunch and then have a smaller dinner," says Dr. Charm. This will help avoid nighttime heartburn.

If it's tight, it's not right. "Abdominal pressure from tight clothing, like a tight belt, can cause heartburn," notes Dr. Gebhard. Even constipation, bending over, or lifting heavy objects can contribute to abdominal pressure and lead to heartburn.

Make meals smaller. If you overeat or indulge in large meals, that, too, can lead to abdominal pressure and heartburn. "The more there is in the stomach, the more there is to go back up the esophagus," says Dr. Charm. So try to eat smaller meals and space them more frequently throughout the day.

Wet your whistle. Drink water with your meals instead of other beverages. Water rinses acid out of the esophagus and helps dilute the acid in the stomach, according to Dr. Gebhard.

Stop the smoke, cure the fire. If there weren't already enough reasons for you to quit smoking, add heartburn to the list. Smoking relaxes the esophageal sphincter, says Dr. Charm, so it can be a major contributor to heartburn.

Mind your table manners. If you swallow too much air, it can lead to belching and burping. During the process, reflux can be released into the esophagus and aggravate heartburn, says Dr. Gebhard. To avoid gulping down air, make sure you chew with your mouth closed. Also, avoid talking while chewing, and be sure you don't gulp down your food. In general, if you take your time during meals, the payoff will be less heartburn.

Switch pain relievers. If taking aspirin seems to kick up your heartburn, try switching to acetaminophen, recommends Dr. Gebhard. All nonsteroidal anti-inflammatory drugs, including ibuprofen, are known to cause heartburn in some people.

Don't worry. "As we get older, we tend to worry too much," says Dr. Charm. If your mind is unable to relax, chances are, your stomach won't be able to either, and that can lead to heartburn. "But with regular relaxation, every meal, every day, can be a celebration."

Try an acid blocker. A new over-the-counter class of acid-reducing drugs called H_2 (histamine-2) blockers actually stops the stomach from producing acid in the first place. Pepcid AC, Axid AR, Tagamet HB, and Zantac are all capable of halting the production of stomach acid. But if you already have heartburn, don't expect relief from an H_2 blocker for about 45 minutes. "These medications should be taken one hour before a meal that you suspect might cause you heartburn," recommends Dr. Charm.

HEART PALPITATIONS

A heart palpitation is really a mild electrical malfunction. Your heart has its own electrical system. Each electrical impulse triggers a heartbeat. If something interferes with the transmission of these electrical impulses, an irregular heartbeat may occur. You'll feel a thumping, pounding, racing, or fluttering sensation in your chest. Or you'll feel as if your heart skipped a beat. But just as quickly as your heart gets off-track, it usually goes back to normal.

Other than the knowledge that your heart is beating to a different drum, heart palpitations are typically nothing to worry about. "Often, there's no treatment necessary. Rarely is it very serious," says Gary Francis, M.D., director of the coronary intensive care unit at the Cleveland Clinic Foundation.

If you have the rare and occasional heart palpitation, assume that you're fine, he adds. If your heartbeat does skip off tempo, you can take a few measures to make it return to its normal rhythm. You can also take a few steps to keep your drum on a steady beat in the first place.

Try This First

Start coughing. Cough during your next heart palpitation episode. The force of the cough will sometimes get a heart back on its regular track, says Robert March, M.D., associate professor of cardiovascular surgery at Rush-Presbyterian–St. Luke's Medical Center in Chicago. "A good cough can break the pattern of the palpitation."

Other Wise Ways

Take a seat. When your heart thumps a little offbeat, sit down, says Michael A. Brodsky, M.D., professor of medicine in cardiology at the University of California, Irvine, Medical Center. Prop your feet up if you can, he adds. Take a few moments to relax and let your heartbeat get back to normal.

Chill out. Splash your face with cold water (not ice water) during your next heart palpitation. The cold water may activate a part of the nervous system that could return your heart rate to normal, Dr. Brodsky says. You can also sip cool water slowly. That may also help stop the palpitations.

Slow your breathing. Many heart palpitations are brought on by stress or anxiety, warns Dr. March. Take a deep breath, and then slowly exhale. Keep repeating this slowly until you calm down. Just the act of relieving tension may bring your heart back in step.

Pump up the pressure. A move called Valsalva's maneuver will derail heart palpitations, explains Dr. Francis. Pinch your nose and close your mouth. Then blow out while keeping your nose and mouth shut. The built-up pressure in your nose and mouth can force your heart back into its normal rhythm, Dr. Francis says.

Get a little help from a friend. While many heart palpitations are temporary and not life threatening, it's a good idea to call over a

MANAGING YOUR MEDS

Although most heart palpitations are mild enough that they don't re-quire treatment, some people need medication. The irony is that some medications given to treat heart palpitations, such as digitalis com-pounds like digoxin (Lanoxin), actually cause palpitations in some pa-tients, says Gary Francis, M.D., director of the coronary intensive care unit at the Cleveland Clinic Foundation.

Other drugs that may cause an irregular heartbeat include:

• Bronchodilators like terbutaline (Brethine)
• Prescription and over-the-counter decongestants containing pseudoephedrine (Drixoral) or phenylpropanolamine (Dura-Gest)
• Prescription antihistamines such as loratadine (Claritin) and astemizole (Hismanal)

Talk with your doctor if you're concerned that any medications you're taking might be causing palpitations.

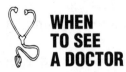

WHEN TO SEE A DOCTOR

For occasional heart palpitations, you don't need to see your doctor, says Gary Francis, M.D., director of the coronary intensive care unit at the Cleveland Clinic Foundation. Your heartbeat usually will go back to normal rather quickly. But sometimes, palpitations may be a sign of another more serious kind of heart problem. At the onset of palpitations, you should talk to your doctor at once if you have a previous history of heart disease. And even if you don't have heart disease, get in touch with your doctor if:

• You also have chest discomfort or chest pains.
• You feel breathless or dizzy.
• The palpitations become more frequent than usual.

friend, loved one, or neighbor during an episode. "That person can sit with you and talk to calm you down while waiting for something to happen," suggests Dr. Brodsky. Your friend could get emergency help if it turns out you need it, he says. And if you don't need medical attention, a friend does a great job of calming you down, which could help offset the palpitations.

Stick with the nonalcoholic brew. For some people, a cocktail sends their hearts aflutter. If you notice heart palpitations after drinking alcohol, put the drinks away, Dr. Brodsky advises.

Some people may experience heart palpitations after one drink, others after a few more, and some people may not have a problem at all. "Everyone has his own threshold," Dr. Brodsky adds. So it's important to remember what your threshold is, and don't go over it, he advises.

Hold back on the coffee. Keep your coffee-cup count to a minimum, Dr. Brodsky says. For some people, coffee or caffeinated products such as soda or chocolate cause heart palpitations, and it may take no more than a smidgen of caffeine to start the arrhythmia. But that's not true for everyone. "Some people smell the coffee and experience heart palpitations," notes Dr. Brodsky. "Others can drink 15 cups a day and have no problems."

Put down the cigarettes. Nicotine can sometimes cause an irregular heartbeat, Dr. March says. For the overall health of your heart as well as for control of heart palpitations, stop smoking.

HEAT EXHAUSTION

A scorcher can be torture, especially for seniors.

"As we get older, our bodies simply don't work as efficiently as they once did," says Stephen Dawkins, M.D., medical director of Hospital Occupational Medicine and Sentry LLC in Atlanta. "A number of factors make it much more difficult for an older person to tolerate heat."

Seniors, for instance, tend to perspire less than younger people, making it difficult to shed body heat, Dr. Dawkins says. Older people also lose much of their sense of thirst. So if you do sweat, you may not feel thirsty until you are severely dehydrated.

In addition, as you age, two of your body's natural insulators—skin and fat tissue—tend to thin and diminish. And without that extra insulation, you're more vulnerable to heat-related problems.

What doctors call heat exhaustion is actually just one in a series of problems that can be prompted by excessive heat. When you have heat exhaustion, you experience excessive thirst, clammy skin, headaches, nausea, weakness, dizziness, or even fainting. But, according to Dr. Dawkins, other things may be happening, too. Some people have mild rashes and cramping. And if the exhaustion gets out of hand on a hot, muggy day, you have to watch out for heatstroke, a dangerous condition that causes your body's temperature control mechanisms to malfunction. When your body can't cool itself, its temperature rises uncontrollably, which can lead to brain damage or death.

Fortunately, as long as you're not in the middle of the Sahara, there are reasonable and fairly easy ways to prevent heat-related health problems, notes Dr. Dawkins. Here are a few ways you can minimize your risk of heat exhaustion.

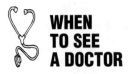

WHEN TO SEE A DOCTOR

Even short-term exposure to high temperatures can cause serious health problems, says Stephen Dawkins, M.D., medical director of Hospital Occupational Medicine and Sentry LLC in Atlanta. See your doctor if you develop muscle cramps, heavy sweating, dizziness, fainting, or nausea. These are signs that you may be developing heat exhaustion.

Try This First

Quench your thirst. Keep your fluids up. It's your best defense against heat-related illness, Dr. Dawkins says. During hot weather, always have a drink of water handy. Take frequent sips. Avoid drinking soda, alcohol, and caffeinated drinks like coffee, because they act as diuretics, pulling liquids out of your body instead of adding them in. They will just make you need to urinate more often, which dehydrates you.

Before you go out, drink an eight-ounce glass of water to ensure that you are hydrated. Then whenever you are outdoors, stop what you're doing and have a six-ounce drink every 15 to 20 minutes, even if you don't feel thirsty, advises Michael Bross, M.D., associate professor of family medicine at the University of Mississippi Medical Center in Jackson.

Even if you're in a cool indoor environment, drink at least six to eight tall glasses of water a day, recommends Dr. Dawkins.

Other Wise Ways

Stay cool. Air-conditioning is your best friend during a heatwave, Dr. Dawkins says. If you have it, use it. Though you may save a few pennies by not turning it on, that's false economizing if you risk heat sickness. If you don't have central air, seal off one room and use a window air conditioner to keep that space livable, Dr. Dawkins advises. In the rest of your home, open windows and use fans to create cross-ventilation.

During a heatwave, if you don't have air-conditioning of any kind, arrange to stay with a friend or relative who does, Dr. Dawkins suggests.

Lie low when the sun is high. Stay out of the sun during the hottest part of the day, usually from 10:00 A.M. to 6:00 P.M., warns Dr. Bross. If you do venture out during these hours, try to spend as much time as possible in malls, movie theaters, and indoor public environments that are air-conditioned.

Get acclimated. Give your body time to adjust to hot weather, Dr. Dawkins says. By acclimatizing to your surroundings, you'll

MANAGING YOUR MEDS

Diuretics such as furosemide (Lasix) or chlorothiazide (Diuril) speed fluid loss and can make it more difficult for you to cope with heat, says Stephen Dawkins, M.D., medical director of Hospital Occupational Medicine and Sentry LLC in Atlanta. Other potential troublemakers in hot weather are high blood pressure medications such as the beta-blockers propranolol (Inderal) and timolol (Blocadren). In addition, the following drugs also can make you more susceptible to heat-related conditions.

- Antihistamines, including diphenhydramine and clemastine, found in over-the-counter products such as Sominex, Benadryl, and Tavist-D
- Antidepressants such as amitriptyline (Elavil) and imipramine (Tofranil)
- Trimethobenzamide (Tigan) and other medications to relieve nausea and vomiting
- Medications containing atropine, such as Lomotil (a drug used to relieve diarrhea and intestinal cramping)
- Bromocriptine (Parlodel), levodopa (Larodopa, Dopar), and other drugs used to treat Parkinson's disease.

If you are taking any of these drugs and develop dehydration or other symptoms of a heat-related condition, talk to your physician. You shouldn't stop taking a medication without your doctor's consent, Dr. Dawkins says. But your doctor needs to be alerted to the heat-related side effects, if you're having them.

sweat sooner but lose less sodium and other minerals that your body needs to stay comfortable in the heat. Begin by spending about 10 to 15 minutes outdoors early in the morning and at dusk. Then gradually increase the amount of time you spend in the heat each day. In a couple of weeks, your body should become acclimatized, and heat-related problems will be less of a concern.

Stay in touch. If you live alone, ask a friend, relative, or neighbor to check in on you at least twice a day during hot weather to make sure you're okay, Dr. Bross suggests. If you're not, they can summon assistance that may save your life.

Turn off the oven. Dr. Dawkins recommends that you eat light, cool meals like salads and sandwiches that don't require cooking. Using the stove or oven just adds unwanted heat to the house. If you must heat your food, try using a microwave.

Take the plunge. A dip in a cool pool, a tepid bath, or a refreshing shower can help lower your body temperature, suggests Dr. Dawkins. Place cool cloths, as needed, on your head, neck, and wrists to help beat the heat.

Go au naturel. Wear light-colored, loose-fitting clothing made from natural fibers like cotton, Dr. Dawkins says. Unlike synthetic nylon or polyester, natural fibers are porous and will help prevent you from overheating. Lighter colors like khaki absorb less heat than darker colors like black.

Reach for the accessories. Wear a broad-brimmed hat to shade yourself in the wilting sun, Dr. Bross suggests. A sunburn will make it harder for your skin to sweat and release body heat. So use sunscreen with a sun protection factor (SPF) of at least 15 whenever you are outdoors.

Shake off the salt tablets. Salt tablets were once believed to speed fluid replacement on hot days. Doctors now know that taking these tablets can actually worsen your reaction to intense heat. In reality, salt tablets actually impede fluids from entering your bloodstream and prevent those fluids from being quickly distributed throughout your body. The excessive amounts of sodium in these pills also can cause kidney damage, Dr. Dawkins notes. Even if salt tablets have been prescribed for some other condition, don't take them unless you have your doctor's permission, Dr. Dawkins warns.

HEMORRHOIDS

If the diagnosis is hemorrhoids, you basically have a problem with swollen veins in and around your anus and rectum. Prolonged sitting, constipation, and hard, dry stools that are difficult to pass are often to blame. Hemorrhoids are a common problem but, still, not simple to deal with, says Amnon Sonnenberg, M.D., gastroenterologist at the Department of Veterans Affairs Medical Center and professor of medicine in the division of gastroenterology at the University of New Mexico School of Medicine, both in Albuquerque. "There are two distinct kinds," he says, "and they should be treated differently, depending on which kind you have."

Least worrisome are internal hemorrhoids, which may cause blood to appear in the stool but are typically painless. If an internal hemorrhoid becomes big enough, however, it may protrude outside the body through the anus, becoming sensitive and painful as a result. Internal hemorrhoids are soft. The swelling of the anal rim makes it difficult to keep this area clean, which can cause itching and irritation. This is known as a protruding hemorrhoid.

External hemorrhoids on the outside of the anus are marked by painful swelling or a hard lump caused by a blood clot in the anal region. "This is called a thrombosed external hemorrhoid, and it can be acutely painful," says Dr. Sonnenberg. "Frequently, the painful swelling of an external hemorrhoid subsides over a period of three to seven days. External skin is more sensitive than the internal lining of the anus, so external hemorrhoids are more painful."

In some cases—with very large or recurring hemorrhoids, for example—medical techniques including surgery may be the best answer for the problem, Dr. Sonnenberg explains, but there are a number of things you can do to ease the discomfort at home. Here are some suggestions.

293

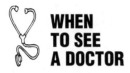

WHEN TO SEE A DOCTOR

When it comes to symptoms that you suspect are caused by hemorrhoids, it's better to be safe than sorry, says Juan Nogueras, M.D., colon and rectal surgeon at the Cleveland Clinic in Fort Lauderdale, Florida. If you detect a lump, blood in your stools, or changes in your normal bowel movement pattern, see a doctor to have it checked out immediately, he says. It may be hemorrhoids, but also it could signify something more serious.

Try This First

Feast on fiber, followed with water. Eating a high-fiber diet with plenty of water may be the best thing you can do to both prevent and defeat hemorrhoids, says Juan Nogueras, M.D., colon and rectal surgeon at the Cleveland Clinic in Fort Lauderdale, Florida. Why? Because an unhealthy low-fiber diet leads to dry, hard stools, which can make going to the bathroom a straining experience. The strain, in turn, can aggravate (and even cause) hemorrhoids.

To add fiber to your diet, just make sure you eat plenty of fresh fruits and vegetables, whole grains, and beans—with the option of a psyllium supplement like Metamucil. If you haven't been consuming a high-fiber diet, start gradually, to avoid problems with gas. Eat at least 15 grams of fiber daily and work up to a total of 25 to 30 grams daily, says Dr. Nogueras. In addition, try to drink at least eight cups of water or other fluids each day. (Caffeinated drinks don't count since they actually deplete your body of fluids.) If you make fiber plus fluids a steady habit, your stools will become much softer and easier to pass. "It takes a lot of strain off your rectum," he says.

Other Wise Ways

Move around and about. Daily exercise plays a vital part in minimizing hemorrhoid outbreaks, according to Dr. Nogueras. When you move around, you reduce the chance of constipation that can cause or irritate hemorrhoids, he says. Try to take a walk or participate in other physical activities at least once a day. Twenty minutes of activity is a good goal to shoot for, he suggests.

Travel to your tub. A good way to ease your symptoms is to take a sitz bath once or twice a day, says Dr. Sonnenberg. Fill your bathtub with three to four inches of warm water and sit in the water for 10 to 15 minutes. The warm water will alleviate pain, provide gentle cleansing, and help to relax your anal sphincter muscles and avoid problems caused by straining to pass stools.

Stop ascending the throne. Sitting on the toilet for long periods of time adds pressure on your anal veins and can therefore put extra pressure on your hemorrhoids and aggravate them, reports Dr. Nogueras. "I tell my patients to move the magazine rack out of the bathroom," he says. If you get restless without something to read, that's probably a good thing; it means you'll spend less time on the toilet and come back when the urge is greater.

Have a pillow, not a doughnut. Many people with hemorrhoids favor inflatable doughnut cushions that enhance comfortable seating at home or the office. But Dr. Nogueras is opposed to them on the grounds that they really don't help hemorrhoids. "It just puts additional pressure on the anus by spreading and stretching the surrounding area of the buttocks," he says. "If you need additional cushioning, use a small pillow instead."

MANAGING YOUR MEDS

The list of medications that cause constipation (and therefore aggravate any hemorrhoid problem) goes on for pages, says Juan Nogueras, M.D., colon and rectal surgeon at the Cleveland Clinic in Fort Lauderdale, Florida. Calcium channel blockers such as verapamil (Isoptin), various psychiatric medicines including tricyclic antidepressants like amitriptyline (Elavil) or lithium (Lithane), and medicines that affect thyroid function, like levothyroxine (Synthroid) are just a few. "Whenever you're prescribed a new medication, it's a good idea to ask your doctor if constipation is a side effect," says Dr. Nogueras. Once you know, you can either ask about alternative medications or prepare for the added pressure on your hemorrhoids.

You should also watch out for multivitamins and supplements that are high in iron, he says. "Iron can cause significant constipation."

Bewitch the problem. Witch hazel also relieves hemorrhoidal pain and itching, says James Duke, Ph.D., botanical consultant, author of *The Green Pharmacy*, and a former ethnobotanist with the U.S. Department of Agriculture who specializes in medicinal plants. Using the witch hazel available at pharmacies, make a compress by saturating some folded gauze or other soft, clean cloth. Apply it to the inflamed area for a minute or two until the pain eases, recommends Dr. Duke.

Paper things over. Wiping the area with scented toilet paper can severely agitate hemorrhoids, says Dr. Nogueras, even if you're using the most expensive brand. Instead, stick with the plain stuff, with no chemical additives whatsoever. And for severe external hemorrhoids that are difficult to keep clean, wet the toilet paper with water to keep irritation to a minimum, he suggests. Make things even more soothing by moistening the paper with witch hazel.

Stop spicing up your life. Eating foods high in strong spices like red pepper and mustard can cause your hemorrhoids to flare up, says Andrew T. Weil, M.D., director of the program in integrative medicine and clinical professor of internal medicine at the University of Arizona College of Medicine in Tucson. Coffee, decaffeinated coffee, or alcohol can also make symptoms worse, as can tobacco. If you can't eliminate these things completely, limit your use of them as much as possible, he suggests.

Take countermeasures. Many over-the-counter remedies are effective, according to experts. Stool softeners containing docusate sodium (Colace) serve to make bowel movements much easier, says Dr. Sonnenberg.

Dr. Nogueras recommends suppositories, which help to lubricate the anal canal, thereby reducing the strain on your hemorrhoids.

One caveat: Avoid gels and lotions that promise to ease pain through topical anesthetics like benzocaine, warns Dr. Weil. "Use Preparation H instead," he says.

Look to the East. If you'd like to try an alternative remedy, two traditional Chinese medicine remedies correct the imbalances that may cause hemorrhoids, says Dr. Weil. Eat an orange three times a day, or eat two bananas as soon as you wake up in the morning. Continue the remedy until your hemorrhoid is gone, he says.

HIGH BLOOD PRESSURE

High blood pressure is the most common chronic illness in the United States and is so rampant among older people that it is often accepted as a normal part of aging. But our bodies are only designed to handle so much sodium, so much extra weight, so much of a subpar diet, believes Paul Whelton, M.D., dean of the school of public health at Tulane University in New Orleans. When you go over those preset limits, you develop high blood pressure. "The genes cock the gun and the environment pulls the trigger," Dr. Whelton says.

High blood pressure goes by the medical name hypertension. That's apt because the condition literally creates too much tension throughout your circulatory system. The condition gets started when your heart begins to work harder either because of stress or because your arteries have been narrowed by fat deposits. It now takes more effort to get blood through the vessels. Pressure increases on the walls of the blood vessels and the heart. Over time, this extra exertion makes your heart stiff and weak, which can cause heart failure.

The two numbers that express the measurement of blood pressure in millimeters of mercury (mm Hg), such as 130/85, represent systolic pressure and diastolic pressure. Systolic, the top number, is measured when your heart contracts or beats. Diastolic, the bottom number, is the minimum pressure and happens when your heart is relaxed between beats. Normal blood pressure is a systolic under 130 mm Hg and a diastolic under 85 mm Hg. William Elliott, M.D., Ph.D., director of the section of clinical research at Rush-Presbyterian–St. Luke's Medical Center in Chicago, recommends an optimal blood pressure less than 120/80 mm Hg.

Simple lifestyle changes can make a big difference, suggests Dr. Whelton. In one study, he found that simply by reducing salt intake

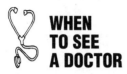

WHEN TO SEE A DOCTOR

There's a reason high blood pressure is considered the silent killer: It typically has no symptoms, says William Elliott, M.D., Ph.D., director of the section of clinical research at Rush-Presbyterian–St. Luke's Medical Center in Chicago. You should get your blood pressure checked regularly. If you have high blood pressure, you should be seeing your doctor for regular visits at least twice a year. If you have high blood pressure and you notice the following, call or see a doctor.

• Frequent or persistent headaches
• Chest discomfort
• Restriction of arm or leg movement
• Change in vision
• Numbness or a strange sensation in your extremities
• Altered state of consciousness leaving you unable to think and talk normally

and losing some weight, older people with hypertension were often able to go completely off high blood pressure medication. "A lot of people could come off their medication safely and they continued to keep their blood pressures down even off the medication," he says.

Make these changes yourself, and you might be able to prevent high blood pressure before it gets a real foothold. And even if you're already taking medications for hypertension, these changes can make the medication work better and increase your chances of beating this silent disease, says Dr. Whelton.

Try This First

Silence your salt shaker. In Dr. Whelton's study, some people could go completely off high blood pressure medications if they reduced sodium and lost weight. For some people, salt or sodium causes their blood pressures to soar.

There's sodium in many canned and packaged foods. You can be better informed about its presence by reading labels and learning to avoid anything with a high sodium content. But the salt we shake on our food is also significant. So ban the salt shaker from your table and your cooking, says Dr. Elliott.

You should limit your sodium content to 2,400 milligrams a day, advises the American Heart Association. Think you'll miss the taste? Don't worry. "After a few weeks, you get pretty used to a low-salt diet," says Lawrence Z. Feigenbaum, M.D., founder and director of the Goldman Institute on Aging in San Francisco.

Other Wise Ways

Stock up on naturally low-salt foods. If you fill your pantry with low-sodium foods, you're bound to cut salt from your diet. Always be sure to have on hand some of the following suggestions from the American Heart Association: fruits, vegetables, fresh or frozen lean meats, poultry, fish, shellfish, unsalted lean pork, eggs for egg whites, water-packed tuna, dried peas, beans, lentils, skim or reduced-fat milk, low-fat yogurt, and whole grains.

MANAGING YOUR MEDS

There are several classes of drugs commonly used to treat high blood pressure, says William Elliott, M.D., Ph.D., director of the section of clinical research at Rush-Presbyterian–St. Luke's Medical Center in Chicago. Diuretics such as hydrochlorothiazide (HydroDIURIL), amiloride (Midamor), and spironolactone (Aldactone) are often used when high blood pressure is your only medical condition. These are very effective in reducing heart attack and stroke in older individuals. A doctor may prescribe beta-blockers like atenolol (Tenormin) and propranolol (Inderal) if you have high blood pressure and other health problems such as a previous heart attack and angina. Angiotensin-converting enzyme (ACE) inhibitors such as captopril (Capoten) may be used if the person also has heart failure or diabetes and kidney problems. Another possible treatment is with calcium channel blockers such as amlodipine (Norvasc).

If you are being treated for high blood pressure, check with your doctor before taking the following:

- Nonsteroidal anti-inflammatory drugs (NSAIDs) such as ibuprofen. These may interfere with high blood pressure medication. Also, most contain sodium.
- Over-the-counter and prescription decongestants like pseudoephedrine (Sudafed). They may raise blood pressure.
- Those over-the-counter and prescription antihistamines that contain decongestants such as diphenhydramine (Bena-D) or chlorpheniramine (Coricidin-D). (The brand name may have a D, but decongestant should appear on the package label.) They may raise blood pressure.

Spice up your life. Salt is usually added for taste, but there are a plethora of spices that can add taste without adding blood pressure points, says May M. Harter, R.D., coordinator of nutrition and weight management programs at New Britain General Hospital in Connecticut. Reach for your spice rack the next time you need to add a little flavor. For instance, use basil for fish, lamb, lean ground meats, stews, salads, and sauces. Try bay leaves with lean meats, stews, poultry, soups, and tomatoes. Dash some rosemary on chicken, veal, lean meat loaf, lean beef, lean pork, sauces, stuffings, potatoes, peas, and lima beans. Use dill on fish sauces, soups, tomatoes, cabbages, carrots, cauliflower, green beans, cucumbers, potatoes, salads, macaroni, lean beef, lamb, and chicken.

Read the labels. When buying products, look for the amount of sodium, Harter says. The red flag should go up if a product has more than 400 milligrams of sodium per serving, she says. If you are eating something that has more than that, make sure the other foods you eat throughout the day are lower in sodium. You don't want to go over 2,000 milligrams a day.

Stalk the produce aisle. Fruits and vegetables are more than just salt-free. They are potassium-rich. "Potassium seems to be an important element in controlling blood pressure. The more potassium one takes in, the lower blood pressure tends to be," Dr. Whelton says. The best way to get the Daily Value of 3,500 milligrams is through fruits and vegetables, adds Dr. Whelton. Food sources include dried apricots, baked potatoes, dried prunes, cantaloupe, spinach, citrus fruits, and most raw vegetables. Don't overdo the dried fruits, however, since they are high in calories.

Be a little lighter. In his study, Dr. Whelton found that older people who reduced the salt in their diets and lost weight reduced their blood pressures so much that about half of them were able to stay off their blood pressure medication. Even obese people who lost as little as eight pounds saw health benefits in regard to blood pressure, he says. His subjects didn't have to go through a brutal regimen either. They were told to do small amounts of exercise like taking the stairs instead of the elevator as well as daily brisk walks. And they were told to make dietary changes like eating more fruits and vegetables and changing a few things in their diets, like switching from whole milk to low-fat or drinking diet soda in place of regular. "Little things can have a big impact. Just cutting out 100 to 150 calories a day will likely result in about a one-pound weight loss in one month," he adds.

Take a walk. Just a brisk walk about a half-hour a day keeps your blood pressure down. You should walk at a pace that will make you a little short of breath but still able to talk to a companion. "When you look at clinical trials, the evidence is very strong that increasing physical activity is overall beneficial. It seems to lower blood pressure and reduce weight," Dr. Whelton says. It is always a good idea to start slowly and increase your activity level over time. Aerobic exercise may keep your blood pressure down by keeping your blood vessels more flexible.

Max out on magnesium. Along with potassium, magnesium is another mineral that may help keep your blood pressure down. The research isn't as conclusive with magnesium as it is with potassium, Dr. Whelton notes. But it is good enough to recommend that you get the Daily Value of 400 milligrams a day. You'll find magnesium in meats, green leafy vegetables, brown rice, legumes, nuts, and whole grains. People with heart or kidney problems should not take supplemental magnesium.

Milk it. Getting adequate calcium in conjunction with standard medication has been shown to be of some benefit in lowering blood pressure for some people, says Ruth Kava, R.D., Ph.D., director of nutrition at the American Council on Science and Health in New York City. Through food or supplements, try to get 1,200 milligrams a day, she advises. The best sources are usually dairy: low-fat and nonfat cheeses, milk, and yogurt.

Along with your 1,200 milligrams of calcium, make sure you also get 400 international units of vitamin D, which can be found in fortified milk; fatty fish like herring, mackerel, salmon, or sardines; and, if necessary, multivitamins. Without vitamin D, calcium can't be absorbed by your body. Your body also makes vitamin D itself with the help of sunlight. Although about 15 minutes of the summer sun gets you a day's worth, older adults may have a decreased ability to produce vitamin D, and sunscreen will interfere with your skin's ability to make vitamin D. This means it may be best to rely on food sources for your daily vitamin D.

High Cholesterol

While lowering cholesterol is the gospel of healthy hearts for people under age 65, there's been some controversy over whether reducing cholesterol means anything in older people. In fact, a few years ago, a major physicians committee didn't recommend cholesterol testing for people over age 65. They didn't think lowering cholesterol in that age group had any benefits.

But before you decide to smother your food in butter and forgo your next cholesterol screening, know that a study by the National Institute on Aging in Bethesda, Maryland, found that high cholesterol was a risk factor for death from coronary heart disease in older men and women. And doctors like Lee Lipsenthal, M.D., medical director of the Preventive Medicine Research Institute in Sausalito, California, still believe that you can increase both the length and the quality of your life by keeping your cholesterol in check, no matter what your age. "There are still health benefits from treating high cholesterol in older people, absolutely," he says.

Lowering cholesterol does improve the quality of life in older people. "We are just now beginning to see that you can reduce angina and the risk of heart attack within a short period of time by lowering a person's cholesterol," says John C. LaRosa, M.D., chancellor of Tulane University Medical Center in New Orleans.

To find out if cholesterol is a problem for you, you have to get tested. When you do, you'll get three sets of numbers: total cholesterol, high-density lipoproteins (HDL), and low-density lipoproteins (LDL). HDLs are the "good" cholesterol and they take cholesterol away from your arteries. LDLs are the "bad" cholesterol and they carry cholesterol to the artery walls.

For total cholesterol, a score under 150 is ideal, less than 200 is desirable, 200 to 239 is borderline high risk, and 240 or more is high risk. An HDL level less than 45 is high risk, according to Dr. Lipsenthal.

When it comes to LDL, a score of less than 100 is desirable if you have heart disease. Less than 130 is acceptable if you don't have heart disease, but when it's 130 to 159, you're at borderline high risk, says Dr. Lipsenthal. Get to 160 or more, and you're in a high-risk category.

Despite its reputation, cholesterol is not evil. Your body actually needs it to build healthy cell membranes and manufacture hormones. But your body makes enough on its own. It doesn't need all the extra cholesterol that results from getting too much fat in your daily diet.

When your body has more cholesterol than it needs, cholesterol starts to stick to your artery walls. That's the beginning of heart disease.

The best way to naturally lower your cholesterol is to cut the fat out of your diet. But besides cutting high-fat foods, you can also reduce your cholesterol numbers by adding certain other foods, Dr. Lipsenthal says. Then combine a healthy diet with exercise, and you'll do your heart a world of good by getting your cholesterol counts in the ranges where they should be. Here's how to get started.

Try This First

Switch to low-fat dairy. Choosing fat-free milk and low-fat cheese over their full-fat counterparts is an easy and relatively painless way to cut fat grams out of your diet, says May M. Harter, R.D., coordinator of nutrition and weight management programs at New Britain General Hospital in Connecticut. "Don't omit dairy to cut out the fat. There are plenty of choices," she says. Pick fat-free yogurt and frozen yogurt, for instance.

Other Wise Ways

Mix up your meats. You don't have to cut meat out of your diet to lower your fat and your cholesterol. You just have to make different meat choices, Harter says. Use extra-lean ground meat or ground turkey breast the next time you make burgers. Look for lean roast beef, or buy cuts such as select-grade eye of round, tip round,

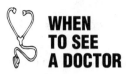

WHEN TO SEE A DOCTOR

If you've been diagnosed with high cholesterol, don't just follow home remedies. Make sure you see your doctor once a year for checkups, says Lee Lipsenthal, M.D., medical director of the Preventive Medicine Research Institute in Sausalito, California. If you have heart disease or high cholesterol, follow your doctor's recommendations.

bottom round, and top sirloin. And when you cook chicken or turkey, remove the skin, she suggests.

Cut down the size. It's not always what you eat that increases your cholesterol—it's how much you eat, explains Harter. "Portion size is important. If you are used to eating two hamburgers for dinner, scale it back to one."

If you get a huge deli sandwich, take off some of the meat or ask the server to trim it a bit and add more vegetables on top. An ideal portion of meat is about two to three ounces, about the size of a deck of cards. You should eat no more than two portions a day, suggests Harter. When you are counting your meat portions, remember to include poultry, pork, and fish in addition to red meat.

Add flavor, not fat. Many people add butter and oils to their cooking to enhance the taste of food. But you can have great taste without the fat, Harter says. Here are just a handful of simple ways to add flavor without adding fat grams and cholesterol points.

- Use no-stick spray such as Pam instead of oils to fry or sauté food.
- Use low-fat, reduced-sodium chicken broth to coat pans and cookware instead of oil or butter.
- Cook food with flavored vinegars.
- Cook or marinate foods in low-fat or nonfat salad dressing.

Spread your oats. Eat two ounces of oat bran a day, says Stephen T. Sinatra, M.D., director of the New England Heart Center in Manchester, Connecticut, and author of *Optimum Health*. Oat bran, found in oatmeal and some cereals such as Cheerios and Life, contains soluble fiber, which is thought to soak up cholesterol and take it out of your system. In various studies, oat bran has shown to lower high cholesterol anywhere from 3 to 20 percent.

Keep the skin on. When you eat a grapefruit, don't cut it in half and scoop out the fruit. Peel it like an orange and eat it in pieces, Dr. Sinatra recommends. Eating it that way, you eat the white stringy stuff on the outside called pectin. Since pectin is another form of soluble fiber, eating more of it may help lower your cholesterol.

Try a Mediterranean taste. The next time you want oil or butter to cook with, reach for olive oil instead. Olive oil is an oil made mostly of monounsaturated fat, which is fat that may actually help raise your HDL, or "good," cholesterol. But fat is fat, and too much will ultimately raise your cholesterol levels, so don't slather it on everything. Dr. Lipsenthal suggests cooking with olive oil instead of other vegetable oils and using a little bit of olive oil on your bread instead of butter. If you have heart disease, however, you should avoid all oils.

MANAGING YOUR MEDS

Your doctor may put you on cholesterol-lowering drugs called statins, such as simvastatin (Zocor) and pravastatin (Pravachol). The best advice if you go on cholesterol medications is take them, says John C. LaRosa, M.D., chancellor of the Tulane University Medical Center in New Orleans. Many people fail to take the medication, at least on a regular basis.

And taking cholesterol-lowering medication isn't a free ride. They only work in conjunction with lifestyle changes, says Lee Lipsenthal, M.D., medical director of the Preventive Medicine Research Institute in Sausalito, California.

Your doctor may also prescribe very high doses of the B vitamin niacin, which has been shown to lower cholesterol. Do not attempt to treat yourself with high amounts of niacin, because it can cause liver damage, Dr. Lipsenthal says. Only do it under the guidance of your doctor.

Meanwhile, diuretic drugs such as indapamide (Lozol) or furosemide (Lasix) may increase triglycerides (another form of fat in your blood that influences your cholesterol level). Talk to your doctor if you take any diuretic medication.

Garnish with garlic. Use garlic when you make your meals. Dr. Lipsenthal says garlic can help neutralize the damage caused by high cholesterol.

To get an effect from garlic, you'd have to eat about a half a clove to a clove a day, notes Dr. Sinatra. If you aren't up to that malodorous challenge, a couple of enteric-coated garlic capsules will provide you with about 1,000 milligrams of garlic a day.

Protect arteries with flax seeds. Take 1½ tablespoons of ground flaxseeds or 1 teaspoon of flaxseed oil a day, suggests Dr. Lipsenthal. To incorporate them into your menu, use either the ground seeds or oil when you make salad dressing. Flaxseeds and flaxseed oil, found at most health food stores, contain omega-3 fatty acids, which are thought to protect the heart from the damaging effects of high cholesterol. "Omega-3's have a role in strengthening the artery walls," explains Dr. Lipsenthal.

Select some soy products. Eating soy products has been shown to lower cholesterol. In a study of 4,838 people in Japan, researchers found that an increase in soy products corresponded to a decrease in cholesterol levels.

In another study, at the University of Kentucky in Lexington, researchers found that eating about 47 grams of soy protein a day could lower total cholesterol 9.3 percent and could lower LDL, or "bad" cholesterol, by 12.9 percent compared to a diet in which the protein is derived from animal sources.

"Soy has a lot of great stuff in it. It is also a wonderful meat substitute as far as protein and nutrition goes. You are substituting a higher-fiber, lower-fat food that is a filling replacement, and it has a lot of benefits," Dr. Lipsenthal says. Here are some of his recommendations for serving soy products.

- Steam a cup of soybeans. "They are real tasty that way. They look like lima beans but taste a lot better," he says. Look for them at your health food store.
- Toss tofu into salads, stir-fries, and pasta dishes. Marinate it in a low-fat sauce or gravy to give it taste, he says.
- Use soy milk instead of cow's milk.
- Look for nutritional supplement shakes with soy in them at your grocery or health food store.
- Try low-fat soy burgers or veggie burgers made with soy.

Shake it up. To get the daily benefits of soy and flaxseeds, try a shake. Dr. Sinatra has one every day. He mixes eight ounces of soy milk with two tablespoons of ground flaxseeds. (You can buy ground flaxseeds in health food stores or grind them yourself in a coffee mill.) He tosses a few strawberries or blueberries into the blender and mixes it all up. The result is a great, nutty, fruit shake that contains a variety of cholesterol-lowering and protective elements: soy, omega-3 fatty acids from flaxseeds, and fiber from the seeds and berries.

Eradicate oxidation. Try to include antioxidants in your diet or take antioxidant supplements, suggests Dr. Lipsenthal. Antioxidants are chemicals that prevent cholesterol from oxidizing. It's the oxidation that causes cholesterol to harden and clog arteries. "Antioxidants don't lower cholesterol but they diminish the damaging effects of cholesterol," he says. He suggests a daily dose of the following.

• Vitamin C. Take between 1,000 and 3,000 milligrams a day. Food sources include broccoli, brussels sprouts, red cabbage, citrus fruits, guavas, parsley, and mustard greens. Over 1,200 milligrams of vitamin C daily may cause diarrhea in some people.

• Vitamin E. Take between 100 and 400 international units per day. Food sources include salad and cooking oils (except coconut oil), seeds, nuts, wheat germ, asparagus, avocado, seafood, apples, carrots, and celery. Watch the fat content of these foods. If you have heart disease, you should be ultra-careful and possibly consider a supplement instead. (Although vitamin E is generally sold in doses of 400 international units, one small study showed a possible risk of stroke in dosages higher than 200 international units. Consult with your doctor if you are at high risk for stroke.)

• Vitamin A. Take 2,500 international units in the form of beta-carotene. Food sources include carrots; dark green, leafy vegetables, such as spinach and collard and mustard greens; yellow vegetables, such as squash, pumpkins, and sweet potatoes; and yellow fruits, such as peaches and apricots.

Stop smoking. Smoking raises your cholesterol and does even more untold damage to your heart, Dr. Lipsenthal says.

HIP PAIN

The twentieth century wasn't kind to the hip. From the hula hoop to hip-hop, boogie-woogie to break dancing, calypso to disco, the joint was jumping, bumping, and grinding at a mind-swiveling pace.

Yet these gyrations and dance sensations were hardly the hip's worst enemies. It's what Americans didn't do in this increasingly sedentary age that really sapped the zap from the hip.

"If anything, swinging your hips on the dance floor, walking to the post office, or just doing a few stretching exercises every day helps keep the muscles and bones of the joint strong. But we've gotten away from doing those things. The vast majority of Americans have become couch potatoes, and they're paying the price for it later in life in the form of thinner, weaker bones and an increased potential for hip fracture," says Jan I. Maby, D.O., director of the Geriatric Medical Home Care program at Mount Sinai Medical Center in New York City.

But it's never too late to make lifestyle changes, including regular exercise, to ease mild hip pain, strengthen weak bones, and reduce your susceptibility to hip fractures, Dr. Maby says. In fact, many of the underlying causes of hip pain in older Americans, such as arthritis, bursitis, and tendonitis, can easily be treated with these home remedies.

Try This First

Seek the heat. Heat is one of your most potent allies against occasional hip pain, says Scott Marwin, M.D., vice chairman of the department of orthopedics at Long Island Jewish Medical Center in New Hyde Park, New York. Try placing an electric heating pad over your hip for 20 minutes three or four times a day, he suggests. If you don't have a heating pad, soak a towel in hot water and wring it out.

Other Wise Ways

Chill out. If heat isn't helping, apply ice where you feel hip pain to help reduce pain and swelling, says Craig Cisar, Ph.D., professor of exercise physiology at San Jose State University in California. To protect your skin, put a towel between your skin and the ice. Ice may be used for 15 to 20 minutes every one to two waking hours.

Reach for reliable relief. Over-the-counter extra-strength anti-inflammatory medications such as ibuprofen can reduce swelling and ease hip pain caused by arthritis, bursitis, and other muscle or joint injuries, says Jacob Rozbruch, M.D., orthopedic surgeon and assistant professor of medicine at Albert Einstein College of Medicine in New York City. If the recommended dosage on the label doesn't help, alert your doctor. You may have a hip fracture or another serious underlying problem that should be evaluated, he says.

Sidestep the ache. When getting out of a car, lift and swing both legs out of the door before standing, Dr. Marwin suggests. By rotating on your rear instead of twisting your pelvis, you'll lessen the strain on your back and hips. "If you step out of the vehicle one leg at a time, you put yourself into a spread-eagle position that is very aggravating to your hips," Dr. Marwin says.

Size up your assistance. A cane or walker is your best friend if it eases your hip pain and helps you stay independent, Dr. Maby says.

If you need a cane or walker for stability, be sure it is the right size, Dr. Marwin says. An ill-fitting assistive device will increase

MANAGING YOUR MEDS

If you are taking anticoagulants, such as warfarin (Coumadin), for your blood vessels, heart, or lungs, do not take ibuprofen or aspirin, urges Jacob Rozbruch, M.D., orthopedic surgeon and assistant professor of medicine at Albert Einstein College of Medicine in New York City. Like anticoagulants, both ibuprofen and aspirin are blood thinners. Taking these drugs in combination could cause uncontrolled bleeding. If you are taking an anticoagulant, ask your doctor or pharmacist about using acetaminophen to relieve your hip pain, Dr. Rozbruch says.

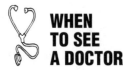

WHEN TO SEE A DOCTOR

In general, any pain in the hip region, particularly if it radiates down into the groin, should be evaluated by a doctor to rule out any serious problem like hip fracture or joint degeneration, says Jacob Rozbruch, M.D., orthopedic surgeon and assistant professor of medicine at Albert Einstein College of Medicine in New York City. In addition, be wary of the following symptoms.

• Your hip pain is caused by a fall or injury, even a minor one.

• The pain persists after a couple of weeks, despite self-care and home remedies.

• You can't bear weight on the hip.

• The pain occurs while you lie in bed at night or disrupts your sleep.

• You have difficulty walking or moving.

• You also have open sores on your feet or leg pain.

your hip pain, not relieve it. Ask your doctor to refer you to a medical supply store where you can be properly measured and outfitted with an appropriate cane or walker.

Be more able with a cane. When you use a cane, hold it in the hand opposite the injured hip, Dr. Marwin says. Move it forward at the same time that you step out with your injured hip, so you're distributing weight away from your bad hip and onto the cane. Then move your good hip forward as you take another stride.

Shed some pounds. Getting rid of excess body weight can help relieve the strain on your hips, Dr. Marwin says. In fact, each pound you lose will take two or three pounds of pressure off your hips.

"As you get older, it becomes more difficult for your muscles to offset your increased weight. As a result, your joints bear more and more of the brunt of the load, and they degenerate," Dr. Marwin says. "So keeping your weight down and staying physically fit are two of the best things you can do to preserve your hips."

Limber up. Stretching exercises often can relieve both hip and back pain by strengthening common muscles and increasing your flexibility, Dr. Rozbruch says.

Over time, Dr. Rozbruch says, loosening your hips will translate into more fluid, graceful, and pain-free movement. You can do the following stretches once a day to coax hip muscles into lengthening gently and slowly. But if you start to feel pain, stop. (And if you have a herniated disk, you should consult your doctor or physical therapist before trying any of these stretches.)

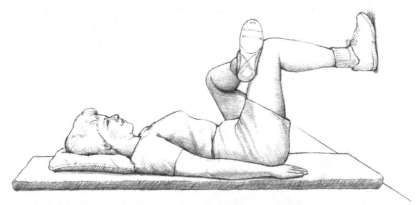

1. Lie down on a bed or on the floor on a mat, with your knees bent and your feet braced about 24 inches high on a wall, letting your head, upper body, and arms relax completely on the floor. (Hint: The farther from the wall you are, the easier this stretch will be.) You can support your head with a pillow or towel. Keep your buttocks on the floor. Keeping your right foot on the wall, cross your left foot over your right thigh, bringing the outer edge of your foot just below your right knee. If you are too stiff to reach that point, let your left leg cross farther over your right leg as much as needed.

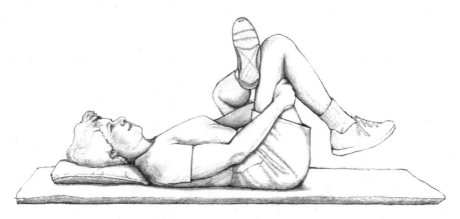

Then, lift your right thigh toward your chest and reach your hands through to interlace around the back of the thigh. Create just the amount of stretch that is good for you by slowly drawing your right leg toward your chest. Hold for up to one minute. (If the reach is too difficult, use a towel to raise your thigh to your chest without lifting your head and shoulders off the floor.) Release and repeat on the other side. Note: You should feel this in the back of your left thigh, hip, or outer buttock, not in your lower back.

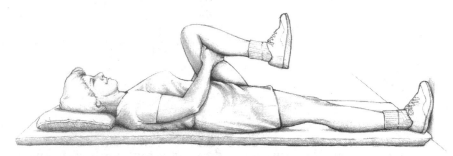

2. Lie down on your back on a bed or on the floor on a mat, with your legs extended and your feet wedged snugly and pressing against a wall. You can support your head with a pillow or towel. Make sure your toes point up toward the ceiling. On an exhalation, slowly draw your left knee toward your chest, interlacing your hands behind your knee/upper thigh. Hold this position for up to a minute, breathing evenly, then release. Repeat with your right leg. Avoid letting your straight leg bend and rise up. The most important part of this stretch is keeping one thigh pressed down onto the floor while you're flexing the other. Getting your knees to your chest is secondary.

HIVES

Unless you're a bee, you want to avoid hives. Unfortunately, evasion is nearly impossible because hives tend to erupt for no apparent reason.

These red, intensely itchy bumps, which may also burn or sting, crop up by themselves or in clusters and afflict 10 to 20 percent of the population at least once in a lifetime. Usually, hives go away within a few days to a few weeks, but occasionally, a person will continue to have hives for many years.

Hives form when a trigger—often something you're allergic to, but not always—sends a flood of immune substances known as mast cells coursing through your blood vessels, squirting an inflammatory substance called histamine into your cells. Histamine makes blood vessels leak fluid, forming the red, itchy bump that you see and feel as a hive.

Medications are the number one cause of hives, says Jonathan Weiss, M.D., dermatologist and assistant clinical professor of dermatology at Emory University School of Medicine in Atlanta. Anti-inflammatory agents like aspirin, ibuprofen, and naprosyn (Aleve)—the sort of over-the-counter drugs commonly taken for muscle strains and headaches—are leading triggers, says Dr. Weiss. In the prescription drug category, antibiotics are another class of medications that can trigger hives.

According to the American Academy of Allergy, Asthma, and Immunology, food is often a trigger. Even exercise or a hot shower can bring on a case of hives.

Unless they cause you to have trouble breathing, form around your eyes, are in or on your mouth, remain for more than 24 hours, or leave bruises, hives aren't serious, but they surely are annoying. Here's how you can avoid getting stung by your hives in the future.

313

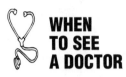

WHEN TO SEE A DOCTOR

Hives are usually a surface problem, but if you develop hives around your eyes or on your mouth or if you have difficulty breathing, seek emergency medical treatment immediately, advises Paul Greenberger, M.D., professor of medicine in the division of allergy and immunology at Northwestern University Medical School in Chicago.

You should also let your doctor know if your hives last longer than 24 hours, says Dr. Greenberger. You should see a doctor if your hives last longer than six weeks or if they cause intense discomfort or bruising. You may have an underlying problem, such as thyroid disease or acute hepatitis, that requires medication.

Try This First

Alleviate with an antihistamine. An over-the-counter antihistamine, like diphenhydramine (Benadryl), can reduce the itch and inflammation of hives and keep them from getting worse, says Dr. Weiss. If this method does not control symptoms, a visit to your dermatologist or primary-care physician is necessary.

Dr. Weiss recommends 25 milligrams of Benadryl up to four times per day. Since Benadryl tends to make you sleepy, he suggests taking a dose at bedtime so you can get the medication's full therapeutic effects without daytime drowsiness.

Other Wise Ways

Keep cool. Heat of any kind makes hives worse. So until your hives subside, you'll be more comfortable if you keep as cool as possible, says Helen Hollingsworth, M.D., associate professor of medicine at Boston University School of Medicine and director of allergy and asthma services at Boston University Medical Center Hospital.

Chill the area. If you get hives from cold weather or cold water, you'll want to skip this next tip. But for most people with hives, ice and cold compresses are about the best things you can put on your hives, says Paul Greenberger, M.D., professor of medicine in the division of allergy and immunology at Northwestern University Medical School in Chicago.

Track the cause. The best long-term treatment for hives is to find and remove the cause of these annoying, itchy bumps, says Dr. Greenberger. But this isn't always an easy task.

Because so many different things can trigger hives, Dr. Greenberger suggests compiling a list of every medication and food item you swallowed in the four hours before an outbreak. Jot down any temperature extremes and anything that may have put physical pressure on your body (like a tight waistband), and note whether or not you exercised.

MANAGING YOUR MEDS

If you're allergic to it, almost any prescription or over-the-counter medication can trigger hives, says Jonathan Weiss, M.D., dermatologist and assistant clinical professor of dermatology at Emory University School of Medicine in Atlanta. If an outbreak occurs, cast a suspicious eye on any new drugs that you've just started taking.

Although any drug can potentially cause hives, Dr. Weiss lists the following medications as likely triggers.

- Antibiotics such as erythromycin (Erycette)
- Oral products for ear infections such as amoxicillin (Amoxil)
- Sedatives such as benzodiazepines (Alprazolam)
- Tranquilizers such as flurazepam (Dalmane)
- Antihypertensives such as ACE inhibitors (Accupril)
- Diuretics such as bumetanide (Bumex)

Nonprescription items can also be potential causes of hives, including these triggers.

- Pain medications such as salicylates (Anacin)
- Vitamins
- Eyedrops such as tetrahydrozoline (Visine)
- Laxatives such as phenolphthalein (Medilax)
- Vaginal douches (Massengill)

If you have an attack of hives, it's important to tell your doctor about all of the preparations that you use. The more he knows, the faster he'll be able to find the cause, says Dr. Weiss.

Rule it out. Once you think you've spotted a cause, try to eliminate it. If you're not sure what caused your hives, you should see a doctor, recommends Dr. Greenberger. If you think a type of food is the culprit, stop eating it and see if the hives clear. Herbs and food additives may also bring on hives, so unless you're sure you won't have a reaction to them, make sure that they are on your suspect list. Once you've pinpointed the offending food, you should refrain from eating even a small portion, he says. A tiny amount can cause a flare-up. If the hives started just after you took a new medication, talk to your doctor about a substitute. You may be able to determine the cause this way and put an end to the misery, says Dr. Greenberger.

Watch your diet. Be cautious about eating tomato sauce, citrus, strawberries, and shellfish while you have hives, advises Dr. Hollingsworth. No one knows why, but these foods frequently aggravate hives.

Cow's milk, eggs, fish, shellfish, peanuts, soy protein, legumes, wheat, and tree nuts such as walnuts and hazelnuts can worsen hives, too, says Dr. Greenberger.

Wear loose clothes. Pressure generated by tight shoes and tight clothes are known to cause hives, and that pressure may aggravate and worsen a case of hives that has already started. So be particularly careful to wear loose clothing and properly fitted shoes when you have hives, warns Dr. Hollingsworth.

Moisturize your skin. Dry skin tends to cause itching, which can irritate hives and make them worse. If your skin tends to be dry, apply a moisturizer to the area around the hives, says Dr. Hollingsworth.

IMPOTENCE

Cary Grant fathered a daughter at age 62. Clint Eastwood had a baby girl at 67. Charlie Chaplin had a son at 73. Tony Randall sired a daughter when he was 77. And Anthony Quinn had his 13th child at age 81.

"Men shouldn't lose potency as a result of getting older. There are age-related diseases that men develop that can lead to difficulty in getting erections. But if men are healthy, they should be able to function all of their lives," explains Drogo K. Montague, M.D., director of the Center for Sexual Function at the Cleveland Clinic Foundation.

Normally, an erection occurs when there is increased blood flow into the penis and penile veins are compressed to make sure that the blood is sealed there, causing stiffness. Nerves in the penis provide pleasurable sensations and help retain the erection until ejaculation, Dr. Montague says.

A man, however, is not a machine. Almost every man fails to achieve an erection rigid enough for intercourse at some point during his adult life, notes Dr. Montague. And for up to 30 million American men, getting and maintaining an erection is a persistent problem. Commonly known as impotence, doctors now call this condition erectile dysfunction.

Estimates of impotence vary so widely that the statistics are nearly meaningless, which says something about truth in reporting when it comes to this delicate subject. By some estimates, only 15 percent of men over the age of 70 are impotent. Other polls put the number nearer 67 percent, which would mean that two out of every three men over the age of 70 are impotent.

Statistics aside, older men do seem to be more prone to erectile problems than younger men. In all likelihood, that's because older men are more apt to have diabetes, atherosclerosis (hardening of the arteries), and other physical ailments that reduce blood flow to the penis. In fact, in men over 50, up to 80 percent of erectile dysfunction is caused by physical problems. But anxiety, depression, and other psychological woes also can contribute to the problem, Dr. Montague says.

Try This First

Fluff up the pillows. Impotence can be triggered by boredom in the bedroom, says Roger Crenshaw, M.D., psychiatrist and sex therapist in private practice in La Jolla, California. Take a few moments to think about your sex life. Are your nightly patterns with your spouse so predictable that it's difficult to get excited about them? Have you

MANAGING YOUR MEDS

For decades, older men whose sex lives were limp, slack, or nonexistent because of impotence faced some pretty grim choices: go without, use cumbersome vacuum pumps, or inject erection-inducing drugs directly into their penises.

Then along came the pill that recharged the sexual revolution among gray-ing Americans. As easy to take as an aspirin, sildenafil citrate (Viagra) quickly became known for its ability to restore a man's erections even after decades of impotence. In its first three months on the U.S. market in 1998, doctors wrote more than two million prescriptions for this "miracle drug," making it the most successful new pharmaceutical on record. Its soaring sales spawned a host of other drugs designed to help men who have erectile difficulties.

The drugs work wonders for about 80 percent of men, stimulating blood flow to the penis and jump-starting long-lost erections. But for nearly one in three men, particularly those with diabetes and other health conditions that damage nerves in the penis, these medications may not help as much.

Viagra has other downsides as well. Doctors say that you should never use Viagra if you are taking nitroglycerin or related nitrate-containing drugs. When combined, Viagra and nitrates can cause a dangerous drop in blood pressure, and some men have died from this side effect, says Roger Crenshaw, M.D., psychiatrist and sex therapist in private practice used the same position for years? How do you feel about kissing and foreplay? Where do you have sex? In the bedroom? In the shower?

Often, just changing when, where, and how you have sex can be erotic enough to revive your potency, Dr. Crenshaw says. So experiment. Try with new positions. Touch your spouse in ways you never have before or try some role-playing games if your spouse is game.

Other Wise Ways

Ask for a healing touch. As men age, they need more physical stimulation to get and maintain erections, explains Dr. Crenshaw.

---

in La Jolla, California. Other drug interactions may emerge as the drug is more widely tested, so be sure to let your doctor know about any drugs you are taking, including over-the-counter products, prior to taking Viagra.

While Viagra is a much-touted cure for impotence, other drugs are notorious for causing impotence as a side effect. In fact, medications account for about one in every four cases of impotence and may be the single most common cause of sexual dysfunction after age 60, says W. Steven Pray, Ph.D., R.Ph., professor of nonprescription drug products at Southwestern Oklahoma State University in Weatherford. Among the common culprits are:

- High blood pressure medications including beta-blockers such as propranolol (Inderal), pindolol (Visken), and metoprolol (Lopressor)
- Digitalis preparations such as digoxin (Lanoxin), used to strengthen weak heart muscles and correct irregular heartbeats
- Antidepressants like clomipramine (Anafranil)

If your erectile dysfunction begins shortly after you begin taking a medication, consult with your physician. You may be able to alleviate the problem by cutting back certain medications or finding substitutes for them. But never reduce or stop your dosage of any drug without your doctor's permission, Dr. Crenshaw warns.

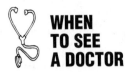

WHEN TO SEE A DOCTOR

If impotence lasts more than two months or is a recurring problem, consult your doctor. Your doctor might also refer you to a sex therapist or physician who specializes in erectile problems, says Roger Crenshaw, M.D., psychiatrist and sex therapist in private practice in La Jolla, California.

More than likely, your doctor will suggest a complete examination and give you a blood test that could rule out physical problems like diabetes and neurological disorders. Blood screenings can also identify low levels of testosterone, the male hormone responsible for sexual response.

Your doctor also may be able to help you cope with stress, anxiety, and other psychological factors that can wilt erections, or refer you to a specialist who can help with these issues.

So ask your spouse to take some time to touch and play with your genitals and other erotic areas of your body.

Turn off the pressure. If you do have difficulty getting an erection, don't dwell on it, Dr. Crenshaw advises. Obsessing about impotence could make you worry so much that you'll have performance anxiety, which leads to impotence, which makes you worry more, which leads to more anxiety. So break the vicious cycle and treat it casually. Shrug it off.

To relieve the tension, avoid having intercourse the next few times you and your partner are intimate, even if you get an erection, Dr. Crenshaw suggests. Instead, hug, kiss, caress, and do other things you enjoy. Satisfy your spouse but avoid touching each other's genitals.

"If intercourse becomes an overarching goal, sex ceases to be fun. And when sex ceases to be fun, that's when you get into trouble," Dr. Crenshaw says.

Clear the smoke. Smoking kills erections, Dr. Montague warns. Each time you light up, you risk damage to arteries; you also restrict blood flow to the penis. And without enough blood, you're not going to be a rocket man. Even if you've been smoking for years, quitting now can help restore your potency.

Stop wine-ing. Alcohol is a depressant that slows down reflexes, including sexual ones. Drink no more than one drink, which is a 12-ounce beer, 5-ounce glass of wine, or 1½-ounce shot of liquor a day if you want to keep your erections as you get older, Dr. Crenshaw says.

Play hard. The fitter you are, the less likely impotence will be a problem, Dr. Montague says. Regular aerobic exercise such as walking and swimming helps keep arteries healthy and that includes the arteries that supply the penis, says Dr. Montague. Better yet, try to fit some running into your schedule, ideally, 15 to 20 minutes three times a week. Remember to check with your doctor before beginning a new exercise program, he adds.

Slice the fat. Dietary fat contributes to clogged arteries all over the body. So what's good for your heart is also good for your penis, Dr. Montague says. To stay potent, trim the fat in your diet down to about 20 percent of total calories. If you eat 2,000 calories a day, that means you can eat up to 44 grams of fat, he explains. To get started in the right direction, read food labels, avoid fried foods, look for low-fat and nonfat products, and switch to fat-free milk.

Snooze. Chronic tiredness is anathema to sex, especially for many older men who have difficulty going to sleep and staying asleep through the night, Dr. Crenshaw notes. Try to get at least six to eight hours of sleep a night. If you're tired, even a 30-minute nap before sex can improve your chances of getting an erection.

Read all about it. There are plenty of tasteful books that can help you learn about sexual techniques, eroticism, and overcoming impotence, Dr. Crenshaw says. For starters, Dr. Crenshaw recommends the timeless classic *The Joy of Sex* by Alex Comfort, M.D. You also may want to check out *A Lifetime of Sex: The Ultimate Manual on Sex, Women, and Relationships for Every Stage of a Man's Life* by Stephen C. George and K. Winston Caine. These and other books can be purchased by mail order or found in a bookstore or library.

INCONTINENCE

If you have a problem with incontinence, it might be a little reassuring to hear that it's a common concern among older people. But is that the kind of reassurance you really want to hear? More likely, you'd like to know that there are things you can do about it.

Well, there are.

"Incontinence is never normal at any age," says Neil Resnick, M.D., chief of gerontology at Brigham and Women's Hospital in Boston and associate professor of medicine at Harvard Medical School. "It's not a function of age nor of gender. Incontinence is almost always treatable and very often curable," he says.

At least 13 million Americans experience urinary incontinence, the involuntary release of urine. And it's not at all fair to both sexes. About 11 million of those 13 million are women. In fact, one out of every three women experiences some degree of urinary incontinence during her lifetime.

In most cases, there are not only solutions your doctor can suggest, there are some methods you can try yourself.

Try This First

Learn Kegels. Pelvic muscle exercises, also known as Kegel exercises, help many women with the most common kinds of incontinence, says Dr. Resnick.

Kegels strengthen the pelvic floor muscle that supports the bladder. When those muscles are stronger, you can tighten up in the area that controls the release of urine.

To do Kegels, you quickly contract your pelvic floor muscles as if you are stopping a stream of urine. Hold the contraction for about three seconds, then relax the muscles for an equal length of time. This pair of movements should be counted as one exercise.

Doing these exercises 45 times each day, divided into three sessions of 15 exercises each for at least six weeks, can help control incontinence, says Dr. Resnick. Just like strengthening biceps or any other muscle-building exercise, it takes time.

The great thing about Kegels is that you can do them anywhere—in the car as you're driving, at a bridge game, while you're washing the dishes—and no one has to know. And they really do work if they're done right, notes Dr. Resnick.

Remember, as with any exercise program, the beneficial effects last only as long as the exercise continues, says Dr. Resnick. One study found that women who practiced Kegels three times a week had the most success, even after five years.

Other Wise Ways

Keep a diary. Before you see your physician, it's a good idea to keep a diary of your urinary habits for two days, advises Dr. Resnick. Write down when you urinate, when you experience leaking, and note activities that may have triggered leaks, such as sneezing, coughing, or exercising. It may also be helpful if you estimate the amount of leakage you experience. Note whether you leaked a few drops of urine, a few teaspoons or tablespoons, or enough to soak a pad or your clothes. Your notes may be able to help your doctor determine what type of incontinence you have and the proper course of treatment.

Time your trips. For people with urge incontinence, bladder drills can help them reassert control, says Phillip Barksdale, M.D.,

MANAGING YOUR MEDS

Some muscle relaxants such as the product dantrolene (Dantrium) can cause incontinence by relaxing the muscles that support the bladder, says W. Steven Pray, Ph.D., R.Ph., a professor of nonprescription drug products at Southwestern Oklahoma State University in Weatherford. Caffeine can be a culprit as well, says Dr. Pray. This includes caffeine in aspirin-based analgesics such as Excedrin.

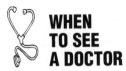

WHEN TO SEE A DOCTOR

Occasionally, incontinence is a symptom of a serious underlying problem, like a brain tumor, urethral blockage, ruptured disc, or multiple sclerosis, according to Neil Resnick, M.D., chief of gerontology at Brigham and Women's Hospital in Boston and associate professor of medicine at Harvard Medical School. In most cases these conditions are treatable if found early, so you don't want to delay diagnosis.

If your health care provider says nothing can be done about incontinence, don't necessarily accept that as the final word, says Dr. Resnick. Since research into new solutions is being made all the time, you may want to find a doctor who's up-to-date on the subject.

urogynecologist with Woman's Hospital in Baton Rouge, Louisiana.

To do them, urinate at set intervals, every hour or two, to keep the bladder from getting too full. After you achieve dryness for a few days, increase the intervals, says Dr. Barksdale. If you pace yourself, you should be able to control urination so you can wait several hours.

Watch what you drink and when. Alcohol and caffeinated beverages like coffee and tea stimulate urine production. Limit your consumption to no more than one or two servings a day or, better yet, eliminate these drinks, suggests Dr. Barksdale. These measures will help you with your bladder drills, reducing the urge to go more often, says Dr. Barksdale. Also, reduce the fluids you have in the evening. Less stress on your bladder will help you remain more comfortable between nighttime bladder drills.

Don't dry yourself out. You may be tempted to drink less throughout the day so you won't have to go as often. But it's important to continue drinking normal amounts of fluids for health reasons, suggests Dr. Barksdale. If you consciously resist drinking when you're thirsty, the deprivation can quickly lead to dehydration, especially when you're a senior.

Timing is everything. Many people with incontinence can be taught by a therapist to contract their pelvic muscles at the moment of physical strain, says Dr. Resnick.

"Usually, you have advance warning that a cough or a sneeze is coming," he says. If you practice doing a Kegel exercise at that exact moment, you can prevent incontinence.

Treat the triggers. Sometimes, treatment of an allergy or cough can "cure" incontinence, says Dr. Barksdale. Once the physical trigger is removed, incontinence often goes away.

Use absorbents wisely. Traditionally, people with incontinence have turned to various absorbent products, like maxipads or disposable adult undergarments.

While absorbent products are still the most widely used means of dealing with incontinence, don't rely on them exclusively. Dr. Resnick and Dr. Barksdale stress that they should be used only in addition to a doctor's treatments and your own restraining measures.

Ingrown Toenails

B ack at the turn of the century, the medical profession had some funny ideas about treating ingrown toenails. But the cures were not so funny for the patient. Using brute force, the doctor would simply rip out the entire nail, root and all.

Thankfully, the days of rip-'em-out nail surgery are behind us. In fact, there are ways you can handle the condition yourself.

Start with an examination. For some reason, the big toe seems to cause the most problems. As the nail grows, the skin near the tip of your toe becomes irritated by pressure, and you'll see redness and swelling accompanied by plenty of pain.

The problem is more common in people with unusually curved toenails, says Kathleen Stone, D.P.M., podiatrist in private practice in Glendale, Arizona. And if you wear tight shoes or stockings or injure your toe, you're more likely to get an ingrown nail.

As you age, you become even more susceptible to ingrown toenails. You're probably less agile than you once were, and that means you're more likely to trip and stub your toe. Also, nails tend to thicken as you age, and thicker nails are more forceful when they nudge their way into your skin. Older people are also more likely to get bunions and hammertoes, foot conditions that make your toes rub together, and with more friction, the skin surrounding your nails can become irritated.

So there are ways to prevent ingrown nails as well as ways to treat them. Here are some tips that cover both angles.

Try This First

Soak your foot. When you have an ingrown nail, the area around it is likely to become inflamed, and that inflammation only makes the condition worse. If you can reduce the swelling, your symptoms will improve, says Loretta Chou, M.D., assistant professor of orthopedic surgery at Stanford University School of Medicine.

To tackle the inflammation, put some hot water in a bucket and soak your foot for 20 minutes. To help prevent infection, add a small amount of mild soap to the water, suggests Dr. Chou. Or use Epsom salts, following the directions on the package. Test the water with your hand to make sure it's not too hot. You can repeat the soak once or twice a day as needed to bring down the inflammation, says Dr. Chou.

Other Wise Ways

Use antibiotic ointment. Ingrown nails easily become infected. Use an over-the-counter antibiotic ointment such as Neosporin or Polysporin. Smear on the ointment after your bath or shower, and be sure to do it again after you've soaked your foot, advises Dr. Chou.

Trim right. When you cut your nail, don't round the edges, or you'll just encourage the skin to be become irritated. Instead, trim your nails straight across when you use a clipper. It's fine to file down the edges slightly to keep them from being so sharp, but don't curve them, explains Dr. Chou.

Wear sandals. Open-toed shoes will keep the pressure off your toes and allow your foot to heal faster. And since the toes are open, there's no chance that you'll accidentally jam your toes into the front of the shoe when you're walking downhill, says Dr. Chou. If you can prevent your toe from being injured, you'll be less likely to develop an ingrown nail, according to Dr. Chou.

Buy shoes that fit. If your shoes are too tight, you'll have more pressure on your nails, says Dr. Chou. Women, especially, are likely to wear shoes that are too small, partly because manufacturers pay more attention to style than to the actual shape of the foot. Since your feet tend to become longer and wider with age, you should get your feet measured each time you buy shoes. And when you select the pair you want, press the toe of the shoe to make sure that

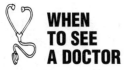

WHEN TO SEE A DOCTOR

A foot infection can spread quickly from an ingrown nail. If your nail is inflamed and pain increases steadily, see a podiatrist as soon as possible. And if you have poor circulation and decreased feeling in your feet due to diabetes, it's especially important that you get treated by a doctor before you try any home remedies, advises Kathleen Stone, D.P.M., podiatrist in private practice in Glendale, Arizona.

Your doctor may prescribe an antibiotic to use when you soak your feet. Or she may perform an office procedure using a local anesthetic, which is no more painful or complicated than having a tooth filled, says Dr. Stone.

there's at least a finger's width from your longest toe to the end of the toe box.

Choose stockings with care. Make sure your socks or stockings aren't too tight, says Dr. Stone. This can be a contributing factor as you age. If too tight, they can cause the thickened nail to be pushed into the skin.

Lace up logically. If you're wearing lace-up shoes, especially for foot-intensive activities like running or walking, you want to prevent your toes from sliding forward into the end of the toe box. To hold your foot in the correct position in the shoe, lace up your shoes so the laces are tightest (but not too tight) near the top of your midfoot, explains Dr. Chou.

INSOMNIA

Older people need just as much sleep as other adults, about eight hours a night on average. However, their ability to sleep can be compromised for a variety of reasons.

As a natural part of aging, you tend to be more easily roused from slumber. Over time, your sleep cycles can change, too, so suddenly you're feeling more tired earlier in the evening. Insomnia enters the picture when you fight the urge to sleep and stay up later in the evening but then cannot remain asleep in the earlier hours of the morning.

Then there are the times when you will experience an occasional bout of sleeplessness because of stressful and worrisome events in your waking life. The changing nature of life, adjusting to retirement, or bereavement may cause situational or transient insomnia. The important thing is to keep these periods in perspective, says Michael Vitiello, Ph.D., professor of psychiatry and behavioral sciences at the University of Washington in Seattle.

Insomnia is wearisome but it's usually not considered a serious hazard to your health. If insomnia lasts for more than two weeks, see your doctor. In the meantime, try practicing these tips to improve your ability to sleep and the quality of the sleep you get.

Try This First

Reset your clock. The circadian rhythm, the body's internal clock that tells it when to sleep and when to be awake, can be influenced by the body's exposure to the sun. This knowledge can be very useful if you start wanting to sleep at 7:00 P.M. and start waking up at 3:00 A.M. That's a sign that your internal clock may be out of whack and needs some resetting.

To get your body clock adjusted, get as much light exposure as

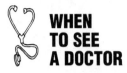

WHEN TO SEE A DOCTOR

If your insomnia persists for more than two weeks or makes you feel so drowsy during the daytime that it impairs your ability to perform important tasks such as driving a car, consult with a sleep specialist, says Michael Vitiello, Ph.D., professor of psychiatry and behavioral sciences at the University of Washington in Seattle. You may have a more serious underlying sleep disorder that needs to be treated by a professional.

you can toward the end of the day, recommends Sonia Ancoli-Israel, Ph.D., director of the sleep disorders clinic at the Veteran's Affairs Health Care System in San Diego, professor of psychiatry at the University of California, San Diego, and author of *All I Want Is a Good Night's Sleep*. This has the effect of moving your body clock ahead a few hours so you feel like going to bed at your more usual hour. Eat lunch outside, go for a walk in the afternoon, and when you have to spend time outside in the morning, wear sunglasses so your eyes are exposed to a little less light. All of these strategies will move your daylight exposure to later in the day, rather than earlier. You should see results in about two weeks, says Dr. Ancoli-Israel.

Other Wise Ways

Don't let your clock get cuckoo. Go to bed and get up at the same time of day seven days a week, and your body will thank you by becoming accustomed to that rhythm and sleeping during those hours, Dr. Ancoli-Israel explains.

Have a real rest room. Keep your room at a comfortable temperature, advises Dr. Ancoli-Israel. And you'll find it easier to sleep as long as you should if you draw the drapes to block out early-morning light.

Leave your worries at the bedroom doorstep. The bedroom is for sleep and sex, period. Leave eating, working, watching TV, even reading for another room in the house, says Patricia Prinz, Ph.D., professor of behavioral nursing and adjunct professor of psychiatry and behavior sciences at the University of Washington in Seattle.

Tune out that TV thriller. Watching scary, violent, or otherwise disturbing movies or TV programs before you go to bed is not a good idea, says Margaret Moline, Ph.D., director of the sleep-wake disorders center at the New York Presbyterian Hospital–Cornell Medical Center in White Plains, New York. They're often too stimulating and will keep you up. And don't trade in your remote control for the latest paperback suspense novel. A good page turner can be just as disruptive to your sleep schedule.

Think routine. Any parent will tell you that setting up a bedtime routine for children is important. Guess what? It's important for adults, too. "Grown-ups forget to do that," Dr. Moline says. "But we need routines just like the little kids do, so that we can relax and get ready for sleep." So take a bath, get in your jammies, and spend some time reading (but not in the bedroom) before you climb into bed.

Dim the lights. Exposure to bright light before you sleep may have a stimulating effect and may keep you up, Dr. Moline warns. Keep the lights in the house low as you get nearer to your bedtime.

MANAGING YOUR MEDS

Certain medications that older people may be taking can interfere with their ability to fall asleep, explains Phyllis Zee, M.D., Ph.D., director of the sleep disorders center and associate professor of neurology at Northwestern University Medical School in Chicago. Check with your doctor if you think your medications may be causing insomnia, but never stop taking them without his consent.

- Antidepressants such as fluoxetine (Prozac)
- Medications for chronic pulmonary disease and emphysema, such as prednisone (Deltasone), theophylline (Respbid), and beta-blockers like propranolol (Inderal) can aid breathing but be so stimulating that they interfere with sleep
- Diuretics for high blood pressure can interfere with sleep indirectly because you'll have to get up in the night to go to the bathroom

Get up and bore yourself to sleep. If you do have trouble sleeping, doctors say, you don't want to wallow all night in bed trying to drop off again. Try for 10 minutes and then get up, leave the bedroom, and go do something quiet and dull until you feel sleepy again.

Turn the clock to the wall. If you do wake up in the night, don't focus on your alarm clock. "It doesn't matter if it's 2:30 or 3:00 A.M.," Dr. Moline says. "The more you pay attention to external stimuli when you're awakened in the middle of the night, the more likely it is that you'll have trouble falling back asleep."

Find some ease with the herb valerian. Have some valerian root to help you sleep, suggests Varro Tyler, Ph.D., distinguished professor emeritus at Purdue University in West Lafayette, Indiana, and author of *The Honest Herbal*. Valerian is an ancient herb that is helpful in adjusting sleep over a period of time, but you don't need to grow it fresh or grind up the root.

Dr. Tyler recommends buying concentrated valerian and using an amount equivalent to two to three grams of root a day. Valerian is also available in capsule form. Look for a standardized extract (0.8 percent valeric acid) and follow the directions on the label. Do not use valerian with sleep-enhancing or mood-regulating medications such as diazepam (Valium) or amitriptyline (Elavil). If stimulant action occurs, discontinue use. In infrequent cases, it may cause heart palpitations and nervousness in sensitive individuals.

Catch some kava. For acute insomnia such as that brought on by jet lag, you may want to try the herbal remedy kava, says Dr. Tyler. This herb is also prepackaged, but you want to check the label to make sure it has the active constituents kavapyrones or kavalactones.

Take between 60 and 120 milligrams before bedtime to help induce sleep. But because kava has a sedating effect, you shouldn't have it if you're already taking a sedative before bedtime, Dr. Tyler warns. Do not take kava with alcohol or barbiturates. Do not take more than the recommended dose. Use caution when driving or operating equipment, as this herb is a muscle relaxant.

Say no to nicotine. Even though some people feel the need for cigarettes to relax them, the nicotine in cigarettes is a stimulant, says Naomi R. Kramer, M.D., associate director of the sleep disorders center at Rhode Island Hospital in Providence. So it's a bad idea to fight insomnia by lighting up. If you smoke, try to avoid doing it at night. "And if you wake up at night and want to go back to sleep, don't have a cigarette," Dr. Kramer advises.

Watch what you drink. Caffeinated beverages interrupt sleep, so don't drink them after noon. And you'll want to avoid alcoholic drinks before bedtime, too. Alcohol initially has a sedating effect, but as your body turns it into energy, it becomes stimulating, causing wakefulness in the night, Dr. Moline states.

Eat lightly. A big meal late at night might make you sleepy, but then again, it might not. If you are prone to heartburn or gastro-esophageal reflux, problems which tend to increase with age, having a huge dinner late will keep you up, says Phyllis Zee, M.D., Ph.D., director of the sleep disorders center and associate professor of neurology at Northwestern University Medical School in Chicago. Try to eat dinner earlier in the evening.

Have some warm tryptophan and cookies. Of course, if you eat an early dinner, it may not be enough to tide you over until you go to sleep. And hunger pangs can certainly keep you awake. Have a light snack to alleviate hunger before bedtime, suggests Dr. Vitiello. He recommends that you include some warm milk in that snack because milk contains tryptophan (a food substance that helps people feel sleepy). Other foods such as turkey, fish, and bananas are also rich in tryptophan.

Plug in a night-light. It's almost inevitable. At some point, you can be pretty sure, you'll have to get up to go to the bathroom. But if you have to turn on a lot of lights, you may overstimulate yourself and find it more difficult to fall back asleep, says Dr. Kramer. If you regularly find yourself in this situation and your eyesight and balance don't cause you any problems, plug in a night-light or even two if it's a long way to the bathroom. Let the small glow light your way.

Limit your sleep. If you are having a difficult time sleeping, you may think that trying to sleep more will help. But this can backfire, making insomnia worse, says Lauren Broch, Ph.D., director of education and training at the sleep-wake disorders center at New York Presbyterian Hospital–Cornell Medical Center in White Plains, New York. "You spend a lot more time in bed where you're not sleeping, and you start learning that bed is not a place to sleep, it's a place to ruminate and a place to be frustrated. You start associating your bed with things other than sleep," Dr. Broch explains. As you age, the amount of sleep you need can become very individualized, so in order to fall asleep efficiently, it's important to limit yourself to only an extra half-hour in bed awake. After that, get up.

Confine your sleep to the night. You might think a nap would be good to help combat the effects of insomnia. But any time spent napping actually takes away from the time you'll spend sleeping at night. That only makes insomnia worse. If you feel tired during the day, try to stay awake until bedtime, suggests Dr. Broch. By then, you may find yourself so tired, you'll fall right to sleep.

Work it out. Exercise has been shown to help sleep, says Dr. Zee. And it doesn't have to be strenuous aerobic exercise, either. In fact, the timing of your exercise is more important than how strenuous it is. Exercise will initially make you more alert. But four to six hours after you exercise, your body temperature and metabolism drop, priming you for sleep, explains Peter Hauri, M.D. co-director of the Mayo Clinic Sleep Disorders Center in Rochester, Minnesota, and author of *No More Sleepless Nights*.

Schedule your workouts for four to six hours before bed, so your body temperature and energy will be declining just about the time you need to get to sleep. Any closer to bedtime and you may be too stimulated to sleep.

INTERMITTENT CLAUDICATION

E ven in bygone days when doctors were scarce and do-it-yourself medicine was all the rage, some ideas were frankly lame. Take, for instance, this oddball cure for leg pain: "Rub leg with turpentine and sit before the fire until leg begins to tingle." Fortunately, this dubious remedy was just a flash in the pan that never really caught fire—so to speak.

Nowadays, there are vastly safer natural remedies for intermittent claudication, a type of persistent leg pain that affects 1 in 10 Americans over age 70. The condition is named for Roman emperor Claudius, who, like many people who have this condition, had a noticeable limp. It is caused by hardening of the arteries supplying blood and oxygen to the lower limbs. High blood pressure, diabetes, smoking, high cholesterol—the very same lifestyle factors that promote heart disease—all contribute to this condition, which can cause a burning, cramplike pain in the legs, feet, hips, thighs, or even the buttocks.

The pain typically strikes after a person has walked a short distance, often as little as a block. After you've stopped and rested a few minutes, the pain usually disappears. When you have intermittent claudication, the pain recurs once you begin exerting yourself again. As the arteries become more clogged, the distance you can walk before experiencing pain gradually decreases.

"Intermittent claudication definitely interferes with living well. But up to 90 percent of people who have it never report it to their doctors. Most people consider it just a part of getting old. They think, 'Oh well, I just can't do what I used to do,'" says Steven Santilli, M.D., vascular surgeon at the Veterans Administration Medical Center and assistant professor of surgery at the University of Minnesota, both in Minneapolis.

That fatalistic attitude is unjustified, Dr. Santilli says. "Lifestyle

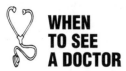

changes like quitting smoking and getting regular exercise can have a huge impact on this condition. There is really no reason you should have to live with intermittent claudication," he says. Here are a few effective ways to put the zing back into your step.

Try This First

Walk away from it. Walking—the very activity that usually induces the pain associated with claudication—also is one of the surest ways to stop it, doctors say.

"Some people look at me like I'm crazy when I tell them they need to get out there and walk more, not less. They want pills. But the truth is, we really don't have a drug that will treat claudication as effectively as walking," says Jay D. Coffman, M.D., chief of peripheral vascular medicine at Boston University Medical Center.

Walking enhances the ability of your leg muscles to extract oxygen from blood, Dr. Santilli says. So if you walk more, not less, your leg muscles will learn to use oxygen more efficiently, and you'll be less apt to develop cramps and leg pain.

Set aside about an hour a day five days a week for walking, he suggests. As you walk, avoid stopping when you feel the first twinges of pain. Instead, let the pain intensify a bit, then pick out a nearby goal, like the next telephone pole, and vow to reach it before you rest. Once the pain subsides, get moving again. When you feel the next surge of pain, set your sights on another goal—say, the length between two telephone poles—

that's just a bit more ambitious than the first goal. Keep going on like this for the full hour.

Don't worry about how many times you have to stop or how fast or far you walk, Dr. Santilli says. In the beginning, some people who try this approach have to stop and rest every two to three minutes. That's okay. If you sustain this effort for several weeks, your pain should subside and the distance between rest stops should increase, he says. In fact, researchers have found that many people with intermittent claudication who use this technique are able to double their walking distance in just two to three months.

Other Wise Ways

Snag a walking buddy. Ask your spouse, a friend, or a co-worker to join you on your strolls, Dr. Coffman suggests. A companion can encourage you to keep moving and reinforce your determination to beat intermittent claudication.

Walk for cover. Rather than ditching your walk on unseasonably hot or cold days, go to an indoor shopping mall where you can do your routine in temperature-controlled comfort, recommends Dr. Coffman.

Corral the Marlboro man. People who smoke are twice as likely to develop intermittent claudication as nonsmokers, Dr. Santilli says. Smoking constricts blood vessels and makes it harder for your leg muscles to work properly. But even if you've lit up for years, quitting now will improve circulation in your legs and help relieve the pain, he says.

Be firm about fat. Eating too much artery-clogging fat will only worsen intermittent claudication, Dr. Santilli explains. That's because a fatty diet can cause hardening of the arteries, which in turn causes intermittent claudication. For every bite of meat, take four bites of fruits, vegetables, beans, and grains. It will help keep you on track for a low-fat lifestyle. If you must, Dr. Santilli says, you can make fatty foods like gravy, bacon, or fried chicken a once-a-month treat.

IRRITABILITY

Irritability sounds far too civilized to most Americans. So we invented slang like cranky, cross, crabby, huffy, touchy, testy, quarrelsome, snappish, snippy, grumpy, surly, sour, vexed, and peeved. You could have a chip on your shoulder, have it in for someone, have had it up to here, have a fit, or have an ax to grind. An irritable person often is called irascible, sullen, thin-skinned, ill-tempered, cantankerous, fire-breathing, or pugnacious. You might fly off the handle, flip your lid, or be fit to be tied.

But no matter what you call it, occasional irritability is simply a part of being alive, says Laura Slap-Shelton, Ph.D., D.Ph., clinical psychologist with a specialty in neuropsychology at Jeanes Hospital in Philadelphia. "No one is perfect. And things will happen in the course of some days that may be upsetting," she says.

Irritability can go hand in hand with almost any illness, including anxiety, diabetes, and arthritis. And certainly, the aches and pains of later life can make us feel more irritable as the years and health problems begin to mount up, says George T. Grossberg, M.D., director of geriatric psychiatry at St. Louis University School of Medicine. But for the most part, older Americans are no more prone to irritability than younger people.

For those times when you feel mildly irritated, try these remedies.

Try This First

Relax, then find the culprit. Whenever you feel irritable, take a few deep breaths and give yourself a mini-break in the action of the day, says Dr. Slap-Shelton. "You may want to take a walk or engage in your favorite form of exercise or your favorite hobby." Then, try to identify the culprit. Take a few minutes to think about what may be bothering you. Worry and fatigue often leads to irritability. If you can identify the cause of your irritability, especially a recurrent problem, it may help you banish it, Dr. Slap-Shelton says.

If you pay all your bills monthly, for instance, and you know that you get edgy on the day you make those payments, change your system so you pay a few bills each week instead of all of them at once. Or, if the weekly bill confrontation is inconceivable, stick to the monthly routine but give yourself plenty of time to get the

MANAGING YOUR MEDS

Caffeine is a major cause of irritability in older Americans, says George T. Grossberg, M.D., director of geriatric psychiatry at St. Louis University School of Medicine. If you find yourself more irritable than usual, try drinking only one eight-ounce cup of regular coffee as part of your morning routine, then switch to decaffeinated coffee for the rest of the day. Eventually, try to eliminate even the one cup of regular morning coffee and avoid other caffeine sources, such as colas and other sweetened soft drinks. Eventually, you will be free of your dependence on caffeine.

In addition to caffeine, almost any medication can trigger grouchiness, says Bruce G. Pollock, M.D., professor of psychiatry and director of the geriatric psychopharmacology program at the University of Pittsburgh School of Medicine. Common drugs that can cause irritability among seniors include:

- Tranquilizers such as benzodiazepines
- Antipsychotic medications such as risperidone (Risperdal) or haloperidol (Haldol)
- High blood pressure drugs like the beta-blockers propranolol (Inderal) and nadolol (Corgard)
- Parkinson's disease drugs like levodopa (Sinemet) or pramipexole (Mirapex)
- Over-the-counter cold- and congestion-relief products like Tavist-D, medications that contain phenylpropanolamine, including Contac, and Comtrex or diet aids like Acutrim and Dexatrim

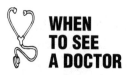

WHEN TO SEE A DOCTOR

Irritability can be a symptom of many diseases ranging from a minor cold or flu to major depression or Alzheimer's disease. If you feel irritable for two weeks or more, let your doctor know about it, says Bruce G. Pollock, M.D., professor of psychiatry and director of the geriatric psychopharmacology program at the University of Pittsburgh School of Medicine. Also consult your physician if in addition to irritability you experience any of the following problems for two or more weeks.

• You have lost your appetite.
• You have difficulty sleeping.
• You withdraw from your usual activities.
• Your mood is adversely affecting your relationships with family and friends.

chore done, and then reward yourself afterward with a fun activity such as a relaxing dinner at a favorite restaurant, Dr. Slap-Shelton recommends. In this way, you can remove or reduce a source of irritability in your life.

Other Wise Ways

Take a break. Try engaging in a task that will distract you from whatever is irritating you, Dr. Grossberg says. Take a walk, dig in the garden, or make your bed. Even if the activity only takes 5 to 10 minutes, it will absorb your attention and give you time to cool off so you don't react impulsively or say something that you'll regret later.

Take a whiff. If you would like to give the ancient healing art of aromatherapy a shot at adjusting your mood, oil of lavender can help relieve irritability, according to John Steele, a worldwide lecturer and aromatic consultant who runs Lifetree Aromatix, a company that sells botanical products and distributes information in Los Angeles. "You can't go wrong with lavender," Steele says. "It's a sedative antidepressant because it has a high number of molecules called esters that are extremely relaxing to the mind and the body."

Apply three or four drops of the oil to a tissue or handkerchief and inhale whenever you feel irritable, he suggests. Lavender essential oil is the concentrated product of steam distillation. It is the most potent therapeutic part of the plant, says Steele. Essential oils are available at most health food stores.

Send out warning signals. Instead of trying to hide your feelings, let others know that you're having a bad day, Dr. Slap-Shelton advises. Simply admitting that things aren't going well and apologizing in advance for being out of sorts that day can help defuse the situation and bring about needed support and understanding.

"Often, older people feel irritable because they feel overwhelmed by everything they need to do, and they don't know how to ask for support," Dr. Slap-Shelton says. Just say how you are feeling. "Friends and family will respond with empathy, humor, and other kinds of support that can go a long way toward getting you out of your bad mood."

JAW PAIN AND TMD

To children, it is an apt name for a 2.6 ounce, 1¾-inch round rock-hard candy. As for the rest of us, well, let's just say that jawbreaker doesn't exactly conjure visions of a sugar-coated delight. If anything, the term serves as a reminder of the foods, stresses, or health problems that can be a real pain in the jaw for older Americans.

"Jaw pain is very common among people over age 60," says Paul A. Andrews, D.D.S., dentist in Maitland, Florida, who practices therapeutic management of head, neck, and facial pain. "Seniors are simply more susceptible to arthritis or falls that can injure the jaw. Often, jaw pain is a progressive problem that sneaks up on you. In fact, even if your jaw was injured in your forties or fifties, the symptoms may not cause noticeable problems until 15 or 20 years later when osteoporosis and other diseases set in and compound the damage done by that old injury."

Once your doctor has ruled out the possibility of a jaw fracture, the prime suspect will probably be TMD (temporomandibular disorder), which is an inflammation or misalignment of the joint that connects the jaw to the head. In studies, up to 75 percent of people have signs of TMD, including muscle pain and clicking, popping, or grating noises in the jaw, Dr. Andrews says.

Often, TMD and other forms of mild jaw pain are temporary and can be relieved by these simple home remedies, Dr. Andrews suggests.

Try This First

Give your jaw a break. Treat your sore jaw as if it were a sore ankle, advises Flora Parsa Stay, D.D.S., dentist in Oxnard, California, and author of *The Complete Book of Dental Remedies*. If your ankle were sore, you'd stay off it. The same rule applies to the jaw.

While your jaw aches, try not to open it too wide. If you're a big yawner, that means you'll have to restrain yourself to avoid stretching your mouth too wide. But even when you're not yawning, you should be conscious of what position your jaw is in. Place your tongue on the roof of your mouth and keep your lips closed. That will help keep your teeth slightly ajar and keep your jaw in a relaxed position. Breathe through your nose. The only time your teeth should touch, Dr. Stay says, is when you are chewing or swallowing.

Other Wise Ways

Hit it with an iceberg. Cold compresses can take the sting out of sore muscles surrounding the jaw, Dr. Andrews explains. Cold helps relax muscle spasms and numbs pain.

After you begin feeling pain, wrap an ice pack in a towel and hold it against your jaw for 20 minutes. Keep it off for 20 minutes, then apply the ice pack once more. Repeat as often as necessary to help ease the soreness.

Then melt it. If the pain persists for more than 36 hours, use a heat pack instead of a cold pack, following the same routine as you did when applying cold. The heat increases blood flow to injured tissues and helps them heal, Dr. Andrews says.

Toss the nuts. Avoid nuts, steaks, hard candies, caramels, and other chewy or crunchy foods when your jaw hurts, Dr. Andrews suggests. Stick with a soft diet that includes foods like macaroni

MANAGING YOUR MEDS

In rare cases, medications for mental problems like depression that contain phenothiazines, such as chlorpromazine (Thorazine) or haloperidol (Haldol), can cause facial twitches and tooth grinding that can aggravate jaw pain, says W. Steven Pray, Ph.D., R.Ph., professor of nonprescription drug products at Southwestern Oklahoma State University in Weatherford. If an antidepressant causes this side effect, ask your doctor if another medication may be more appropriate.

WHEN TO SEE A DOCTOR

Seek medical care if the following symptoms persist for more than seven days.

• Your jaw muscles feel tender and achy.

• You have a dull aching pain in front of your ear.

• You notice a clicking sound or grating sensation when you open your mouth or chew food.

• You have a persistent headache that seems centered behind your eyes.

• Your teeth or dentures don't come together normally.

and cheese; meat loaf; steamed vegetables; bananas; and other tender fruits; juices; and water until the pain subsides.

Unplug the coffeepot. Caffeine increases muscle tension and makes the nervous system more sensitive to pain. So steer clear of coffee, teas, colas, chocolate, and other caffeine-laden beverages and foods if your jaw aches, Dr. Stay recommends.

Stoke up on C. Take vitamin C supplements. They'll help your body repair connective tissue surrounding the jaw and hasten healing, Dr. Stay says. She recommends taking 2,000 milligrams of vitamin C daily. (Vitamin C in doses above 1,200 milligrams per day may cause diarrhea in some people.)

Use your noggin'. Meditation may help relax muscles and relieve jaw pain, according to Dr. Andrews. "Many older people have carried strains and tensions in their jaw joints all of their lives, and now all that stress is beginning to show up as pain," he says.

Focus on your breath as a simple, powerful way to meditate, he says. To try it, sit in a comfortable position, close your eyes, and take a couple of deep breaths. Inhale slowly through your nose for a count of 4, then slowly exhale through your mouth as you count to 10. Once you get accustomed to that pattern, stop counting breaths and focus all of your attention on the rhythm of your breathing as you inhale and exhale. To help you stay focused, try this: As you breathe in, think to yourself, "Calm mind." As you exhale, think, "Peaceful body." If your mind begins to drift, simply refocus your attention on your breath. Do this for 10 to 15 minutes a day or whenever your jaw pain seems worse, Dr. Andrews advises.

Glide into slumber. Devote your last waking hour each day to enjoyable activities like pleasurable reading, listening to soothing music, or soaking in a warm bath, suggests Gretchen Gibson, D.D.S., director of the geriatric dentistry program at the Veterans Administration Medical Center in Dallas. These routines will help relax your facial muscles and lessen the chances that you'll clench your teeth while you sleep.

"Don't do laundry, clean the kitchen, or take out the garbage at 9:45 P.M. and then hop into bed at 10:00. Your body won't be relaxed and you'll be more apt to wake up with jaw pain the next morning," Dr. Gibson says.

Straighten up and chew right. Poor posture forces your shoulders and head to pitch forward in order to maintain your balance, Dr. Andrews says That can put extra strain on your jaw muscles and pull your teeth out of alignment, so chewing is more difficult.

To alleviate this problem, lie on a carpeted floor so that your back, shoulders, and the back of your head all touch the floor at the same time. Remain lying in that position for 15 to 20 minutes a day, Dr. Andrews suggests. If you like, you can prop your legs up on a pillow or chair.

Eyeball your dentures. Jaw pain can be a sign that your dentures are worn out and need to be replaced, Dr. Andrews warns. Check with your dentist.

LARYNGITIS

Y ou may have heard that as you age, the muscles in your body can get weaker over time. That's not just true of the muscles in your arms and legs, but in all of your muscles, even the ones you don't think about, such as the ones in your throat.

Your larynx or voice box, for instance, is made up of muscles. As you age, they can weaken and change shape. The same is true for your vocal cords. Consequently, when you get laryngitis (an inflammation of the larynx that makes your voice go hoarse and raspy), your weaker throat muscles may take longer to bounce back from the inflammation. Doctors even have a name for this problem. They call it presbylaryngis, which simply means an aging larynx.

"In general, older people will get problems with their cords more easily than other age groups and the problems might last longer. As people get older, the cords themselves are a little bit weaker and a little bit bowed," says Gregory Grillone, M.D., otolaryngologist and director of the voice center at Boston Medical Center.

Some diseases that can affect seniors' voices are Parkinson's disease and diabetes. But for most people, laryngitis has common-sense causes. If you get a simple viral infection such as a cold, it can affect the larynx. If you let loose with a holler at your granddaughter's soccer game, your vocal cords may get the sensation that you're out to beat them. And then there are people who chronically abuse their voices because they overuse them professionally, such as some teachers, singers, or lawyers.

A surprisingly common cause of laryngitis that is not as well known is gastrointestinal reflux (heartburn), which happens more frequently as you age. Reflux occurs when some contents of your stomach—including very harsh digestive acids—back up into your esophagus. The acids from the stomach cause irritation and laryngitis. "It's the most common reason I see for voice problems," Dr. Grillone says.

Whatever has made you hoarse, though, doctors recommend the following strategies for getting your voice back in shape.

Try This First

Liquefy your larynx. A phrase used among voice doctors and professional singers is "pee pale," Dr. Grillone says. Singers know that if their urine is not clear like water, they're not drinking enough water. And drinking enough water is a major part of good vocal hygiene. Drinking water keeps the secretions in the throat thin and mobile as well as helps the whole body with the healing process. So polish off at least eight, eight-ounce glasses of water a day.

Other Wise Ways

Keep mum. Getting through a day without talking can be difficult. But when you have laryngitis, what you need is a respite for your larynx and vocal cords, states Marshall Postman, M.D., allergist in private practice in Reno, Nevada. "If you had tendonitis, you would try not to use the joint that tendon was affecting, so with laryngitis, really the best thing is to get vocal rest," Dr. Postman advises.

Don't even whisper. People think that whispering doesn't count as talking. But whispering is very straining and in no way saves the voice, warns Florence B. Blager, Ph.D., professor in the department of otolaryngology at the University of Colorado School of Medicine and chief of speech pathology and audiology services at National Jewish Medical and Research Center, both in Denver. When you whisper, your larynx tightens with a great deal of effort as your breath comes through a very constricted laryngeal area. This causes strain, and the louder you try to whisper, the greater the constriction and the more the strain on your vocal cords.

Write it down. Carry a pad and pen or pencil with you so you can still communicate, Dr. Blager says.

Avoid irritating environments. Don't go to places where smoke or fumes that you inhale may irritate the larynx further, Dr. Blager recommends.

Be smart about cheering the home team. Dr. Blager has studied the strain and damage that cheerleaders can cause to their voices.

WHEN TO SEE A DOCTOR

If you've been having laryngitis for more than two weeks, see your doctor. You should also give your doctor a call if you have laryngitis but can't remember when you had a cold or any other obvious reason for the problem. Hoarseness can be a symptom of laryngeal cancer, which seniors are at greater risk for, especially if you have a history of smoking or drinking, says Gregory Grillone, M.D., otolaryngologist and director of the voice center at Boston Medical Center. Also, see your doctor if you suspect the cause of your laryngitis may be heartburn, especially if it's accompanied by coughing, throat clearing, or difficulty swallowing.

"You overuse the cords, and, yes, you can ruin the vocal cords forever," Dr. Blager says. She advises people to not shout themselves hoarse at a sporting event. If you want to cheer for your team, give your voice some support. "Roll up your program and use it as a megaphone so you get a lot of intensity increase without shouting. It lets you feel that you're really contributing," Dr. Blager says.

Put your voice in the right place. With an illness such as flu, you can become tired and weak, and your breath can become shallow. When this happens, it takes effort to keep your voice forward. Even after the illness is gone, the shallow breathing pattern can remain, causing you to speak from deep in your throat, Dr. Blager says. That can cause hoarseness after just a couple of weeks. It may be necessary to relearn how to breathe and get your voice forward again, Dr. Blager says. Focus on breathing from your abdomen, not from your chest, and focus your voice in the front of your face, not in your throat.

Strengthen your voice. One way to strengthen your voice, Dr. Blager suggests, is to practice extending your exhale up to 15 to 20 seconds. Two or three times a day, make a conscious effort to breathe out steadily on an "s" sound, while you time yourself or silently count the seconds. And concentrate on talking while you exhale. This helps you avoid straining your throat by speaking after all your breath is exhaled.

Get a little humidity. Using the power of humidity is also a good way to keep your airways moist and your secretions moving, says Anne L. Davis, M.D., associate professor of clinical medicine at New York University in New York City. You can give yourself a humidity treatment with simple kitchen equipment. Heat a large open pan of water until it's boiling, and remove it from the stove. While it's still busily steaming, take it to the table, drape a towel over your head, hang your head over the pot, and inhale deeply. Keep your eyes closed and don't get so close that you burn your skin. Steam for 5 to 15 minutes.

Go for a soothing feeling. Suck on a hard candy or drink warm lemon and honey. These remedies can soothe a raw throat, Dr. Davis suggests.

Take an antacid. If you suffer from reflux, a common cause of laryngitis, take antacids such as Mylanta and Maalox and acid reducers such as Tagamet and Pepcid AC. These can help reduce nighttime gastroesophogeal reflux, a backing up of the stomach's contents into the esophagus, Dr. Grillone says.

Eat wisely. If reflux laryngitis is your problem, there are some things to consider about when and what you eat. "There are a lot of things that people do in their diets or their day-to-day habits that make reflux worse," Dr. Grillone explains. Make your last meal of the day light and eat it at least three hours before bedtime.

Guard against reflux producers. Avoid alcohol, tobacco, caffeine, and mint or menthol, which all stimulate gastric acid and encourage reflux, says Dr. Grillone. Stay away from carbonated beverages, because the carbonation bloats your stomach and as it does, it puts pressure on the valve between your stomach and esophagus that is supposed to keep reflux from occurring.

MANAGING YOUR MEDS

Many types of drugs can affect the voice and cause hoarseness, says Gregory Grillone, M.D., otolaryngologist and director of the voice center at Boston Medical Center. The most common are steroids. Taken in pill form such as prednisone (Deltasone) or in inhalers such as flunisolide (Nasalide). Many steroids can start to atrophy the vocal cords' mucous membranes, affecting the quality of the voice. But be sure you don't give up these drugs without your doctor's consent.

LOWERED

SEXUAL DESIRE

When she was 30, Eleanor Hamilton, Ph.D., asked a woman in her seventies, "At what age does sexual desire stop?" The woman's eyes twinkled with amusement as she replied, "I'll let you know."

Of course, the woman never did. And Dr. Hamilton, a retired sex therapist now in her late eighties, thinks she knows why.

"Her answer surprised me at the time. But now it doesn't at all. I know full well now that sex can go on until you die," says Dr. Hamilton of West Linn, Oregon.

In fact, studies suggest that up to 74 percent of married men and 56 percent of married women over age 60 are still sexually active. And, even after age 80, 63 percent of men and 30 percent of women report having intercourse regularly, researchers say.

"One of the unfortunate myths of our society is that older people aren't sexual and shouldn't want sex anyway. Well, obviously we are sexual and we do want sex," Dr. Hamilton says.

But sexual desire is also fragile. "It's a real blow to your sex drive when you have problems in the bedroom. Failure doesn't exactly make people want to come back for more," says Fran Kaiser, M.D., adjunct professor of geriatric medicine at St. Louis University and senior regional medical director for Merck pharmaceuticals, based in Irving, Texas.

Drops in testosterone production and other hormonal changes, for instance, do decrease sex drive and make it more difficult for older men to get and maintain erections. And without the certainty of success, many older men become skittish about sex, Dr. Kaiser says. As for women, menopause triggers a decline in estrogen production. Without estrogen, vaginal lubrication needs some help because the vagina doesn't get quickly and naturally moistened when foreplay begins. Unless you and your spouse are aware of this, you might attempt intercourse despite vaginal dryness, and that can make the experience painful and, ultimately, less desirable.

Sexual desire also can be derailed by arthritis, heart disease, stroke, osteoporosis, and other ailments associated with aging. "Any chronic disease that causes pain, discomfort, anxiety, or shortness of breath is going to sap your libido. If your body hurts, why would you want to have sex?" Dr. Kaiser asks.

In addition, unreasonable expectations can transform sex into an avoided chore rather than an anticipated pleasure, points out James Semmens, M.D., sex therapist and professor emeritus at the Medical University of South Carolina College of Medicine in Charleston, South Carolina.

"Some older people still think that sex has to be an explosive achievement. If they don't have orgasms, they feel as if they've failed their partners somehow. So they back away from sex altogether. That can place a heavy burden on their relationships," Dr. Semmens says. "It's important to keep sex in proper perspective as you age. Your sexual performance may not be the same as it was in your thirties or forties, but it still can be fun, rewarding, and novel as you get older."

Here are a few ways to keep your sexual flames burning.

Try This First

Broaden your horizons. Sex is about much more than intercourse. Explore new ways to express your sexuality, Dr. Semmens says. Be sure to give each other lots of hugs, kisses, gentle caresses, and other displays of tenderness. Just the physical act of holding hands can be as fulfilling as traditional sexual activity.

"Learning new ways to play in the sexual sandbox is important in later life," Dr. Semmens says. "Remember, the goal of sex is not always a physical one, it's emotional, too."

Other Wise Ways

Let the hands roam within limits. For a few minutes or longer each day, lend your body to your partner, suggests Karen Martin, program coordinator of the sexuality center at Hillside Hospital of

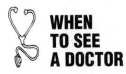

WHEN TO SEE A DOCTOR

If you think that lowered sexual desire is a problem, you may want to seek counseling from a sex therapist, says Eleanor Hamilton, Ph.D., retired sex therapist in West Linn, Oregon. In particular, seek help if:

• You feel angry about or disappointed with your sex life.

• You and your partner disagree about how often you ought to have sex, to the point that it is eroding mutual respect or hindering communication.

• You have physical problems that make sex difficult or undesirable but you don't know how to overcome these barriers.

Northshore–Long Island Jewish Health System in New Hyde Park, New York. Your partner can touch you in any way that provides pleasure to either of you, but during this time, the breasts and genitals are off limits. That will free your spouse to explore different parts of your body without feeling obligated to arouse you. It can also help you feel good about yourself. If a particular touch, such as running a finger down your back, hurts or bothers you in any way, ask your partner not to do it. Allow enough time for each partner to take turns.

This exercise can be emotionally gratifying and can redefine your sexual feelings for each other, Martin says.

Make it a priority. Upgrade the importance of intimacy, Dr. Semmens suggests. Instead of suppressing your desires until all your daily chores are completed, allow lovemaking to be more spontaneous. If you let the moment pass, fatigue, stress, and other pressures of life will extinguish your passion.

Let life imitate art. Provocative television shows, movies, magazine articles, or novels are wonderful icebreakers for older couples, especially for those who are reluctant to discuss their lack of sexual intimacy, Martin says.

"If you're watching television together and a sex scene occurs, you might say to your spouse, 'Gee, that looks like fun. Would you like to try that?' or 'You know, if you touched me like that, I would love it.' You might be surprised by how a simple suggestion like this can spark communication and re-ignite your passion for each other," Martin says.

Rediscover romance. Remind your spouse of your love, Dr. Hamilton says. Read a poem, write a love letter, take a moonlit walk, scatter rose petals on the bed. Little romantic gestures can have a big impact on sexual desire.

"My husband always brought me my breakfast in bed and, very often, on the tray there was a love letter, a flower, a pretty seashell, or something else that he thought was delightful," Dr. Hamilton says. "It was those kinds of things that made me desire him all the more."

Give birth. Plant a garden, build a piece of furniture, make a loaf of bread, paint a landscape, write a novel, or get involved in some other creative activity. It may help rev up your love life, Dr. Hamilton says.

"There is no doubt that creativity and sex are teammates on the vital side of living," Dr. Hamilton says. "Having someone admire something you've done really warms your heart and soul."

MANAGING YOUR MEDS

Medications used to treat high blood pressure, including diuretics such as hydrochlorothiazide (HydroDIURIL) and beta-blockers like timolol (Timoptic), commonly decrease sex drive, says W. Steven Pray, Ph.D., R.Ph., professor of nonprescription drug products at Southwestern Oklahoma State University in Weatherford. In some cases, estrogens such as estradiol (Estraderm) used in hormone replacement therapy also can lower libido. And there are dozens of other medications that also can crimp your sexual desire, including:

- Antidepressants such as imipramine (Tofranil)
- Haloperidol (Haldol) and other drugs that relieve anxiety and agitation
- Allopurinol (Zyloprim) and similar drugs used to treat gout

If your sex drive plunges shortly after you begin taking a medication, consult with your physician. Cutting back on or substituting certain medications often can alleviate the problem. But never stop or reduce your dosage of any drug without your doctor's permission, Dr. Pray warns.

Help Mother Nature with some lubrication. Since vaginal dryness is predictable among older women, you probably need some help with lubrication during sex, Dr. Semmens explains. Use a water-soluble lubricant such as Astroglide, K-Y Jelly, or Lubrin to relieve vaginal dryness and pain.

If there's pain, explain. Your spouse can't intuitively know what's painful for you, so you need to tell each other if something makes you uncomfortable. Be sensitive to your partner's physical limitations, Dr. Semmens says. Maybe a sexual position that you used to enjoy is now painful for one of you. If so, experiment and find new sexual positions, Dr. Semmens urges.

If necessary, use pillows to support and protect joints while making love. If the man has arthritis, for instance, the woman should sit astride him or lie beside him, supported by pillows. If the man is on top and the woman has arthritis, he should support his weight with his hands and knees, Dr. Semmens suggests. These simple changes can bring pleasure back into your sex life.

Clean up your act. Poor personal hygiene can make sex less appealing, Dr. Semmens says. Bathe, wash your hair, and brush your teeth or clean your dentures, and your spouse will likely be more receptive to your advances.

LYME DISEASE

E arly in the twentieth century, the picturesque countryside surrounding Old Lyme, Connecticut, was, as one artist put it, a landscape waiting to be painted.

Today, much of the landscape is still pastoral, but within this alluring scenery lurks an insidious danger unheard of when Old Lyme was a turn-of-the-century art mecca. The trouble was recognized in the early 1970s, when a group of children in Old Lyme who lived near wooded areas developed puzzling arthritis-like symptoms. It took researchers seven years and the dissection of thousands of minuscule prime suspects to unravel the mystery. But when they did, the town earned a dubious distinction. It became notorious for being the site of the first outbreak of Lyme disease, a serious infectious condition spread to humans by deer ticks.

Although southern Connecticut still has the highest incidence of Lyme disease in the United States, more than 99,000 cases of the ailment have been reported nationwide since 1982, making it the most common tick-borne disease in the country, according to the Centers for Disease Control. The disease is caused by a bacterial infection that is spread by the bite of infected deer ticks, tiny reddish-brown eight-legged bugs that can be no bigger than a poppy seed. The more time you spend outdoors in the wooded, brushy, and grassy areas that these ticks prefer, the greater your risk of contracting the disease, says Edwin J. Masters, M.D., primary-care physician and Lyme disease expert in Cape Giardeau, Missouri.

Typically, in its initial stages, Lyme disease looks an awful lot like the flu, causing chills, fatigue, muscle and joint pain, fever, and headache. About 60 to 80 percent of people also develop a red, round rash around the bite within 30 days. The center of this rash can become clear as it gets larger and can begin to resemble a bull's-eye.

If detected early, Lyme disease can be cured with antibiotics. If

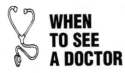

WHEN TO SEE A DOCTOR

If you develop symptoms of Lyme disease, it is important to seek treatment as soon as possible, to prevent any serious complications. Even though you may not remember being bitten, see a doctor if you have one or more of the following symptoms within 30 days of being in a tick-infested area.

• You develop a red circular skin rash that resembles a bull's-eye.
• You have chills and fever.
• You feel unusually fatigued.
• You have headaches or a stiff neck.
• You develop muscle and joint pain.

untreated, the disease can lead to a multitude of severe complications, including arthritis, memory loss, walking difficulties, high blood pressure, and heart problems. Although seniors are at no greater risk of getting Lyme disease than other age groups, they tend to get sicker when they do get it, says Anthony L. Lionetti, M.D., an internist in Hammonton, New Jersey, and a medical consultant to the Lyme Disease Foundation in Hartford, Connecticut.

Here are a few ways you can protect yourself from Lyme and other tick-borne diseases.

Try This First

Be fashion conscious. When you are walking in tick-infested areas, wear light-colored clothing. It will make it easier for you to spot any ticks, Dr. Lionetti says. Wear a hat, a long-sleeved shirt, and long pants. Tuck your shirt into your pants and your pant legs into your socks so ticks can't crawl under your clothing. Wearing calf-high rubber boots also may discourage ticks from latching on to you.

Other Wise Ways

Eliminate the loading zones. While properly clothed and wearing gloves, clear brush, cut tall grass, and remove leaves around your house and at the edge of gardens, Dr. Lionetti urges. Ticks lurk in these shady, moist areas, waiting to attach themselves to anything that happens to brush by. So if you eliminate the unkempt places in your yard, you'll greatly lessen the chance that you'll be a tick's next meal.

Take a detour. If you can, avoid walking through grassy, wooded, or marshy areas, especially during May, June, and July when ticks are the most active, Dr. Masters says. A short stroll in a meadow or even on shaggy roadside grass can increase your risk of getting bitten. If you must go through a tick-prone area, walk in the middle of well-established trails so you'll be less likely to brush up against vegetation.

Give clothing a good scrubbing. Wash your clothes in hot soapy water and dry them in a hot dryer immediately after you finish any outdoor activity, Dr. Lionetti says. The heat will kill any ticks hidden in your shirt sleeves, socks, or pants before they have a second chance to bite you.

Give yourself a once-over. Do a complete body check immediately after gardening, walking, or other outdoor activities in tick-infested areas, Dr. Lionetti says. Disrobe, and be sure to check your hairline, ears, behind your knees, armpits, and groin areas, where ticks like to hide. Give your pets a thorough once-over as well.

Evict them. If you find a tick attached to your body, remove it immediately, Dr. Lionetti says. It can take up to 24 hours of feeding for an infected tick to transmit enough bacteria into your system to cause Lyme disease. So prompt removal can prevent you from becoming sick. Here's how to safely get a tick off your body.

• Grasp the tick with a pair of tweezers as close as possible to its mouth (the part that is imbedded in your skin).

• Pull straight back with a slow, steady force. Avoid jerking.

• Avoid crushing or squeezing the tick. When it is squeezed, a tick acts like a tiny syringe, injecting a dose of bacteria into your bloodstream.

• After removing the tick, wash the bite with warm soap and water to disinfect it.

• Place the removed tick into a small tightly sealed container. If symptoms develop during the next 30 days, take the tick with you when you see your doctor. The tick may help your doctor identify the problem.

MACULAR DEGENERATION

About one in four Americans over age 65 and one in three over age 75 will get macular degeneration, the most common cause of vision loss in people over the age of 65, according to the Association for Macular Disease in New York City.

The disease is caused by a breakdown of the macula, a dot-sized part of the retina that allows a person to read, thread a needle, and see other fine details clearly, says Anne Sumers, M.D., ophthalmologist in Ridgewood, New Jersey, and a spokesperson for the American Academy of Ophthalmology. When the macula doesn't work properly, it causes blurriness or darkness in the center of vision.

Macular degeneration may be linked to aging, since it most often strikes in later life. But what really triggers this malfunction is still a mystery, Dr. Sumers says. Some of the suspects include diabetes, family history, atherosclerosis (hardening of the arteries), and ultraviolet light.

There is no cure for macular degeneration. In a few instances, laser surgery can prevent progression of the disease, but it can't restore vision that has already been lost, Dr. Sumers says. Because side vision is usually not affected, people often can continue many of their favorite activities by using low-vision aids such magnifying glasses.

"Many people with macular degeneration have functional vision for many years, which enables them to see well enough to complete household tasks such as cooking and laundry but may not allow them to read regular print in a newspaper. They might even continue to drive with their doctor's approval," Dr. Sumers says. "It is not necessarily a sentence of blindness. People should not get depressed when they get the diagnosis. There are lots of things you can do to continue living a full and active life despite this disease."

Try This First

Gaze in the shade. Avoid direct sunlight exposure, which places an additional strain on the retina and damages the light receptors in the eye, says James G. Ravin, M.D., author of *The Eye of the Artist* and a clinical associate professor of ophthalmology at the Medical College of Ohio in Toledo. When you're outside, wear a pair of sunglasses that filters out ultraviolet (UV) rays. "Try to avoid exposure between 10:00 A.M. and 2:00 P.M., when the UV rays are most intense. The closer you live to the equator, the more you need to protect your eyes."

Other Wise Ways

Reach for Popeye's favorite dish. Eat five to nine servings of fruits and vegetables daily, including at least one serving of dark green leafy vegetables, says Dr. Sumers. Dark green vegetables, particularly spinach, are the ideal food for the eyes, she says, because they contain an array of nutrients, including zinc, beta-carotene, and magnesium, that may improve blood flow to the eye and protect the retina from the worst effects of macular degeneration.

Normal chemical reactions caused by the effect of light on the macula may activate oxygen and cause macular damage over time.

MANAGING YOUR MEDS

Antimalarial drugs such as chloroquine (Plaquenil), which are also used to treat lupus and rheumatoid arthritis, can spark chloroquine retinopathy, a condition that has many of the same symptoms as macular degeneration, says Samuel L. Pallin, M.D., ophthalmologist and medical director of the Lear Eye Clinic in Sun City, Arizona. The difference is that chloroquine retinopathy is reversible, while macular degeneration is not. If you are on one of these drugs and develop signs of macular degeneration, consult your doctor. In most cases, once you stop taking the offending medication, the symptoms will disappear and your vision will return to normal.

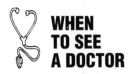

WHEN TO SEE A DOCTOR

See your doctor immediately if:

• You notice irregular patches of dimness in your vision.

• You have a sudden loss of vision, even if fleeting.

• You have trouble reading or words appear blurred on a page.

• You notice a dark or empty area in the center of your vision.

All are possible symptoms of macular degeneration and need to be checked out right away.

Some vitamins and minerals like beta-carotene function as antioxidants, chemicals that work against this activated oxygen, and perhaps protect the macula from damage. In addition, zinc, one of the most common trace minerals in your body, is highly concentrated in the eye, particularly in the retina and tissues surrounding the macula.

"There's a reason why Popeye always says, 'I'm strong to the finich 'cause I eats me spinach,'" says Stuart P. Richer, O.D., Ph.D., chief optometrist at the Department of Veteran Affairs Medical Center in North Chicago. "Dark green leafy vegetables are very important to the overall health of your eyes. I tell my patients to eat the equivalent of 2½ to 5 ounces (one-half to one cup) of frozen spinach a day." That's the same as one-quarter to one-half of a 10-ounce box. For variety, he suggests trying collard greens, kale, or romaine lettuce.

Bigger is better. Large-print books and playing cards, television remote controls with large readable buttons, and other over-sized products can help you continue doing activities you enjoy, Dr. Sumers says. Some companies even sell telephones with large numbers and extra-large wall clocks and calculators. Ask your ophthalmologist if these products are available in your area, or for a catalog of items designed to make life a little easier for people of low vision, write to Lighthouse International, a nonprofit agency for people who have partial sight or are blind, at 111 East 59th Street, New York, NY 10022. The catalog is available in large-print, braille, and audiotape versions.

Zoom in. A high-quality magnifying glass is a must if you want to read, says Charles R.

Fox, O.D., director of vision rehabilitation at the University of Maryland School of Medicine in Baltimore. You don't have to purchase it from a vision rehabilitation center or mail-order service; buy it at Brookstone, the Nature Store, or another gizmo and gadget store. It can be just as good as one you would get from a low-vision center and often will be cheaper, he notes. To make sure that you get a high-quality magnifier, put the magnifier flat on a piece of lined paper and raise it up until the lines look bigger. It helps to use just one eye for this. The lines should look bigger, but just as sharp. Make sure that there are no distortions, no waves, and no breaks.

Cozy up to your TV. If you have trouble watching television because of macular degeneration, try sitting as close as you can to the set, Dr. Fox suggests. "If the television is far away from you, the black hole in the center of your vision may cover the whole screen. Bring the television closer and closer, and the black hole covers less and less of the screen. So if it helps to sit three feet away from the television, do it."

Light up your life. Switch to 100-watt soft lightbulbs. They will brighten your living space and cut down on glare, Dr. Fox says. Make sure that your lamps or light fixtures can handle the additional wattage. Many have a maximum safe rating of 60 watts, which is usually labeled on the lamp, near the socket that holds the bulb. Get a goosenecked or swing-arm adjustable lamp from a home center or office supply store so you can shine the light directly onto the material you are reading.

Listen to passenger protests. You may feel offended if friends and relatives are reluctant to ride along when you drive. But don't ignore their protests, particularly if their warnings are repeated on a regular basis. Macular degeneration erodes sight slowly, so you may not be aware that your driving skills are impaired because your vision betrays you at times. Consider their concerns about your safety to be a warning sign that it may be time to relinquish the car keys and let someone else slip behind the wheel, Dr. Ravin says.

Weed out cigs before they blindside you. Snuff the smokes, urges Dr. Sumers. People with macular degeneration who continue to smoke are three times more likely to go blind than those who quit, she says. Over-the-counter nicotine patches and gums can help you kick the habit and retain your usable sight.

MEMORY LOSS

Elvis lives. Sasquatch roams the forest. Aliens have landed. Yes, modern myths abound. But few are as pervasive or damaging as the misconceptions about aging and memory. Just take a gander at these tall tales.

- You lose 10,000 brain cells a day, and one day you just run out.
- Your memory gets worse as you get older, and you can't do anything about it.
- Forgetfulness is a sign that something is wrong with your brain.

Not one of these statements is true, yet thousands of people over 60 continue to believe them, says Barry Gordon, M.D., Ph.D., behavioral neurologist at Johns Hopkins University School of Medicine in Baltimore and author of *Memory: Remembering and Forgetting in Everyday Life*.

"These myths about memory give people over 60 a fatalistic attitude about these problems that is often quite harmful to self-esteem." Dr. Gordon says. "While it is true that many people will have a worsening of memory with age, it is also true that some of these problems are reversible. They can be helped with a few simple coping strategies."

If a person has a mild memory loss, it doesn't necessarily mean his brain is rotting, says Dr. Gordon. It could be a simple problem that is easy to remedy. Here's a look at few simple ways to sharpen your recall.

Try This First

Keep on listing. Regular mental exercise like memorizing names, shopping lists, and other important information is vital if you want to keep your memory sharp as you age, says Alan S. Brown, Ph.D., author of *How to Increase Your Memory Power* and professor of psychology at Southern Methodist University in Dallas.

"People in their sixties, seventies, and eighties tend not to practice using their memories as much as they did when they were younger," he says. "Many people in this age group, for instance, rely on lists, and that's a fine technique if it isn't overused. But if you become overly dependent on lists, that can actually diminish your ability to concentrate and recall."

So at least once a week, try making a mental rather than written list to help do your shopping, housecleaning, or daily errands. Memorizing these tasks is one of the best and simplest brain-stretching exercises you can do, according to Dr. Brown.

Other Wise Ways

Sweat it out. Aerobic exercises like brisk walking or swimming can improve memory 20 to 30 percent, Dr. Gordon says, although he recommends checking with a physician before beginning any exercise program.

Snooze and you won't lose. When you're tired, you'll have more trouble focusing your attention and your recall will suffer, says Janet Fogler, co-author of *Improving Your Memory* and clinical so-

MANAGING YOUR MEDS

Many over-the-counter sleeping pills and cold remedies like Benadryl and Tylenol PM contain diphenhydramine and other ingredients that can cause confusion and temporary memory loss. So avoid using them, warns Juergen Bludau, M.D., geriatrician and instructor at Harvard Medical School. Here are a few other drugs that commonly affect memory in older people.

- Alcohol
- High blood pressure medications like methyldopa (Aldomet) or propranolol (Inderal)
- Antidepressants like amitriptyline (Elavil)

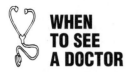

WHEN TO SEE A DOCTOR

See your doctor if you:

• Get lost while driving a familiar route

• Completely forget important appointments

• Tell the same stories over and over to the same person in a single conversation

• Have periods when you are confused about the time of day or where you are

• Are unable to manage simple finances (like balancing your checkbook) that you've always done with ease in the past

• Experience a personality change

• Have language difficulties like being unable to name an object

• Notice a sudden change in your artistic or musical abilities

All are possible early warning signs of Alzheimer's disease.

cial worker at Turner Geriatric Services at the University of Michigan Health System in Ann Arbor.

A good night's sleep also will help your brain process and store new information, Dr. Gordon says. Although most people get six to eight hours of sleep a night, the amount you might need will vary. Try to get enough sleep so that you feel well-rested when you wake up, he suggests.

Toss chaos. If you randomly scatter bills, car keys, and glasses around your home or office, you're going to have trouble finding them simply because you probably weren't paying attention when you set them aside, Fogler says. Designate a hook for your keys and always hang them there. Toss old magazines and newspapers at least once a week. Keep a wastebasket near where you sort through your mail, and throw away unwanted mail immediately, Fogler suggests.

Take a moment. Most of us have experienced at least one anxious instant when we couldn't remember if we fed the cat or turned off the iron. Usually, that's a sign that we were distracted. So always pause, take a deep breath, and relax before you dash out the door, says Danielle Lapp, author of *Don't Forget: Easy Exercises for a Better Memory* and memory training researcher at Stanford University. Take a moment to ask yourself some questions. Where am I going? What am I doing? What do I need? Have I forgotten anything important?

Talk the walk. Talking to yourself as you do a task can help focus your attention and make things easier to remember, Fogler says. As you straighten up your house, for instance, literally talk your way through the process. You could say, "I'm putting these old clothes in a white cardboard box marked with a red X. Now I'm carrying the box down to the basement. I'm placing the box on the floor behind the blue lounge chairs that we use on the patio during the summer." When you want to find the box, talk your way back through what you did, and you'll probably have no trouble finding it, she says.

Make the ordinary extraordinary. A good reminder can be unconventional or even weird, Fogler says. The next time you need to remember an errand, try placing a sock in the refrigerator. You can be sure the sight of that sock will jog your memory the next time you open the fridge.

Make the connection. It may take more effort to retrieve information as you get older, but don't give up, Lapp says. Try to organize your thinking. Keep your memory scanner in the area of the subject. If you can't think of a movie title, for example, keep talking about the movie. Name as many actors and actresses as you can. That may trigger the recollection you want, she says.

Catch a wave. Relaxation techniques like deep breathing can reduce stress and boost your ability to recall, Lapp says. To try it, sit comfortably, without tensing your muscles, and close your eyes. Let your arms and legs rest limply. Keep your mouth closed and inhale deeply and gradually through your nose until your lungs are full. Now exhale slowly, again through your nose, until all of the air is out.

As you continue breathing deeply, listen to the rhythm of air rushing in and then slowly seeping out. Notice how it sounds like waves crashing gently against the shore. Visualize the motion of the waves, their sound, and the smell of the sea breeze. Enjoy the sensations. Use this visualization technique as often as you can, particularly when you feel tense and are having difficulty remembering things, Lapp says. Try it while at work or while waiting in line. The visualization part of the exercise is enough to lessen anxiety when you have trouble remembering a piece of information.

MOBILITY PROBLEMS

Mobility is freedom. Each step is a declaration of independence. Each time you stand, you become a statue of liberty.

"Without mobility, your quality of life is greatly diminished," says Sandy O'Brien-Cousins, Ed.D., professor of exercise gerontology at the University of Alberta in Edmonton. Stiffness in your joints doesn't necessarily stop you in your tracks. But it definitely takes more energy to do things; eventually, you will have trouble getting around and may lose your independence.

"We're taught that it is okay to take it easy when you get older," says Wayne Phillips, Ph.D., professor of exercise science at Arizona State University in Tempe. "It's considered the reward for working hard throughout your life. But taking it easy after age 60 isn't a reward. It turns out to be a penalty. It causes much of the loss of mobility that we attribute to aging. You can reduce your risk of these problems if you just stay active. It truly is a matter of move-it-or-lose-it." Staying active helps you maintain all of the components—your muscles, bones, flexibility, and balance—that you need to remain mobile, he says.

"Studies have shown that people well into their nineties can improve their mobility. Some of these people were using walkers, canes, and wheelchairs. But when they added strength training and other activities to their daily lives, they were able to rehabilitate themselves and set these assistive devices aside," says Bryant Stamford, Ph.D., director of the health-promotion and wellness center at the University of Louisville in Kentucky.

Try This First

Be active. Look for ways that you can use more energy and become more active in your life, either by doing things a little faster or a little longer than normal, Dr. Phillips says. "You'll be doing your body a world of good."

For example, if you want to do things faster than normal and it usually takes you 20 minutes to vacuum your house or rake up leaves in your yard, try doing it in 15 minutes, he says.

If you want to use more energy by taking longer than normal to do things, look for ways in which you can break a single task into many. Instead of piling folded clothing on the stairs and letting it sit there until you can carry them up in one trip, take each piece up the stairs as you finish folding it. When you're putting away groceries after shopping, put each item on the table, then move each one to a counter, and finally put it where it belongs. If you garden, kneel down and stand up each time you dig up a weed. Painting the house? Go up and down the ladder more times than necessary.

Other Wise Ways

Be self-reliant. If you have difficulty doing a task, you should be doing it more, not less. So if a friend or relative offers to assist you

MANAGING YOUR MEDS

A cornucopia of over-the-counter and prescription drugs can make it harder for you to move about safely, says Helen Schilling, M.D., medical director of HealthSouth-Houston Rehabilitation Institute in Texas. So check with your doctor or pharmacist before taking any drug or drug combinations, she suggests. Be particularly cautious when you are using propoxyphene, acetaminophen, and other prescription pain relievers. These drugs can cause drowsiness and make you less sure-footed. In addition, be wary of:

- Alcohol
- Prescription antianxiety medications known as benzodiazepines (Valium, Xanax)
- Phenothiazines (Thorazine), which are used to treat nervous, mental, and emotional disorders
- Antihistamines, including diphenhydramine (Benadryl)

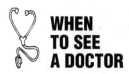

WHEN TO SEE A DOCTOR

Any mobility problem, including walking difficulties, should be evaluated by a physician because it could be a sign of a more serious, underlying condition, says Helen Schilling, M.D., medical director of HealthSouth-Houston Rehabilitation Institute in Texas. It is particularly important to see your doctor as soon as possible if:

• You have fallen.
• You have difficulty getting in to and out of chairs.
• You balance yourself on furniture and chairs in order to avoid falling.
• You are reluctant to go outside without someone to hold on to for balance.

in getting around, politely refuse, Dr. Stamford suggests.

"Too many people want to rescue older people from difficult situations. If a grandchild sees you struggling with something, she might say, 'Don't worry about carrying those groceries from the car, Grandma. I'll do it for you.' Don't let her do that to you. The only way you're going to get better at lifting and carrying things is to do it," Dr. Stamford says. "If you let others do too many things for you, you'll get weaker. As you get weaker, more things will be a challenge for you."

Take a hike. Walking is moving at its finest, according to Dr. Stamford. It works out all of your muscles and strengthens bones. The more you can do it, the better, he says. Even if you can only walk two to three minutes a day, you'll be moving in the right direction.

Try the bookworm workout. Get in the habit of carrying a box of books from room to room. It will help build the muscle strength you need to stay mobile, Dr. Stamford recommends. Put enough books in the box so that it weighs about as much as a sack of groceries. Every time you leave a room, lift the box from the bottom with two hands, making sure to keep your back straight. Hold the box close at chest level, with your elbows at a 90-degree angle.

Get out of that chair. Here's a mobility exercise that requires a firm chair with sturdy armrests. Have a seat. Grasp the armrests and push off with your arms and legs, rising to a standing position. Then slowly lower yourself to a sitting position.

Do this exercise at least twice each time you sit down, Dr. Stamford suggests.

Hit the floor. Lie with your back flat on the floor and try to get up any way you can. You'll work out virtually every muscle in your body, Dr. Stamford says. Do that three or four times a day.

"Most people turn over on their stomachs and do a pushup. It's a great exercise. You're using your hands and knees. You have to balance yourself," he says. "It's really one of my favorites."

Pump some creamed corn. Lift everyday household objects. You'll strengthen your upper body and promote mobility, Dr. Stamford says. Start with an object that you can comfortably lift 10 times, like an 18-ounce jar of peanut butter. Add one lift each day until you reach 25. Then try a slightly higher weight at 10 repetitions and repeat the cycle.

Relax and lengthen your muscles. Stretching can improve your flexibility and make getting around easier, Dr. O'Brien-Cousins says. Try doing the following stretches twice a day, she suggests. Hold each stretch for 15 to 20 seconds. These exercises are adapted from her book *Exercise, Aging, and Health: Overcoming Barriers to an Active Old Age*, which she co-authored with Art C. Burgess, Ph.D., former director of the campus fitness and lifestyle programs at the University of Alberta in Edmonton.

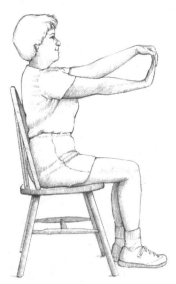

◄ WRIST STRETCH

Sitting on a sturdy chair with one arm straight out in front of you, pull the fingers of that hand toward you with your other hand until you can feel the stretch in your fingers and palm. Stretch your other hand the same way. Then repeat the exercise with each hand.

SHOULDER STRETCH ▶

Sit on the edge of a sturdy chair. Interlace your fingers behind your back with your palms facing away from your body. Bend forward at your waist, as far as you can, keeping your head above your hips with your eyes looking forward, not down at the ground. You'll feel the stretch in your shoulders.

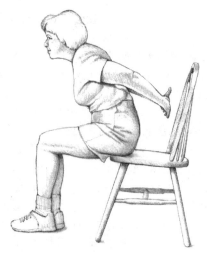

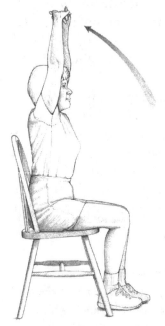

◀ UPPER-BODY STRETCH

Sit on a sturdy chair. Intertwine your fingers in front of you, palms facing outward, and stretch your arms straight forward until you can feel pressure in the back of your hands, wrists, and arms. Keeping your fingers intertwined, raise your arms above your head briefly. You'll feel the stretch in your upper back and shoulders.

CALF STRETCH ▶

Stand with your feet flat on the floor and your legs straight, a few feet away from a countertop or sturdy, immobile piece of furniture. Lean forward until your palms are resting against the edge of the furniture. Your toes should be facing directly forward, and your hips should also be pressing forward. Don't arch your back. You'll feel the stretch behind your lower legs at your calves.

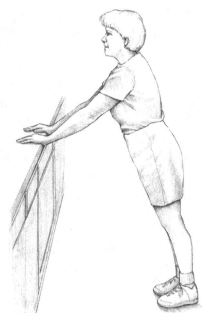

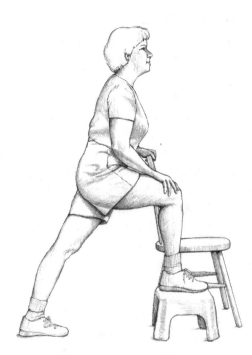

◄ HIP STRETCH

Stand to the side of a sturdy chair with one hand resting on the back of it for balance. Place one foot on a sturdy stool or low step. Step back with your other foot so that your feet are a few feet apart but not so much that you find it hard to keep your balance. Keep both feet facing forward while you shift your weight forward onto your bent knee. Place your other hand on your bent knee. Feel the stretch above your flexed knee, and at the front of your hip and in the calf area of your rear leg. Switch your position and repeat with the opposite leg bent.

SWING STRETCH ►

Stand a few feet away from a sturdy piece of furniture such as a hip-high desk. Rest your hands on the desktop for balance. Shift your weight to one foot, then gently swing your other leg backward 10 to 12 times until you feel more limber. Switch your position and repeat with the opposite leg.

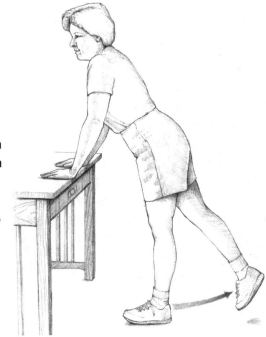

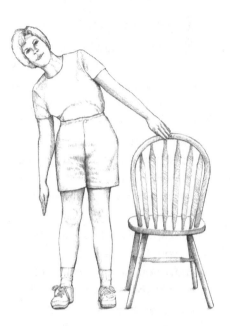

◄ TRUNK STRETCH

Stand tall with your feet shoulder-width apart, your feet flat on the floor, and your left hand resting on the back of a sturdy chair for balance. Slowly bend sideways to your right, sliding your right hand down your leg toward your knee. Try to keep your body aligned—don't lean forward or backward. Repeat with your other side. You should feel the stretch along the side of your trunk.

WARM-DOWN STRETCH ►

Stand with your feet shoulder-width apart, with your feet flat on the floor behind a sturdy chair. With your hands on the back of the chair for balance, slowly bend your knees, keeping your back straight and your feet flat. Lower yourself a few inches while you breathe out and relax. Then return slowly to the upright position and relax again. Repeat about five times.

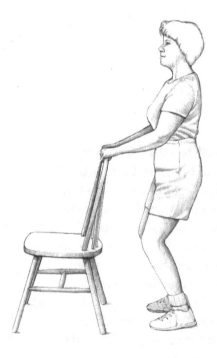

Morning Aches and Pains

Jack LaLanne doesn't feel your pain. "You gotta get up in the morning, count your blessings, and get moving. That's the key to living pain-free," he says.

"I don't even think about morning pain. I just get up and begin living. I kick my butt out of bed every morning, go work out for a couple of hours, and then just do what I have to do," says the octogenarian fitness guru. "Too many people dwell on their aches and pains. Well, don't dwell on them. Get up and do something about it. If you give in to your aches and pains, pretty soon you'll be a goner. Anything in life is possible if you make it happen. God helps those who help themselves. Help the most important person in this world—you!"

Okay, so it may be a lot easier for a real-life man of steel like Jack LaLanne to get going in the morning. And certainly Jack, who once swam 1½ miles while handcuffed, shackled, and towing 70 boats, is more gung ho than most people his age. But his message about being active every day, experts say, is right on target.

"An older person doesn't necessarily have to jump out of bed, dash to the gym, and do a workout every morning. But certainly, if you become more active in your daily life and have a positive attitude about what you are doing, you'll be less prone to joint pain and muscle stiffness," says Wayne Phillips, Ph.D., professor of exercise science at Arizona State University in Tempe.

Researchers aren't certain how prevalent morning stiffness is among older Americans. If you have it, it could be a sign of overactivity and injury or an underlying illness such as rheumatoid arthritis or other inflammatory conditions of muscles or joints. But in many cases, morning stiffness is merely a stern warning from your body that you may be, in fact, underusing your body in daily activities, says Maria A. Fiatarone Singh, M.D., associate professor

373

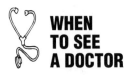

WHEN TO SEE A DOCTOR

Morning pain and stiffness that persist more than an hour after you awaken or that aren't relieved by over-the-counter pain medications like aceta-minophen should be brought to your doctor's attention, says Daniel Fechtner, M.D., assistant professor of rehabilitation medicine at Albert Einstein College of Medicine of Yeshiva University in New York City. In addition, seek medical care if:

• You have symmetrical pain in both hands or both feet.
• You have morning pain accompanied by feelings of fatigue or tiredness.
• You awaken with numbness or tingling that travels down your arms or legs.
• You have loss of appetite or unexplained weight loss.

of nutrition at Tufts University and a scientist at the Jean Mayer USDA Human Nutrition Research Center on Aging at Tufts in Boston.

In fact, the sedentary lifestyles that many seniors lead can provide an open invitation to morning aches and stiffness. As we age, many of us become less active. As a result, bones become more brittle, tendons lose flexibility, range of motion decreases, and muscles shrink and become weaker. These changes in the musculoskeletal system can make it difficult to do simple activities of daily living that require stretching, bending, or turning, making you feel like you are stiff all over at times. If your neighbor spends her days lounging by the pool instead of swimming in it, then sleeps on a worn-out mattress all night, you shouldn't be too surprised when she complains about aches and pains in the morning, says Dr. Singh.

Sometimes, simply taking a warm shower or having a massage can ease an occasional morning ache, she says. But if dawn's early light heralds the onset of persistent pains, you'll want to advise your doctor of this symptom. If nothing serious can be found after a medical examination, check out these remedies.

Try This First

Uncoil tight muscles. Stretching or flexibility exercises can reduce body pain and increase muscular relaxation, which can improve blood circulation, Dr. Phillips says.

Start your day with a gentle stretch in

bed. Raise your arms over your head as you curl your toes toward the footboard, Dr. Phillips suggests. Then, roll up on your side and sit on the edge of the bed, take a couple of deep breaths, and stretch your hands over your head again. For a more prolonged morning stretch routine that will do your joints, muscles, and bones a world of good, see "Waking Up Your Flex Life" on page 376.

Other Wise Ways

Get a bungee cord. Some seniors have difficulty doing stretches properly because it is hard for them to bend their arms or legs into certain positions. If you have this problem, try using a bungee cord, suggests Louis Sportelli, D.C., chiropractor in Palmerton, Pennsylvania, and former public affairs spokesperson for the American Chiropractic Association. These cheap elastic cords, available at most hardware stores, can make it easier for you to stretch without overtaxing your muscles and joints. You can also buy specially designed stretch cords for exercising, available at sporting goods stores, he says.

(continued on page 380)

MANAGING YOUR MEDS

If you consistently wake up feeling as if you've just fallen off an eight-story building, chances are, the pain medication you took at bedtime wore off long before dawn's early light, says W. Steven Pray, Ph.D., R.Ph., professor of nonprescription drug products at Southwestern Oklahoma State University in Weatherford.

"If someone, for instance, takes regular-strength ibuprofen or acetaminophen for arthritis pain, it's probably not going to last through the night," Dr. Pray says. "But a longer-acting anti-inflammatory drug like naproxen (Aleve), which you only need to take every 8 to 12 hours, should do the trick."

You also might ask your doctor if long-acting prescription pain relievers such as piroxicam (Feldene) or sulindac (Clinoril) might help, Dr. Pray says.

WAKING UP YOUR FLEX LIFE

The following rise-and-shine stretching routine was developed by Janie Clark, exercise physiologist and president of the American Senior Fitness Association in New Smyrna Beach, Florida, and was adapted from her book *Full Life Fitness: A Complete Exercise Program for Mature Adults.*

Doing this routine at least three times a day—morning, mid-afternoon, and just before bed—should help keep your muscles and joints limber and pain-free, adds Wayne Phillips, Ph.D., professor of exercise science at Arizona State University in Tempe.

These stretches can be done while seated in a sturdy, armless chair or while standing. If you have back problems, consult your physician before beginning new exercise activities. Although the following gentle stretch routine is especially designed to be easy on the back, not all positions are comfortable for everyone. If any stretch causes you pain, omit it from your routine. It will probably take most people about 10 minutes to complete the routine.

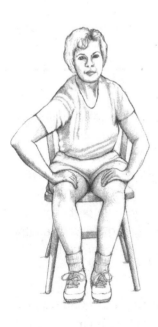

◄ SHOULDERS FORWARD

Bend at your hips and rest your hands on the fronts of your thighs in a comfortable position. Your fingers should be pointing toward each other. Press one shoulder gently forward toward your opposite knee. Hold for about 15 seconds then gently bring it back. Repeat with your other shoulder. Do three repetitions of this stretch, holding each shoulder forward for about 15 seconds. If desired, relax for a count of five between repetitions. You'll feel this stretch in the sides of your back.

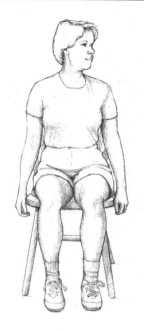

◄ HEAD TURN Gently and slowly turn your head to look to one side. Hold for three seconds before slowly turning to look to the other side. Turn toward each side twice. Relax for a few seconds between each stretch. You'll feel this stretch in your neck.

SHOULDER LIFTS ►

Slowly hunch your shoulders up toward the ceiling and hold for 15 seconds. Lower your shoulders back to their normal position and relax for a count of five. Do five repetitions. You'll feel this stretch in your upper and mid back.

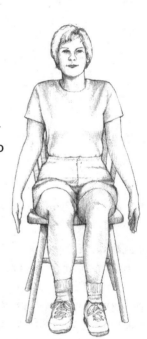

◄ BENT STRETCH

With your fingertips touching your head behind your ears, gently direct your elbows backward. Hold for 10 seconds, then repeat. If desired, relax for a count of five between repetitions. You'll feel this stretch in your chest.

WAKING UP YOUR FLEX LIFE—Continued

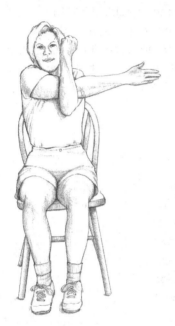

◄ STRETCH ACROSS

Stretch one arm across your chest. Place it in the bend of your opposite elbow. Hold for 15 seconds, then stretch your other arm. Do two repetitions with each arm. Avoid slumping or slouching. Think of yourself as "sitting tall in the saddle." If desired, relax for a count of five between repetitions. You'll feel this stretch in your upper arms and shoulders.

CAT CURL ►

Bend at your hips and rest your hands on the fronts of your thighs in a comfortable position, with your fingers pointing toward each other. Your knees should be bent, your feet separated for good balance, and your back straight. Round your back upward while contracting your buttocks and abdominal muscles. Hold for about 15 seconds, then return to the starting position. Do this stretch three times. If desired, relax for a count of five between repetitions. You'll feel this stretch in your mid and lower back.

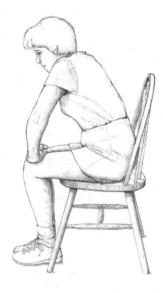

FORWARD STRETCH ▶

Slowly allow your upper body to bend forward from your hips as far as feels natural and comfortable. Hold for 15 seconds, then repeat. To make certain that your spine is properly supported at all times during this stretch, walk or slide your hands down your legs as you lower your body. As you relax into your stretch, rest your torso on your upper legs and place both hands on your ankles. As you rise, slide your hands up your legs. Relax in an upright position for a few seconds between stretches. You'll feel this stretch in your buttocks and lower back.

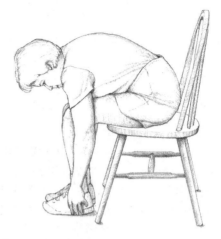

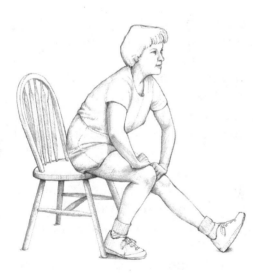

◀ HAMSTRING/ GLUTEAL STRETCH

With your hands on your thighs, extend one leg forward with your heel on the floor. Gradually bend forward at your hips until your body is at roughly a 45-degree angle. Hold for 15 seconds, then extend your other leg forward and repeat. You'll feel this stretch in your hamstrings at the back of your calves and buttocks.

To stretch your hip muscles, for instance, sit in a sturdy chair and make a loop with a bungee cord, interlocking the J-shaped metal loops around a chair leg. Slip your right foot into the circle formed by the bungee. Keeping your thigh flat on the chair seat, press your right foot against this restraint, moving your lower leg outward and away from your body until your leg is straight out and parallel with the ground. Hold for a count of 10, then return to the starting position.

Repeat this stretch five times, then switch to your left foot, Dr. Sportelli suggests. Try to do this exercise three times with each leg several times daily. People with arthritis of the knee or ankle, or with hip, knee, or ankle replacements, need to consult their doctors before beginning any exercise program.

To stretch your shoulders, attach the bungee cord to a doorknob and stand with your body perpendicular to and 6 to 18 inches from the door. Pull the cord across your body with your right hand. Hold the cord taut for a count of 10, then return to your starting position. Repeat this stretch five times, then switch to your left hand, Dr. Sportelli says. This exercise also should be done three times with each arm. People with arthritis of the shoulder or with shoulder replacements should check with their doctors before trying to do this exercise.

Rock on. Get a rocker, Dr. Sportelli says. Rocking in a chair helps increase circulation to your legs and may prevent muscle cramps in the morning. The rocking motion from the toe to the heel helps create a milking action that helps return blood to the heart. People who have blood clots should first check with their doctors.

Toss your pillow. If you consistently wake up with neck aches or headaches, your pillow may be the culprit, suggests Dr. Sportelli. If your pillow is too thick, your head and neck might be slightly flexed while you're sleeping. This position straightens your neck and pulls on the muscles and ligaments that support it, causing pain and often morning stiffness and headache. A thin pillow that you can curl under your neck so it supports both your head and neck is a better choice, according to Dr. Sportelli.

Bounce the bed. If your mattress is more than seven years old, consider getting a new one, advises Dr. Sportelli. Even if the covering still looks okay, the springs are probably worn out and not supporting your body as well as they should. So you're more susceptible to morning pain.

When you shop for a new mattress, look for one that has individually wrapped coil springs. It will provide better support than other mattresses, Dr.Sportelli says. It is important to also change your box spring when you change your mattress.

Stretch your imagination, too. Visualizations or imagery are alternative approaches that may help your mind and body work together to conquer morning pain, says Dennis Gersten, M.D., who practices psychiatry and metabolic medicine in the San Diego area and is the author of *Are You Getting Enlightened or Losing Your Mind?* and publisher of *Atlantis: The Online Imagery Newsletter*.

When you awaken, picture your morning pain as a ball that has a particular size, shape, color, and texture, Dr. Gersten says. It may be as small as a marble or as large as a basketball. Allow the ball to grow larger and larger. As it does, your morning pain may momentarily increase. Now let the ball shrink smaller than its original size, but don't let it disappear. As the intensity of the pain changes, allow the ball to change color, too.

Now imagine that the ball turns into a liquid that flows down your arm, drips on the floor, and reforms as a ball. Kick or throw the ball out into space. Watch it disappear. Most of your pain should dissipate as the ball soars off into infinity. Dr. Gersten suggests doing this imagery for 10 minutes twice a day—when you wake up and just before bed.

MOUTH SORES

For a long time, Janet Segall thought it was just another ordinary mouth sore. "There was this one particular spot on the right upper part of my gums that kept blistering and tearing. It hurt, but then it would go away. The doctor just said I should ease up on my brushing," says Segall, a Berkeley, California, woman in her fifties.

But within a year, she began developing blisters all over her body, including a renewed onslaught on the inside of her mouth. Eventually, she was diagnosed with pemphigus vulgaris, an obscure skin disorder that begins in the mouth and causes stinging wounds that will not heal.

"It's similar to a canker sore, except it lasts forever. It feels like you have first-degree burns all over your mouth, tongue, and throat," says Segall, founder and president of the National Pemphigus Foundation.

Although rare, affecting less than 1 percent of all Americans, pemphigus and two other ulcerative conditions—mucous membrane pemphigoid and lichen planus—become increasingly prevalent after age 50, says Michael Siegel, D.D.S., associate professor of oral medicine and diagnostic sciences at the University of Maryland School of Dentistry in Baltimore.

"These sores can be very severe. They can get to the point where they are extremely disabling. They can prevent people from eating, swallowing, or even talking. They're extremely painful and can get very large. They run from small spots about the size of a pencil eraser up to the size of a quarter in some people," says Brad Rodu, D.D.S., professor in the department of pathology at the University of Alabama School of Medicine in Birmingham.

Lichen planus, which can look like little interlocking threads of white lace on the cheeks, gums, and tongue, is usually considered a mere annoyance, says Grant J. Anhalt, M.D., acting chief of dermatology at Johns Hopkins University School of Medicine in

Baltimore. But severe cases of lichen planus, pemphigus, and pemphigoid can lead to oral cancer and other life-threatening complications.

Some researchers suspect that these conditions are triggered when, for some unknown reason, the body's immune system mistakenly begins attacking the cells in the mouth and skin, Dr. Rodu says.

Because lichen planus, pemphigus, and pemphigoid have similar symptoms, it is important to see a dentist or dermatologist for proper diagnosis and treatment, Dr. Anhalt says. For long-term relief, steroids, immunosuppressants, and other prescription drugs are the only effective answers. But even if you are on medication, the home remedies below may help you avoid intensifying these mouth rashes.

Try This First

Pamper your mouth. Avoid mouth rinses made with alcohol, and harsh toothpastes like products containing calcium pyrophosphate.

MANAGING YOUR MEDS

More than 30 prescription drugs can cause rashlike outbreaks in the mouth that mimic lichen planus, says Michael Siegel, D.D.S., associate professor of oral medicine and diagnostic sciences at the University of Maryland School of Dentistry in Baltimore. Among the prime offenders are:

- High blood pressure medications like thiazide diuretics such as chlorothiazide (Diuril) and hydrochlorothiazide (HydroDIURIL)
- Antibiotics such as tetracyclines (Vibramycin, Sumycin)
- Medications used to treat rheumatoid arthritis, such as auranofin (Ridaura), penicillamine (Cuprimine, Depen Titratable), and hydroxychloroquine (Plaquenil)

If you develop a mouth rash, take all of your medications, including any over-the-counter drugs, with you when you go to your physician or dentist. It will help him determine if your rash is drug-induced.

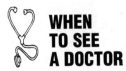

These ingredients will only aggravate your mouth rashes, Dr. Siegel says.

For brushing, use a soft toothbrush with a pinch of baking soda or a mild children's toothpaste like Kid's Crest, says Dr. Rodu.

Other Wise Ways

Rinse frequently. Mix a teaspoon of salt into a quart of water to create your own soothing mouthwash, Dr. Rodu suggests. Use as needed to relieve mouth rash discomfort.

Keep spices in the rack. Cinnamon, curry, and other zesty spices can aggravate mouth rashes, so it is best to avoid any foods made with these ingredients until your rash disappears, Dr. Rodu says.

MUSCLE SORENESS

You used to be able to run around all day and wake up the next morning without the faintest trace of muscle soreness. These days, however, overdoing it on the tennis court or even in the garden can cause some unpleasant consequences like sore muscles, a restricted range of motion, or general all-over achiness. These symptoms can make the exercise motto "No pain, no gain" seem like something best left for the grandkids.

But sore muscles actually have a bright side. If you weren't active, you wouldn't get them. It's perfectly normal, says William J. Evans, Ph.D., director of the nutrition, metabolism, and exercise laboratory at the University of Arkansas for Medical Sciences in Little Rock. But, he adds, your symptoms will be much worse if you've exercised too much too quickly.

Since there are so many health benefits to exercise, such as lowering cholesterol and helping to prevent bone and muscle loss, you don't want aches and pains to prevent you from keeping active. The trick is to make sure that exercise doesn't leave you groaning every time you move the day after. And for that, there are plenty of things you can do before, during, and after your workout.

Most of these suggestions apply to dull aches and pains experienced during or after a workout. If you're experiencing acute pain, that's a signal from your body that something is not right. See your doctor if you have sharp pains, says Dr. Evans. Don't try to exercise right through it.

Try This First

Have an ice day. You may be able to recover from muscle pain more quickly by icing the muscles that are complaining, says Dr. Evans. "Your muscles swell somewhat when you damage them from

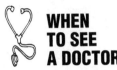

WHEN TO SEE A DOCTOR

Some muscle soreness is routine after a vigorous workout or overdoing it with a new activity, says William J. Evans, Ph.D., director of the nutrition, metabolism, and exercise laboratory at the University of Arkansas for Medical Sciences in Little Rock, but you should be concerned if the pain doesn't go away relatively quickly. "You should report any pain that persists for more than a week to your doctor."

You should also be concerned if the pain is acute, he says. If the pain is sharp or stabbing, you might have a muscle tear or joint injury. This is the sort of thing that can be quite painful and lead to further injury, says Dr. Evans, so you'll want to get checked out right away.

overuse. Ice can help to reduce the inflammation." Wrap a frozen ice pack in a thin towel and place it on the affected area for no more than 20 minutes each hour. You can repeat as often as necessary until the area is no longer sore. If an ice pack isn't handy, you can use a bag of frozen peas wrapped in a towel instead.

Other Wise Ways

Ask for acetaminophen. Other over-the-counter medications will probably reduce pain, but acetaminophen (Tylenol) is the best choice for muscle pain, says Dr. Evans. Why? Other possible painkillers on the pharmacy shelf—aspirin, ibuprofen, ketoprofen, and naproxen—all share a single drawback. These anti-inflammatory drugs block your body's production of chemicals that cause swelling and pain, but in so doing, they interfere with your body's muscle-repair process.

Acetaminophen, on the other hand, blocks pain impulses within the brain itself, allowing the muscle-repair process to proceed normally, says Dr. Evans. It's also the pain reliever that causes the least number of side effects when taken in normal amounts. Just make sure to follow the directions on the label, and never take more than 12 of the 325-milligram pills in a single day.

Turn up the heat. When the aches and pains are particularly bad the day after you've exercised hard, take a warm bath, says Priscilla Clarkson, Ph.D., professor and associate dean in the department of exercise science at the University of Massachusetts

School of Public Health and Health Sciences in Amherst. You can soak for as long as you like, she says. "The warm water helps your muscles relax and promotes circulation, which will have a soothing effect. The pain will come back 15 minutes or so after you get out, but it still makes for a nice break."

Rub it out. Massage can significantly reduce muscle soreness, and it's a safe alternative if you don't want to take over-the-counter medication. In addition, it may decrease levels of cortisol (the stress hormone) and increase production of serotonin, a compound produced in the brain that has a calming, pain-killing effect, says Maria Hernandez-Reif, Ph.D., director of the massage therapy research program and senior research associate at the University of Miami School of Medicine's Touch Research Institute. Here are some self-massage tips from Dr. Hernandez-Reif.

• Use a massage oil or lotion to make the experience a lot more pleasant. Put a little oil or lotion on the palm of your hand, then rub your hands together to warm it before beginning the massage. The heat helps loosen muscles more quickly.

MANAGING YOUR MEDS

Over-the-counter painkillers can have harmful interactions with some other medications, and they're not good for people with certain health conditions, says William J. Evans, Ph.D., director of the nutrition, metabolism, and exercise laboratory at the University of Arkansas for Medical Sciences in Little Rock. "Acetaminophen has fewer side effects than any other analgesic," he says, "but taken with alcohol, it can have a toxic effect on the liver." Other than that, acetaminophen has been shown to be remarkably safe, but it shouldn't be taken in doses higher than that recommended on the label.

Dr. Evans emphasizes that anti-inflammatory drugs such as aspirin, ibuprofen, ketoprofen (Orudis KT), or naproxen (Aleve) should be avoided since they interfere with muscle healing. But there are other reasons to avoid them as well. They can occasionally lead to stomach problems, says Dr. Evans, as well as complications with a bleeding condition, kidney disease, or liver disease.

• Don't skimp on the pressure. You'll know that you're not applying enough pressure if the rubdown feels like light tickling. Ideally, you should cause some muscle stimulation but not so much that you feel pain.

• Rub the right way. Cup your hand and glide it along the skin's surface. This is most effective when you can massage a large surface all at once, like the side of your leg from the ankle to the knee. "It's taught in massage therapy classes to rub in one direction toward the heart," says Dr. Hernandez-Reif.

Note: Never apply pressure to any joint area, says Dr. Hernandez-Reif. You might injure that joint.

Eat an orange after exercise. Vitamin C after heavy exercise may reduce day-after swelling and pain, reports Dr. Clarkson. When your muscles are damaged by overuse, she says, they produce free radicals, the wide-ranging, highly charged atoms that can damage tissue and age your cells. Antioxidants such as vitamin C may absorb the free radicals before they can cause too many problems, according to Dr. Clarkson. So make sure you're getting the Daily Value (60 milligrams a day) of vitamin C, she says. You'll find more than that amount in the average orange.

Distract yourself. Another simple way to handle muscle soreness is to just do your best to ignore it until it goes away, says Dr. Clarkson. "Unless you seriously overdid it, the pain will go away within three days." This means that every time you distract yourself with a favorite book or CD, or by taking the dog for a walk, you may return from that activity to find that the pain has diminished just a little bit more. (See a doctor if your pain lasts for more than a week.)

Start up slowly. The easiest way to avoid severe muscle pain after exercise is to start slowly any time you try a new activity, says Dr. Evans. Even if it's an activity you're used to, start slowly if you haven't done it in awhile, he adds. "Muscle soreness occurs primarily when you force your body to do something it's not accustomed to doing," he says. "If you know you're going to be playing tennis a week from now, do some jogging and light exercises a few days beforehand."

Keep your exercise on an even keel. The key is to keep yourself at a baseline level of fitness where an occasional game or weight-lifting session is no huge shock to your system. If you sit around all winter long and then throw yourself into a day's worth of heavy-duty gardening, you're just asking for trouble, notes Dr. Clarkson. Try to get 30 minutes of aerobic activity such as walking, jogging, or swimming at least three times a week.

Conditioning your body in this way should significantly reduce muscle pain after exercise, says Dr. Evans.

Follow the 10-percent rule. One of the best ways to not overexert yourself is to obey what's called the 10-percent rule, says Dr. Clarkson. Quite simply, it means that you never increase the difficulty of your workout more than 10 percent from week to week. "Because muscle pain usually hits 24 hours after exercising, it's easy to do a lot of damage to your muscles without realizing it at the time," she says. "This rule prevents you from doing that."

How does this translate into your regular exercise routine? Easily. For example, if you take 30-minute power walks three times a week, try to add three extra minutes, but go no further until you're used to the new time frame.

Get ready with a home stretch. When you stretch before exercising, you warm up your muscles, which may help prevent the tiny muscle tears that lead to morning-after pain, says Dr. Clarkson.

Before your next round of vigorous activity, perform this all-around stretching routine, suggests Barbara Sanders, Ph.D., chairperson of the physical therapy department at Southwest Texas State University in San Marcos. Keep in mind, these stretches should be slow and gradual, not bouncy. Don't try to complete any stretch that causes pain.

• Shoulder rolls. Stand straight with your head high, your chin in, and your arms at your sides. Rotate your shoulders up, back, down, then forward. Repeat five times.

• Side bends. Stand with your right arm above your head, your left arm across in front of your stomach, your knees bent slightly, and your feet about shoulder-width apart. Lean to the left as far as you comfortably can. Hold for five seconds, stand up straight again, then repeat. Now reverse the arm positions and follow the same process, leaning to the right.

• Hip stretch. Lie on your back with your lower back snugly resting against the floor. Keeping your left leg extended, clasp your right leg with your right hand under the knee and bring it to your chest, letting your knee bend double. Hold for five seconds, release your leg, straighten it, and lower it to the floor. Repeat once, then do the same stretch with your left leg and left hand.

• Hamstring stretch. Sit on the floor with your right leg relaxed and your right knee bent so that your foot is flat on the floor. Extend your left leg straight in front of you. Now reach for the toes of your left leg with the fingertips of both your hands, feeling the stretch in that hamstring (the long muscle on the back of your thigh). If you can't reach your toes, grab onto your ankles. Stretch for 20 seconds, relax, and then do it again. Now change the position to extend your right leg, and repeat the stretch.

• Calf and Achilles tendon stretch. Stand three to four feet from a wall and lean toward it, supporting yourself with your hands at roughly shoulder level on the wall. Bring your right leg forward, bending at the knee. As you lean forward, keep your left leg straight with your left foot flat on the floor, while pressing your right knee toward the wall until you feel a comfortable stretch in the straight left leg. (Don't arch your back.) Hold for 20 seconds, then repeat with your left leg forward with your knee bent, and your right leg extended behind.

• Shoulder stretch. Stand straight with your arms extending straight behind your lower back. Grab your left wrist with your right hand and slowly pull both arms back from your spine as far as possible without causing pain, all the time staying as upright as possible. Keep your neck straight, not arched. Maintain the stretch for a few seconds, relax, then repeat with your left hand grabbing your right wrist.

NAUSEA

Nausea is not a disease. From your body's point of view, it's not even a problem, really, but a safety mechanism. Nausea usually strikes as a kind of distress signal. If you swallow something that your digestive system doesn't like or that it even suspects is bad for you, it sends out an alarm through the complex system of nerves that connects your stomach to your brain.

If your body is experiencing other stresses like motion sickness, emotional distress, or even unpleasant sights or odors, your body may again use this distress signal to get your attention and register a problem. And it's an effective signal. Say what you want about nausea, but it's certainly hard to ignore.

If you've long suffered from problems like motion sickness or the nausea that sometimes accompanies migraine headaches, you're all too familiar with the conditions that may be your nemesis. But as you leave middle age behind, new causes can crop up.

For people over 60, medication is a common cause of nausea, says Robert Charm, M.D., gastroenterologist and internist in Walnut Creek, California, and professor of gastroenterology and internal medicine at the University of California, Davis. Sometimes, you may simply be sensitive to one type of medicine. Or a combination of different medicines may be interacting to make you ill.

Even if the cause isn't obvious, there are ways to spot the source of your nausea and ease that queasy feeling whenever it strikes—especially if it's caused by a motion that your body doesn't like.

Try This First

Take a break. Your tummy will feel calmer if you rest a bit when a wave of nausea hits. Put your feet up and sit a spell. If you're in a car, pull over, roll down the window, and get some air. While you're

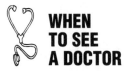

WHEN TO SEE A DOCTOR

If nausea is temporary, linked with a probable cause (like the flu), and home remedies have reduced the discomfort, then you're probably okay, says Martin Brotman, M.D., gastroenterologist at California Pacific Medical Center in San Francisco.

But persistent nausea lasting more than three days for no apparent reason should by checked by your doctor. It could be a sign of any one of a number of problems, including ulcers or problems of the gallbladder, liver, or pancreas, says Robert Charm, M.D., gastroenterologist and internist in Walnut Creek, California, and professor of gastroenterology and internal medicine at the University of California, Davis. "Nausea can also be the first sign of a heart attack."

resting, gaze out the window, says Roger L. Gebhard, M.D., gastroenterologist at the Veterans Affairs Medical Center and professor of medicine in the division of gastroenterology at the University of Minnesota, both in Minneapolis. "People with nausea often feel better if they can look outside and focus on the environment."

Other Wise Ways

Change your meal plan. In the midst of a nausea spell, don't eat anything. Wait a couple of hours in order to give your stomach time to settle, says Dr. Charm.

Give nausea the sip. If you have nausea, sip—don't gulp—some clear liquid. Flat soda, water, a fluid replacement drink like Gatorade, or some clear broth are all good choices. Take a sip once or twice every five minutes, suggests Dr. Charm. Hydration is especially important if you are also experiencing some vomiting, he says.

Snack a little. If the nausea has passed and you haven't eaten anything for a couple of hours, then it's okay to eat something light. Just be sure to make it a low-fat snack of plain foods. Spicy and fatty foods are hard to digest and can make a queasy stomach feel even worse. "Some white rice, toast, or crackers can help," says Martin Brotman, M.D., gastroenterologist at California Pacific Medical Center in San Francisco.

Swallow some relief. Pepto-Bismol, Mylanta, or other over-the-counter antacids can help calm an unsettled stomach.

For nausea linked with dizziness and motion sickness, take dimenhydrinate (Dramamine). But be aware that anti-motion sickness medicines won't do much good if the nausea is from a flu or something you ate, says Dr. Brotman.

Chew on some ginger. For a natural nausea reliever, chew candied crystallized ginger, which you can find in natural food stores or the spice aisle of your supermarket.

MANAGING YOUR MEDS

Nausea is one of the most common adverse reactions to medications. In some cases, the medication irritates the stomach. In others, it may affect the brain directly. Older adults do not tolerate these medications as well as when they were younger.

So many drugs can cause nausea that a comprehensive list could probably fill a good-size book on its own, according to W. Steven Pray, Ph.D., R.Ph., professor of nonprescription drug products at Southwestern Oklahoma State University in Weatherford. Even when limited to the most commonly prescribed drugs for seniors, the list can be exhaustive.

If you have excessive nausea or queasiness and you're taking any of these drugs, don't stop taking them, but do see your doctor, says Dr. Pray. Your doctor may recommend dosing instructions that will ease the discomfort, or he may prescribe a substitute. Just some of those drugs that cause nausea are:

- Antiangina drugs such as atenolol (Tenormin) and verapamil (Calan)
- Digoxin (Lanoxin), which is prescribed as a heart stimulant in congestive heart failure
- Estrogen (Premarin) prescribed for relief of hot flashes and night sweats that are sometimes experienced during menopause
- Drugs such as furosemide (Lasix) and thiazide diuretics such as hydrochlorothiazide (HydroDIURIL) that act as diuretics and treat mild cases of high blood pressure
- Lisinopril (Zestril) and metoprolol (Lopressor), which are prescribed to control high blood pressure
- Warfarin (Coumadin), a blood thinner that is prescribed to prevent clogged arteries

Or add some fresh ginger to your meals. "Grate the ginger into sauces or food, such as chicken," says Mike Cantwell, M.D., clinician and coordinator for clinical research at the Institute for Health and Healing at the California Pacific Medical Center in San Francisco. "You can also make ginger tea."

Shop for capsules or tinctures. Take one or two ginger capsules three times a day while the nausea lasts, advises Dr. Cantwell. Ginger in capsule form is at its most potent and may offer you a greater medicinal effect.

You can even mix yourself a ginger cocktail with some tincture of ginger, also found at the health food store. Stir 30 drops into a few ounces of water or juice three to four times a day, until the nausea goes away.

Stop the ills with ale. There may not be much, if any, ginger in the soft drink, but it may still help soothe your stomach. "Anything that's worked in the past or from childhood, like ginger ale, has the added benefit of being comforting and reassuring," says Amy Saltzman, M.D., internist at the Institute for Health and Healing at the California Pacific Medical Center in San Francisco.

Press here. If your nausea comes from motion sickness, you may be able to relieve it with an acupressure wrist band (Sea-Band), which is specially designed to apply pressure to a pressure point on the inner wrist that can actually help ease nausea. You'll find these bands in some drugstores and in the sporting goods area of some department stores.

NECK PAIN

Imagine a jelly doughnut that's been in the microwave oven too long. While still warm and gooey on the inside, it has lost some of its springy resilience. Now imagine a stack of these doughnuts supporting a 14-pound bowling ball on top. Doesn't sound like too promising a situation for the doughnuts or the bowling ball.

Your neck and head have been in that situation since adolescence. The human head weighs about the same as the bowling ball and—as we get up there in years—the row of supporting disks are much too much like jelly doughnuts. As people age, disks lose a lot of the fluid that gives them their strength and shock-absorbing ability, says Karen Rucker, M.D., professor in the department of physical medicine and rehabilitation at Virginia Commonwealth University in Richmond. That alone can make people over 60 more prone to stiff, crampy necks.

Couple this with increases in arthritis, osteoporosis, and poor posture, and it's no wonder that neck pain tends to increase as we get older.

Being gentle to your neck and following the rules of good posture go a long way toward lessening neck cricks, twinges, and stiffness. Try these doctors' recommendations.

Try This First

Give your neck a break. Whatever you're doing, whether it's sitting at a desk or working on a hobby, if you stay in one position for a long period of time, your neck can get stiff and pain can creep up on you. To prevent this, get a kitchen timer, says Mary Ann Keenan, M.D., director of neuro-orthopedics at Albert Einstein Medical Center in Philadelphia. Set it to go off every half-hour or so to remind you to stand up, do a little stretch, and take a little break.

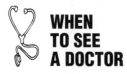

WHEN TO SEE A DOCTOR

If you have neck pain that persists even when you change position and that is also accompanied by any of the following complaints, be sure to call your doctor immediately, says Karen Rucker, M.D., professor in the department of physical medicine and rehabilitation at Virginia Commonwealth University in Richmond.

• Pain shooting down your arms or hands

• Numbness or tingling in your fingers or arms

• Sudden or significant muscle weakness, such as the inability to lift your legs or extend your arms

• Dizziness

• A feeling of pain when you move your jaw, which may be a sign of an abscess or infection

• Onset of fever with a new onset of neck pain and stiffness

Other Wise Ways

Get your neck stretched. If tension is causing your pain in the neck, you can relieve it with a little bit of stretching. "Just start by tilting your head from side to side, then rolling it around, first to the right and then to the left," Dr. Keenan says. Next, take your hand, put it on top of your head, and help the stretch by pulling your head gently halfway down toward your shoulder on each side. Be sure to perform these stretches with slow, smooth movements. "Any quick stretch is more likely to tear a muscle or ligament. You need to do it more gradually," Dr. Keenan warns.

Stand and sit up straight. "When you're not using good posture—specifically, you're slumping—all of a sudden your muscles are having to work hard to hold your head up," Dr. Rucker says. But you can take some of the workload off your neck. Whenever you're sitting or standing, make sure that your shoulders are over your hips and your ears are over your shoulders. Your head should never be tucked under, like a horse in a bridle.

"Think about the top of your head," Dr. Rucker advises. "Try to visualize the top of your head trying to touch the ceiling. You will lengthen, elongate your neck and get as tall as possible."

Get a chair with a better back. The old clerical chair had nothing more than a seat cushion and an oval pad that you could position somewhere in the middle of your back. If you're still using one of those, retire it in favor of a chair with a back that goes up to shoulder level. With the high-backed chair, your head, neck, and back are kept vertical, and you can lean your head back periodically to give your neck a chance to relax, says Don Chaffin, Ph.D., professor in the center for ergonomics at the University of Michigan in Ann Arbor.

Apply heat or cold. You can apply a hot-water bottle or an ice pack to relieve your neck pain, Dr. Keenan states. It's really your preference. "They both work the same way by increasing the circulation to the area."

Talk on a speakerphone. Wedging a phone in the crook between your tilted head and your shoulder can strain your neck. Even phones with headrests can cause pain, Dr. Keenan says. If you have long phone conversations, use a headset or speakerphone. You'll find both at electronics stores or office supply stores.

Buy an athletic bra. If you're a woman with a large bosom, you may not be getting enough support from your bra, and that can surely cause neck, back, and shoulder pain. Try an athletic or jogging bra, Dr. Keenan recommends, because they give more support and have wider straps. Athletic bras are designed to distribute weight more evenly.

Use a fanny pack. Carrying a weighty shoulder-strap purse can put strain on your neck, Dr. Keenan says. A better option would be to switch to a fanny pack, which fits around your waist and doesn't

MANAGING YOUR MEDS

It's not a common reaction, but some blood pressure medications like nifedipine (Procardia) and some anticholesterol medications such as cholestyramine (Questran) can cause muscle aches—including achiness in the neck area. More commonly, if you have stopped taking a sedative drug like diazepam (Valium) or sleep medications such as chlordiazepoxide (Librium) or temazepam (Restoril), you can have an achy neck. "The withdrawal aspect of those medicines will often cause increased pain and muscle tightness all over," says Karen Rucker, M.D., professor in the department of physical medicine and rehabilitation at Virginia Commonwealth University in Richmond. Take these medicines only with close physician supervision, she advises.

put any strain on your neck at all. You can change to a handheld purse for more dressy occasions.

Sleep with your neck in line. If you have an old pillow that has become droopy through years of use, throw it out, advises Dr. Keenan. It's time to get a good supportive pillow, she says. You want one that will keep your head in straight alignment with your mid back (the line from the center of your head down your back to the crease in your buttocks) and your spine when you lie on your back or side. Although pillows have firmness labels that can help, your best bet is to try them out before buying. Throw one on a bed display and lie down on it. Keep testing until you find the right one.

Set up your computer correctly. If you use or own a computer, make sure it's set up correctly, says Dr. Chaffin. Place the monitor at a distance that is comfortable for reading and at a level where your head is not bent forward or tilted back. Some experts suggest placing the monitor so you are looking at it straight ahead. The keyboard should be positioned so your elbows are at your sides, bent at about a 90-degree angle, with your wrists straight and level.

Favor the gradual movements. Quick, sharp movements can injure your neck or back. But often, we're reckless about our neck movements until we start to feel pain, notes Dr. Rucker. Treat your neck gingerly, she urges. When you get out of bed in the morning, roll gently onto your side first, rather than sitting bolt upright. And be careful when you're getting in and out of the car. Sit on the car seat first and then rotate your body, bringing your legs around and into the car. Reverse this process when you get out. "We should be using those techniques all the time" to minimize the daily damage that can lead to a big pain in the neck, says Dr. Rucker.

Neuroma

If you're a woman with sleek black heels in your closet, you may be tempted to put them on again—perhaps many times—if they look good with your outfits.

But maybe those shoes don't belong on your feet again. In fact, you may want to consider offering them for sale with your next batch of yard-sale items. Or, at least, relegate them to the back of the closet and trot them out only on special occasions.

Sometimes, shoes are saboteurs. They may be the very shoes that are causing or contributing to a painful foot ailment called Morton's neuroma, says Wilford K. Gibson, M.D., assistant professor of orthopaedics at Eastern Virginia Medical School in Norfolk.

If you've been wearing high heels or ill-fitting shoes for a long time, you may already be familiar with the symptoms, which afflict more women than men, Dr. Gibson says. Don't be surprised if you've had cramping, pain, numbness, tingling, or burning in your forefoot, often between the third and fourth toes. The reason is that those troublemaker shoes compress or squeeze the nerves between the toes, causing the nerves to swell.

Neuromas can occur between your other toes, too, says Donald G. Hovancsek, D.P.M., podiatrist in Olympia, Washington, and a spokesperson for the American Podiatric Medical Association.

Your chances of developing the condition increase with age, whether you are a man or a woman, Dr. Hovancsek says. That's because the fat pads on the bottoms of your feet become thinner as the years pass, leaving you less protected from knocks and bumps. Also, your Achilles tendon, which attaches to your heel, often shortens over the years, putting more daily pressure on the front of your foot, which can also cause neuroma pain, he says. Water retention or other causes of swelling, such as arthritis, can also put pressure on the nerves in the foot.

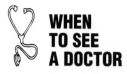

WHEN TO SEE A DOCTOR

If numbness, burning, or pain in your feet and toes becomes unbearable, don't suffer—talk to your doctor, advises Donald G. Hovancsek, D.P.M., podiatrist in Olympia, Washington, and a spokesperson for the American Podiatric Medical Association.

Symptoms may come and go depending on your activities and choice of footwear, Dr. Gibson says. But those symptoms are more likely to linger and scar the nerves if you just limp along and ignore them. Some people require physical therapy, steroid injections, or even surgery if the neuroma is allowed to get its way. So check out the following simple tips for preventing or easing Morton's neuroma. And then take a peek in that closet.

Try This First

If the shoe doesn't fit, don't wear it. In most cases, symptoms will subside when you change your shoe, Dr. Gibson says. "Go for comfort over looks for daily wear." Choose a shoe with a well-cushioned sole and heel, wide toe, and sturdy arch. A lace-up provides more support than a slip-on, he says.

Consider wearing an athletic shoe, something with a woven leather toe, or a thick-soled earthy-style walking sandal, Dr. Hovancsek says.

Other Wise Ways

Try stretching. If you're developing a neuroma or have a neuroma with numbness and tingling but not too much pain, these three simple stretches, each performed for a minute or so several times a day, can help, Dr. Hovancsek says. If done correctly, you should feel a stretch in your Achilles and leg muscles.

• While holding on to a sturdy railing, stand with your toes and the balls of your feet on a bottom step (never a higher one), with your heels over the edge. Slowly rise on your toes and then descend until your heels are below the step.

• When you're in your kitchen after washing dishes, take a couple of steps back from your work, dry your hands, and then lean forward while holding on to the sink. Bend one knee, raising your heel off the floor, and then the other, and continue in a peddling motion. Keep your head up, looking toward the window or wall.

• For an exercise that's more challenging, sit on a straight-back chair. Raise one leg until your thigh is not supported by the chair and your knee is locked. With your toes pointed toward the ceiling, move your foot in a circle, as if your big toe were a hand on a clock.

Revive your routine. If you have pain during exercises like running or walking, shorten or change your activities until your discomfort subsides, Dr. Gibson says. But don't use the pain as an excuse to stop exercising. Switch to swimming or bicycling. When you return to walking or running, stay off hard surfaces, which can aggravate pain.

Do a shoe survey. Make sure your athletic shoes aren't the cause of your discomfort, Dr. Gibson says. Don't wear thin-soled shoes when walking or jogging, even if symptoms subside when you stop or remove your shoes.

Choose looser legwear. Tight-fitting or support hosiery can worsen pain in a foot that's already been tortured by being stuffed in an ill-fitting shoe, says Dr. Gibson. Wear appropriately sized socks with athletic shoes.

MANAGING YOUR MEDS

Ergot alkaloids such as ergotamine (Cafergot), which are used to treat migraine and cluster headaches, can cause side effects such as numbness or tingling in the toes and weakness in the legs, says W. Steven Pray, Ph.D., R.Ph., professor of nonprescription drug products at Southwestern Oklahoma State University in Weatherford. If these symptoms last for more than one hour, check with your doctor.

Turn to the bottle. Over-the-counter medicines can be helpful. If your doctor says it's okay, try ibuprofen, enteric-coated aspirin, or acetaminophen for temporary pain relief and swelling, Dr. Hovancsek says.

Go for the chill of it. Apply an ice pack wrapped in cloth to your foot for up to 20 minutes at a time. This may reduce pain and swelling, especially if it's related to activity, Dr. Gibson says. But be careful, especially if you have numbness, he warns. Some serious medical conditions, such as diabetes, may cause loss of feeling in the feet.

For a convenient ice pack that molds to your foot, freeze a bag of unpopped popcorn and place it on the affected area, Dr. Hovancsek says. Elevating your foot may also help reduce swelling.

Lighten up. Your painful foot is going to be a lot more uncomfortable if you are carrying more weight than you need to, Dr. Gibson says. As your foot strikes the ground when you walk, it carries the full weight of your body. If you run or jump, the burden can be four or five times your body weight. And since your little toes aren't made to endure that kind of force, you'll need to lose a few pounds to give them a holiday.

Examine your soles. Every six months, look closely at your shoes for signs of wear, especially in the soles. Worn-down soles or uneven wear might be inviting neuroma. "It may be time for a new shoe," Dr. Gibson says.

Shoe shop toward dusk. When buying shoes, shop at the end of the day, when your foot is larger. "Your foot tends to swell with activity," Dr. Gibson says. Also, take along the socks or hosiery that you'll wear with the shoe to make sure that you have a good fit. And be sure to try on both shoes since one of your feet may be larger than the other.

Put your foot in the other shoe. Don't wear the same pair of shoes every day. Instead, alternate your favorites with others in your closet, Dr. Gibson says. Not only will your shoes last longer, but you'll be giving your feet a welcome break.

Night Vision Problems

Blinded by an explosion, Charles McNider believed that his promising career as a physician and researcher had been hopelessly derailed. Then one evening as he sat alone in his darkened living room, an owl crashed through a window. McNider tore off his bandages and found that he could see in the dark!

Soon he transformed himself into Dr. Mid-nite, a 1940s comic book hero who wore special goggles to see in the light. Armed with blackout bombs that released a pitch-black cloud in which only he could see, Dr. Mid-nite battled evil foes like the Baleful Banshee and the Sky-Raider. "I am blind, yet I can see," Dr. Mid-nite declared. "The city is draped in night, but to me it is always day. There are no dark corners for evil to hide in, no shadows too deep for the ever-vigilant eyes of Dr. Mid-nite to penetrate!"

But in the real world, midnight is hardly prime time for aging eyes. "There are plenty of reasons why virtually every 20-year-old wants to go on a road trip at night and virtually every 60-year-old doesn't," says Anne Sumers, M.D., ophthalmologist in Ridgewood, New Jersey, and a spokesperson for the American Academy of Ophthalmology. "First, as you age, your eyes need more light to work properly. Second, the lenses in your eyes aren't as clear at 60 as they were at 20. Third, as you get older, your pupils don't dilate as well as they used to. And in order to see well at night, your pupils have to get very large. So the overall result is that you have a lot more difficulty focusing on objects and seeing at night as you age."

While none of us will ever match the nocturnal prowess of the fictional Dr. Mid-nite, there are plenty of simple ways to bolster your night vision even at 60, 70, or 80. Here's how.

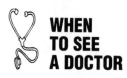

Try This First

Lighten up. The average 60-year-old person needs seven times as much light as a 20-year-old to see well in the dark, according to the American Optometric Association. So brighten up the rooms of your home with 60- or 100-watt neodymium lightbulbs, suggests Bruce Rosenthal, O.D., chief of low-vision programs at Lighthouse International, a vision rehabilitation organization in New York City. These bulbs provide higher contrast and produce less glare than regular lightbulbs, so you should be able to see better at night. Neodymium bulbs are available at specialty lighting stores and from some mail-order catalog companies.

For walking in the dark, try using a portable camping lamp to illuminate where you are stepping, says Charles R. Fox, O.D., Ph.D., director of vision rehabilitation at the University of Maryland School of Medicine in Baltimore. Camping lamps, which are available at most sporting goods stores, are better than flashlights because they provide a wider arc of light and make it easier for you to get around, he says.

Other Wise Ways

Bend and tilt. Adjustable floor or table lamps that swivel and bend so you can fine-tune the lighting to your needs can help overcome night vision problems, Dr. Rosenthal says.

If you are reading, for instance, adjust the lamp so that it's about 12 inches from the page yet not causing an annoying glare, Dr. Rosenthal suggests. Look for lamps with built-in reflectors that will help increase illumination.

See yourself seeing well. Imagery may help improve your night vision, says Robert-Michael Kaplan, O.D., author of *The Power behind Your Eyes*. Twice a day when natural light is dim—within two hours of sunrise and two hours of sunset—take a moment to close your eyes and move your head slowly to the left and then to the right. As you do this, take 5 to 10 deep breaths and visualize beams of light streaming into your eyes and activating the portions of your vision that are responsible for seeing well at night. This exercise can be done in less than two minutes a day.

Ease off the gas pedal. Many night vision problems aren't obvious until you get behind the wheel, says Gary Mancil, O.D., adjunct professor at Southern College of Optometry in Memphis.

On low beam, for instance, your headlights illuminate about 100 feet in front of your vehicle, says Steve Creel, California

MANAGING YOUR MEDS

Pilocarpine (Isopto Carpine, Pilocar), beta-adrenergic blocking agents (Betagan), and other medications used to treat glaucoma can cause temporary night vision problems for up to four hours after use, says W. Steven Pray, Ph.D., R.Ph., professor of nonprescription drug products at Southwestern Oklahoma State University in Weatherford. If this dimming of vision is bothersome, ask your doctor if you can switch to another medication that might not cause this side effect. Other drugs that can affect night vision include:

- Nasal and eyedrop steroids such as beclomethasone (Vancenase)
- Antidepressants containing trazodone (Desyrel), imipramine (Tofranil), or amitriptyline (Elavil)
- Antihistamines including over-the-counter products like doxylamine (Nyquil), diphenhydramine (Benadryl), and chlorpheniramine (Chlor-Trimeton)

Highway Patrol public affairs officer. And at 65 mph, you're traveling about 100 feet per second. So at that speed, even if you had perfect vision and were driving in perfect conditions, your headlights wouldn't be much help. That's why it's important to slow down at night, particularly in poor weather. As a self-check, pick out an object in the distance and begin counting until you reach the object. A four- to six-second count is an indication that you are driving at a safe speed. If you reach that point in less than two seconds, you would not have been able to stop safely if that sign were in the middle of the road, Creel says. So ease up on the throttle.

"Just because the speed limit is 55 or 65 doesn't mean you have to go that fast. That might not be the safe speed for you, particularly if you have trouble seeing at night," Creel says.

See and be seen. Regularly clean all the lights on your car, especially your headlights, because at night these lights are the only way you can communicate with other drivers, Creel says.

"If you have night vision problems, you're probably driving slower than some other people on the road. So it's just as important to be seen," Creel says. "One good rule of thumb is if the portions of your windshield that aren't cleaned by your wipers are covered with gunk, it's time to clean all your lights."

Look for landmarks. Street signs are harder to read at night, so when traveling to someplace unfamiliar, get detailed directions that include lots of gas stations, grocery stores, and other landmarks, Dr. Mancil suggests. Check out a reliable road map before you start out, and take the map with you. If you find yourself on darkened streets, you can always pull over, turn on the overhead light, and check the map.

Don't be a deer in the headlights. When you encounter oncoming traffic, look toward the right and follow the shoulder of the road until the other cars pass, Creel suggests. Diverting your eyes like this will reduce the blinding glare from the approaching headlights.

Break out the shades. Whenever you stop at a gas station, restaurant, or other well-lighted place, put on a pair of sunglasses before getting out of your car, Dr. Fox says. That way you'll have less trouble re-adapting to the darkness once you get back behind the wheel again. Of course, be sure to remove your shades before driving off.

Get a pair of night glasses. Sometimes, poor night vision is merely a sign of increasing nearsightedness, Dr. Sumers says. Ask your optometrist or ophthalmologist if a new pair of glasses that is specifically prescribed for nocturnal activities like driving will help you see better after sundown.

Slash the glare. Ask your vision-care specialist about getting an antireflective coating on your glasses, Dr. Rosenthal suggests. These coatings cut down on glare, increase the amount of available light coming into your eyes, and can improve your night vision.

NOSEBLEEDS

og owners know that a moist nose is a healthy nose. The same is true for people, mostly. We don't have slippery, leather-like muzzles on the ends of our faces, but our noses produce a lot of moisture, about a quart of mucus a day, says Louis D. Lowry, M.D., professor of otolaryngology at Thomas Jefferson University Hospital in Philadelphia. The mucus, which is about 95 percent water, humidifies the air we breathe for the lungs.

As we get older, though, that moisture in our noses can dry up. The delicate membrane inside becomes dry and brittle, exposing a delicate network of veins and arteries that can break open and cause a nosebleed at even the slightest sneeze or sniff.

Unless they last for a long period of time, nosebleeds aren't terribly serious, but they are annoying and a little scary. You can stop or prevent them with these simple measures.

Try This First

Stem the flow. There are three basic steps to follow to stop a nosebleed, says Jack B. Anon, M.D., otolaryngologist at Peach Street Medical in Erie, Pennsylvania, and chairman of the Nasal and Sinus Committee for the American Academy of Otolaryngology—Head and Neck Surgery.

1. Sit up straight with your head tilted slightly forward so that the blood doesn't run down your throat.
2. Gently blow out of your nose any clots that could prevent a blood vessel from sealing.
3. Put the squeeze on. Pinch the soft part of your nose between your thumb and forefinger for 10 minutes. "Sometimes, people don't know where to squeeze. The nose is designed so that your

fingers fit right in the soft part on the outside of your nose," says Dr. Anon. Some blood will come out when you squeeze— but just hold a folded-up tissue at the base of your nostrils to catch the drips.

Other Wise Ways

Spray the vessels shut. If your nose does not stop bleeding after 10 minutes of steady squeezing, use a nasal spray, such as Afrin or Neo-Synephrine, to constrict the vessels in your nose and stop the blood flow. Put four or five squirts in the bleeding nostril and pinch the soft part of your nose for an additional 10 minutes, says Dr. Anon.

Don't dry out. If you are developing nosebleeds from a dry nose caused by a lack of mucus production, moisten the membrane in your nasal passage with a saline spray to prevent it from cracking and rupturing. Spray the saline in your nose in the morning and evening, says Dr. Lowry.

MANAGING YOUR MEDS

Any medication that thins the blood will make it more difficult to stop a nosebleed, says Jack B. Anon, M.D., otolaryngologist at Peach Street Medical in Erie, Pennsylvania, and chairman of the Nasal and Sinus Committee for the American Academy of Otolaryngology— Head and Neck Surgery. It may also make your nose bleed more frequently. Here are a few common drugs that can slow the time normally required for your blood to clot.

• Aspirin, which is often prescribed in low doses to prevent heart attacks
• Nonsteroidal anti-inflammatory drugs (NSAIDs), such as ibuprofen
• Anticoagulants, such as warfarin (Coumadin), prescribed for clotting problems

If you have a nosebleed that has been induced by anticoagulants, try to slow the blood flow with the tips in this chapter and see a doctor right away.

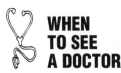

WHEN TO SEE A DOCTOR

If your nose does not stop bleeding after 20 minutes of applying pressure, then you should head to the emergency room, says Jack B. Anon, M.D., otolaryngologist at Peach Street Medical in Erie, Pennsylvania, and chairman of the Nasal and Sinus Committee for the American Academy of Otolaryngology—Head and Neck Surgery.

You also need to seek medical help as soon as possible if you feel blood running down the back of your throat when you are sitting or standing up or after you have pinched your nostrils. This could be a sign of a posterior nosebleed, which occurs more frequently in older people. You can lose blood quickly with a posterior nosebleed because the larger vessels behind your nose are affected.

Humidify your home. Breathing heated air in the winter or cooled air in the summer can dry out your mucous membranes and make you more prone to nosebleeds. Use a cool-mist humidifier to add moisture back into the air and your mucous membranes, says Dr. Lowry. To make sure the level of moisture in your home stays at or above 40 percent relative humidity, buy a gauge at a home-electronics store like Radio Shack.

Avoid heavy lifting or bending. Although direct pressure on the blood vessels will make them stop bleeding, pressure from within the vessels will start the flow again, says Dr. Anon. Avoid straining the vessels by lifting anything heavy. And keep your head above the level of your heart to avoid putting pressure on the vessels.

Take your vitamins at night. If you are prone to nosebleeds, be sure you are getting enough vitamin C, which is important in the maintenance of the blood vessels, and vitamin K, which is necessary to control bleeding. The Daily Value for vitamin C is 60 milligrams per day, and 80 micrograms per day of vitamin K. To get the most out of nutritional supplements, you should take them at night, says John A. Henderson, M.D., otolaryngologist and assistant professor of surgery/otolaryngology at the University of California, San Diego, School of Medicine.

"Only take your nutritional supplements at bedtime. If you take them at breakfast, they'll be in the urine within seven minutes," he explains. "Your kidneys slow down when your body is horizontal and sleeping, and vitamins will remain in your system longer and be absorbed."

NUMBNESS
AND TINGLING

Imagine a four-year-old girl who's sound asleep. Her left arm is contorted behind her neck. Her right hand is twisted into the small of her back. Her head is pinched up against her right shoulder, and her legs are crossed at the ankles.

Yet when she awakens, she won't feel numb. She'll have none of the tingling pins-and-needles sensations that many adults would experience. But give her time—say, 60 years—and her mangled nerves probably won't be so forgiving.

Numbness and tingling become more common as you get older for at least a couple of reasons, says Mark E. Williams, M.D., author of *The American Geriatrics Society's Complete Guide to Aging and Health* and director of the program on aging at the University of North Carolina at Chapel Hill School of Medicine. First, your body's nerves are an intricate road map comprised of superhighways, side roads, and a maze of intricate paths. These tortured and tangled avenues lead through tiny tunnels between muscles, tendons, and microscopic holes in bone. As you age, many of these spaces shrink, compressing the nerves and making you more susceptible to numbness and tingling. In addition, many seniors tend to develop bone spurs (tiny, hard outgrowths on their bones) that press on nerves and aggravate them, says Dr. Williams.

If a minor problem like pressure on nerves is clearly causing your arm or leg to fall asleep, here's what you can do to wake it up and prevent it from happening again.

Try This First

Fidget. Okay, so you don't have to be a Rhodes scholar to figure out that if a body part falls asleep, you need to reposition yourself

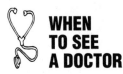

WHEN TO SEE A DOCTOR

so there is less pressure on the pinched nerve. But what you may not know is how to prevent it from happening in the first place.

The key? Don't allow your arms, legs, and other vulnerable body parts to remain in one position for too long, says Linda Morrow, M.D., medical director of Alexian Brothers Senior Health Center in San Jose, California.

If you're watching television, for instance, take a few moments during each commercial break to uncross your legs, curl your toes, stretch your arms over your head, twirl your wrists, and slowly bend and unbend your fingers into your palms. This routine can prevent compressed nerves and lower your risk of numbness and tingling.

Other Wise Ways

Move the wallet. If you have numbness in a leg, maybe you've been carrying a thick wallet in your back pocket and its bulk is contributing to the problem, Dr. Williams says. Every time you sit down, that lump in your back pocket puts pressure on the sciatic nerve that runs along your buttocks and continues down the back of your leg. The solution? Find another way to carry your cash and credit cards.

Pop a multivitamin. A variety of vitamin and mineral deficiencies can cause nerve damage in older adults, Dr. Williams says. Take a multivitamin daily that includes zinc, chromium, folic acid, and vitamin B_{12} to help make up for any subtle deficiencies in your diet that may leave you vulnerable to numbness and tingling.

Quit smoking. Smoking reduces blood flow to your extremities and increases the likelihood that you'll feel numbness and tingling in your arms, hands, legs, and feet, Dr. Williams says.

MANAGING YOUR MEDS

Over-the-counter nasal decongestants such as Sudafed, Dimetapp, Contac, and other products containing phenylpropanolamine can cause tingling, says W. Steven Pray, Ph.D., R.Ph., professor of nonprescription drug products at Southwestern Oklahoma State University in Weatherford. Excessive amounts of vitamin B_6 also can cause numbness and tingling in some people. If you take B_6 supplements, the National Research Council recommends taking no more than 100 milligrams a day.

In addition, the following prescription medications also can make you feel numb.

- Chloroquine (Aralen), used to treat arthritis and lupus
- Auranofin (Ridaura), used to treat rheumatoid arthritis
- Nitrofurantoin (Macrodantin), used to treat kidney infections
- Isoniazid (Rifamate), used to treat tuberculosis
- Anticonvulsants such as phenytoin (Dilantin)

OSTEOPOROSIS

"Drink your milk, then go outside and play." Good advice when you were six. Good advice at 46. Turns out, that's even good advice at 60 or 86, if you want to stave off osteoporosis.

Osteoporosis, which literally means "holes in the bones," occurs when the loss of bone tissue exceeds its replacement, a process that begins in your midthirties. A silent disease in that there are no symptoms or pain until a fracture occurs, osteoporosis robs bones of their strength over many years. Once this silent thief has done its work, bones can be so fragile that everyday actions like sneezing or lifting a bag of groceries can cause a fracture.

While women are four times more likely to develop the disease, men also suffer from osteoporosis. Women lose bone mass rapidly in the years following menopause, because their bodies produce less estrogen; yet by age 65 or 70, women and men lose bone mass at the same rate, experts say, and calcium absorption decreases in both sexes. Osteoporosis in men has been recognized as an important public-health issue, given that the number of men over 70 is estimated to double between 1993 and 2050.

Fractures resulting from osteoporosis typically occur in the hips, spine, and wrists, frequently costing an individual her independence. Yet although it affects nearly half of all people over the age of 75, doctors say osteoporosis is not an inevitable part of aging.

Bone tissue renewal continues throughout life. So with proper diet and lifestyle changes, you can slow, or even stop, osteoporosis, says James Webster, M.D., director of the Buehler Center of Aging at Northwestern University in Chicago. The time to combat osteoporosis, he emphasizes, is before your bones start to break.

Try This First

Up your calcium. You might not like milk, but you have to get enough calcium. Up to age 65, doctors recommend 1,000 milligrams of calcium a day for all men and for women on estrogen replacement therapy (ERT). Women who are past menopause but who are not receiving ERT should consume 1,200 milligrams of calcium daily, as should everyone over age 65.

To reach or surpass the goal of 1,000 milligrams through diet alone, strive for drinking 2½ to 3 eight-ounce glasses of fat-free milk a day. The rest you'll get through a healthy, balanced diet, says Robert P. Heaney, M.D., professor of medicine with the osteoporosis research center at Creighton University in Omaha, Nebraska.

Milk is fortified with vitamin D, which your body needs to assimilate calcium, so it's really the best source. But there are other foods that supply calcium alone. You can get 1,000 milligrams from eating 2½ cups of nonfat yogurt or five ounces of Cheddar cheese. Other good sources of calcium are sardines (with bones), collards, tofu, and calcium-fortified orange juice.

Other Wise Ways

Consider supplements. It's best to get calcium through food, but if you can't get enough in your diet, supplements offer the elemental calcium your body needs, says Dr. Webster. If you're ill or if you've had kidney stones, however, talk to your doctor before taking any supplements.

For best absorption, take supplements in divided doses of 500 to 600 milligrams at a time, and 1,000 to 1,200 milligrams per day, advises Elizabeth Lee Vliet, M.D., founder and medical director of HER Place: Health Enhancement and Renewal for Women and clinical associate professor in the department of family and community medicine at the University of Arizona College of Medicine in Tucson. "Your body will absorb a smaller amount better than taking your daily dose all at one time."

Calcium carbonate and calcium citrate are two common supplements available over the counter. Dr. Vliet says calcium car-

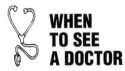

WHEN TO SEE A DOCTOR

To avoid becoming one of the women who first learn that they have osteoporosis while their doctors are setting their broken bones, have a DEXA (dual energy x-ray absorptiometry) scan now. This simple 15-minute test will measure your bone density and tell whether you're at risk for osteoporosis. In general, you're especially at risk for osteoporosis if you:

• Are thin and small-boned
• Have a history of eating disorders
• Have family members with osteoporosis
• Have generalized bone pain and tenderness
• Take corticosteroids, anticonvulsants like phenytoin (Dilantin), thyroid medication, or blood thinners

bonate can cause bloating or gas; calcium citrate doesn't, but these tablets contain less calcium, so you'll have to take more. Do not use bone meal or dolomite supplements, she warns, because they may contain lead and other toxic metals.

Maximize with magnesium. Magnesium is another crucial mineral to help build strong bones as well as help bowel function, prevent leg cramps, and improve sleep, according to Dr. Vliet. "But the sad fact is that most American women's diets are seriously deficient in magnesium." She recommends taking 250 milligrams in the morning and another 250 milligrams at night. Try a capsule formulation since it's better absorbed. For women with significant bone loss, problems with constipation, or nighttime leg cramps, the dose may need to be increased to 400 milligrams twice a day, suggests Dr. Vliet. Talk to your doctor first before taking supplemental magnesium. It may cause diarrhea. Also, people with heart or kidney problems should not take it.

Get Ds every day. To absorb calcium and build strong bones, your body needs vitamin D. Several studies have shown that when vitamin D and calcium are taken together, bone mineral density increases and the number of fractures decreases. Unfortunately, there aren't many good sources. Milk is fortified, as we've mentioned, and so are some cereals—so read labels to see how much of the Daily Value you're getting. Apart from that, your best source is sunlight, which triggers vitamin D production in your body. As little as 10 minutes of summer sun exposure on your hands, face, and arms is enough, says Dr. Vliet. Sunscreens with sun protection factors (SPF) of eight or above prevent vitamin D synthesis, so apply them immediately after your 10 minutes for vitamin D.

If you can't get outdoors, dietary vitamin D intake should be at least 400 international units (IU) but not more than 600 IU a day, recommends Dr. Vliet. One cup of fortified milk—whole, low-fat, or fat-free—has 100 IU, and most multivitamins provide 400 IU. Too much vitamin D can have harmful effects, including kidney damage, so don't decide to take supplements above the DV of 400 IU without first consulting your doctor.

Make room for "fit-bits." Weight-bearing exercise helps bones grow stronger. Start doing any exercise—walking, running, aerobics, pumping iron—that forces your bones and muscles to work against gravity.

Exercise stimulates bones to lay down new tissue, says Dr. Webster. Ideally, everyone should follow the American College of Sports

MANAGING YOUR MEDS

While an occasional antacid containing aluminum may settle the stomach after a spicy feast, excessive use of these stomach-soothers can have the unwanted effect of weakening bones. Certain medications can also add to your risk for developing osteoporosis and can even accelerate bone loss, says W. Steven Pray, Ph.D., R.Ph., professor of nonprescription drug products at Southwestern Oklahoma State University in Weatherford. They include:

- Long-term use of corticosteroids such as dexamethasone (Decadron) and prednisone (Deltasone), which are prescribed for many diseases, including arthritis, asthma, Crohn's disease, and lupus
- Anticonvulsants used to control seizures, such as phenytoin (Dilantin), carbamazepine (Tegretol), and divalproex sodium (Depakote)
- Barbiturates that are prescribed to relieve anxiety and tension or control seizures, such as phenobarbital (Barbita)
- Gonadorelin (Factrel), a hormone used to treat endometriosis

Medicine's suggested minimum of 20 minutes of aerobic exercise a day at least three times a week, but for some older people that much exercise at one time is not realistic, explains Dr. Webster.

If you can't handle 20 minutes of walking or weight-lifting, he recommends breaking it down into "fit-bits." Any exercise that has you carrying your own body weight, lifting weights, or pressing against some resistance is going to help, notes Dr. Webster. Easy fit-bits are exercises like a 10-minute stroll around the block or 5 minutes of biceps curls using one-pound weights. Just do enough fit-bits in a day to total 20 minutes of aerobic exercise.

But don't take it too easy on yourself, says Dr. Webster. "Doing as much as you can handle is going to give you the best results." Walking will strengthen the bones of your hips and lower back, he says, but if you can add light leg weights, that's even better.

Don't strain. Exercise is an effective means of combatting osteoporosis, but the exercise you choose shouldn't put any sudden or excessive strain on your bones.

Dr. Webster says to take care when lifting heavy objects and to avoid exercises where you bend forward or twist your spine. These movements tend to encourage compression fractures in the spine. Instead, lift with your thigh muscles by squatting.

Not surprisingly, doctors often suggest that patients with brittle bones give up golf, tennis, and basketball because of the twisting motions associated with these sports and their impact upon joints. Ask your doctor what type of exercises you can do safely to preserve bone, or ask for a referral to a physical therapist who specializes in osteoporosis.

Whatever activity you choose, keep in mind that you want to minimize your chances of breaking a bone. And remember, says Dr. Webster, that the benefits of exercise last only as long as you maintain the program.

Increase protein. Bones are not made of calcium alone. In fact, the matrix of your bone—the close weave of tissue that holds the calcium—incorporates a great deal of protein. Too often, experts say, the diets of older Americans are short on protein, which adds to the osteoporosis risk.

Dr. Webster suggests adding a packet of instant breakfast or another protein supplement to a glass of low-fat or fat-free milk twice a day to increase bone strength. Protein should make up 30 to 40 percent of your diet, he says, noting that skinless chicken breasts are a good source of inexpensive protein.

Stand tall on a wall. Doctors believe that exercises for persons with osteoporosis should emphasize balance, flexibility, and upper-body strengthening. Choose an exercise that improves balance, like tai chi, suggests Kay Solar, M.D., board-certified obstetrician/gynecologist in Baton Rouge, Louisiana. Or do simple posture exercises at home, she says, like shoulder blade squeezes or pressing your spine against a wall until your back is as straight as possible.

Take fall-safe measures. With osteoporosis, bones break more easily when you take a tumble. If you want to decrease your risk of debilitating fractures, you have to prevent falls, say doctors.

Remedying unsafe situations is an important part of changing the way you do things, Dr. Solar says. The best way to do this is to evaluate your everyday routine. Take a moment to think about what you're about to do, whether it's washing dishes or getting the newspaper, and consider if it may cause extra stress on your bones. You want to avoid sudden movements. Learn to move slowly and wisely.

Think about your surroundings at work or home. Is there anything that could cause you to trip or fall? If so, correct the problem, says Dr. Solar. In the kitchen, store frequently used items within easy reach. Avoid using step stools. Put handrails on both sides of a staircase. Get rid of throw rugs.

Don't smoke your bones. Smoking accelerates bone loss both in men and in women, according to Dr. Vliet. For women on ERT, it poses an extra threat, she says. Smoking speeds the rate at which the body burns estrogen, the hormone that helps prevent rapid bone loss. Since women get good doses of estrogen when they have ERT, the therapy could be a big benefit. But if you smoke, the bone-preserving properties of estrogen are quickly diminished.

Don't booze away bone. If you drink more than two ounces of hard liquor a day, cut back. In large amounts, alcohol hinders the formation of bones, Dr. Solar says, not to mention the adverse effect it can have on your equilibrium. Limit yourself to one standard alcoholic beverage a day, which is a 12-ounce beer, 5-ounce glass of wine, or 1½-ounce shot of liquor.

Limit the calcium flushers. If you drink coffee, tea, or soft drinks with caffeine, limit yourself to two to three cups of liquid per day, says Dr. Solar. Beyond that, caffeine acts as a diuretic, flushing calcium from the body.

Hold the salt. As with caffeine, too much salt causes your body to excrete calcium. Check food labels, advises Dr. Solar. Avoid products with more than 300 milligrams of salt per serving, and limit your daily sodium intake to 2,400 milligrams a day.

Choose the right shoes. Preventing falls starts from the ground up. Choose athletic shoes because they provide good balance and support. For dressy occasions, choose flat shoes with a broad, flexible sole. Avoid high heels or clogs, says Dr. Vliet. Not only are you more likely to fall but also these types of shoes aren't good for your back.

Build bone if you're blue. Researchers at the National Institute of Mental Health (NIMH) in Bethesda, Maryland, have found decreased bone mineral density in women with past or current depression. Researchers speculate that the link may be due to hormonal changes, changes in physical activity, or other changes associated with depression.

While the link is being investigated, NIMH researchers suggest that women who've been diagnosed with depression take steps to maximize bone building.

OVERWEIGHT

In the modern era, when the ever-present, unforgiving television camera records every presidential bumble, stumble, and misstep, William Howard Taft would have been cannon fodder for the media.

Taft, who weighed more than 300 pounds, was America's twenty-seventh and, let's just say, most well-rounded president. By the last year of his life, the former president frequently experienced dizziness, shortness of breath, and heart palpitations caused by severe hardening of the arteries. He died in his sleep at age 72 after suffering a massive heart attack.

The moral of this story is probably one that you have already heard. Namely, aging and serious weight problems are a nasty, and often fatal, duo.

"There is clearly a relationship between aging and weight problems. You can almost think of one helping the other to hurt you," says Robert Di Bianco, M.D., director of cardiology research at the Washington Adventist Hospital and associate clinical professor of medicine at Georgetown University School of Medicine in Washington, D.C.

About 20 percent of all Americans over age 65 are overweight, according to David A. Lipschitz, M.D., Ph.D., chairman and professor of geriatrics at the University of Arkansas for Medical Sciences in Little Rock. If you're one of them, here's a glimpse at just some of the havoc those excess pounds may be causing in your body.

Blood. People who are overweight are more prone to high blood pressure, a risk factor for stroke and heart attack, says Jan I. Maby, D.O., director of the Geriatric Medical Home Care program at Mount Sinai Medical Center in New York City. Every pound of excess weight drives your systolic blood pressure (the top number

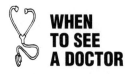

WHEN TO SEE A DOCTOR

If you have a chronic health problem like diabetes or high blood pressure, see a doctor before starting a weight-loss program.

If you're more than 20 pounds overweight, your risk of developing serious health problems is higher than normal. See your doctor for regular checkups.

in a blood pressure reading) up 4.5 millimeters.

Heart. The more overweight you are, the harder your heart has to work to pump blood and supply nutrients to all of the cells in your body. Excessive body weight also contributes to atherosclerosis (hardening of the arteries). Being overweight may quadruple your chances of having a heart attack or stroke.

Lungs. Although your body can keep getting bigger, your lungs can't. The same two lungs that did so well when you were thinner now have to supply oxygen to a much larger body. That puts a lot of strain on your respiratory system, Dr. Maby says. In addition, thick pads of fat in the abdomen can interfere with your ability to breathe well.

Abdomen. Your stomach isn't causing that potbelly. It's fat that has accumulated under the skin and within your abdominal cavity. Harvard researchers found that men with waist circumferences of 43 inches or more are 2½ times more likely to develop colon cancer than those whose waists are less than 35 inches.

Pancreas. Diabetes is three times more common among people who are overweight.

Reproductive system. Endometrial cancer is two to three times more common in overweight women than in those who are lean.

Joints. Excess weight causes greater wear and tear in joints and can aggravate symptoms of arthritis. The strain is particularly hard on the knees and lower back.

Although you may have tried losing weight several times in the past, here are a few reminders and several fresh ideas that can help you shed the pounds and keep them off this time.

Try This First

Get a new lifestyle. Don't focus just on your diet, suggests Maria Simonson, Sc.D., Ph.D., director of the health, weight, and stress clinic, and professor emeritus at Johns Hopkins Medical Institutions in Baltimore. In most cases, diets won't do the job for you. By their very nature, diets imply temporary denial or sacrifice. Once you go off the diet, you'll likely fall back into the very eating habits that got you into trouble in the first place.

Your best bet is to fine-tune your eating habits as part of a comprehensive strategy that includes getting regular exercise and developing a positive attitude, Dr. Simonson says. Remember, this is a lifestyle makeover that will help you add life to your years. Start by making small changes. For breakfast, have a one-ounce slice of

MANAGING YOUR MEDS

Relying on appetite suppressants and quick-fix over-the-counter weight-loss products will lighten your pocketbook but do little else, says Jan I. Maby, D.O., director of the Geriatric Medical Home Care program at Mount Sinai Medical Center in New York City.

Many prescription medications such as dexfenfluramine (Redux) and phentermine (Adipex-P), which you may know as Fen-Phen, did help some people lose weight. But these products caused severe side effects, including serious heart problems, and some, such as Redux, were quickly withdrawn from the market, notes W. Steven Pray, Ph.D., R.Ph., professor of nonprescription drug products at Southwestern Oklahoma State University in Weatherford.

As for over-the-counter medications, forget about it, Dr. Pray says. Many nonprescription weight-control products such as Dexatrim and Acutrim contain phenylpropanolamine, a substance that can dangerously elevate an older person's blood pressure and cause heart problems or even stroke, Dr. Pray says.

Canadian bacon instead of four slices of regular bacon. You'll save more than 100 calories if you do. Park a few extra spaces away from the supermarket so you'll walk a bit more. Take a moment each day to concentrate on an aspect of your body that you like, such as your smile, and take pride in the features that are improving.

These small but important lifestyle changes can make big differences in your weight, Dr. Simonson says.

Other Wise Ways

Make many moves toward weight loss. Get moving and keep moving as much as you can, suggests Marilyn Cerino, R.D., marketing director for Allegheny University Executive Health and Wellness Program in Philadelphia.

"If I'm trying to help an overweight senior, the first thing I'm going to do is get him moving," says Cerino. "Maybe he can only walk a block; fine. We can build from there. But you're simply not going to get your weight under control without some form of exercise."

A person over 60 can easily cover a mile a day by doing errands on foot or walking from room to room cleaning house, Dr. Simonson says. If you do it every day and combine your exercise program with a healthy high-fiber, low-fat diet, you can lose up to 11 pounds a year. You should aim for walking a minimum of three miles a week or doing some other exercise for 30 minutes three times a week, she suggests.

Pass the convenience store. Many seniors like shopping at mini-markets because they're conveniently close to home. But they offer little to help you lose weight, Cerino says. "Many of the foods at these stores are premade. Unfortunately, a lot of them are snack-type things that are high in fat, sodium, and sugar. You might find some healthy sandwiches there, and you can certainly find fat-free milk, margarine, and some low-fat snacks. But your choices are very limited if you're looking for a good selection of foods that are low in fat or calories."

Try to shop at larger grocery stores where there is greater variety so you can make healthier food choices. If you have difficulty shopping or are intimidated by traffic, you may want to hire a neighbor's teenager to shop for you, Cerino suggests.

Make your kitchen less cozy. If your kitchen is your living room—the place where you watch television, chat with friends, and spend most of your time—make some changes. A kitchen that is too comfy is dangerous if you're overweight, because you'll be tempted to spend more time there nibbling on snacks and other foods. So move the rocking chair and television back into the living room, where they belong, Cerino says.

Then rearrange your kitchen so snacks, cookies, and other high-calorie temptations take more effort to get to than healthy and tasty foods like grapes, carrots, rice cakes, and whole-grain crackers.

Cook it, serve it, store it, eat it. If you put foods into serving bowls and place them on the table, you'll be tempted to take seconds, Cerino says. Instead, take modest portions—so they don't overlap on your plate—right from pots and pans in the oven or on the stove. Then quickly wrap up any leftovers and put them away before you eat. That way you'll end up with a spare meal in the freezer instead of a spare tire around your belly.

Savor the experience. Take your time and enjoy eating, Cerino suggests. A meal should last at least 20 to 30 minutes because there is a lag time between when you take your last bite and when your stomach lets your brain know that it is full. If you eat too fast, you may be going beyond that point without even knowing it, particularly after age 60, when it begins to take more time for your digestive system to react.

Put your fork down between bites and chew carefully. Note the time before you begin eating. If you're finished within 5 minutes, try to stretch that out to 8 minutes during the next meal. Gradually increase the time it takes you to eat, until you reach 20 minutes, Cerino says.

Throw your stomach a bone. If you have trouble controlling your appetite, have a 100-calorie snack, like one ounce of low-fat cheese and a few crackers, or two cups of warm air-popped popcorn, 30 minutes before eating. That way your stomach will already have something in it, and you won't need to eat as much to feel full, Cerino says.

Drinking an eight-ounce glass of water about 10 minutes before you eat can also have the same effect, Dr. Simonson says.

Take in fuel at a steady pace. If you eat smaller meals more frequently, you'll gain better control of your appetite, Cerino says. After breakfast, have a midmorning snack like yogurt or an apple. Have a hearty lunch entrée such as low-fat stew, baked chicken breast, or spaghetti. Then have a late-afternoon snack like low-fat cheese and crackers, and a small dinner like three ounces of skinless chicken or lean beef with rice, two vegetables, and a little bit of margarine or olive oil. And you can finish off the day with a light evening snack such as a scoop of fat-free frozen yogurt.

"A person who only eats one or two times a day is probably going to weigh more than someone who has five or six smaller, calorie-controlled meals a day," Cerino says. "When you eat fewer meals, you end up starving by the time you do eat, and you tend to eat a greater number of calories than if you kept the hunger to a minimum by eating frequent meals."

Ultimately, whether you gain or lose weight depends on the kinds of foods you eat, Dr. Simonson says. Cutting down on fat and sugar will go a long way to helping you reach your goal.

Don't sweat the small stuff. Some older people ultimately sabotage their efforts by dwelling on the little defeats in their struggles with weight control rather than focusing on their many achievements, Dr. Simonson says. Don't be one of them.

Instead of focusing on your overall goal, set your sights on a modest weight target that you can easily achieve, like losing half a pound a week, Dr. Simonson says. If you don't reach your goal in one week, try to think of it not as a failure but as a learning experience. Jot down the things you did and didn't do that will help you make a better effort in the next seven days.

Don't get discouraged, she says. It may take longer to lose pounds than it did in the past. As you age, your metabolism slows down, which simply means it takes your body longer to burn up food calories or turn them into energy. If you're someone over 60 and you can lose a half-pound to a pound a week, you're doing great, Dr. Simonson says.

PHLEBITIS

It's been dubbed "economy-class syndrome" by British researchers studying airline travelers, but you may know it by its more common name: phlebitis (an inflammation of veins, usually in the legs). It tends to happen to a lot of healthy people who sit through long flights or travel by car, says Gabriel Goren, M.D. vascular surgeon and director of the Vein Disorders Center in Encino, California.

With little leg room, you certainly can't kick up your heels. Leg circulation is constricted and that impedes blood flow. "When blood is pooling and stagnating in veins, it can clot," says Dr. Goren. "The clot triggers the inflammation, and phlebitis is born."

But you don't have to fly coach to spark a phlebitis attack. Any period of immobility can trigger an episode, and that includes times when you're recovering from an injury, illness, or surgery. As you get older, especially during episodes of debilitating diseases, your risk of developing phlebitis increases.

"There are two types of phlebitis: superficial, and deep vein phlebitis (DVT) or thrombosis," says Dr. Goren. Superficial phlebitis is generally seen in people who have varicose veins. Just beneath the skin of the leg, you may notice a red cordlike vein that feels hard, warm, and painful to the touch and is accompanied by redness of the skin around the affected vein.

In the case of DVT, you may feel an overall heaviness in the leg, mainly in the calf, and occasionally ankle swelling.

An estimated 30 percent of DVT cases go undiagnosed and go away on their own, says J. A. Olivencia, M.D., vascular surgeon and medical director of the Iowa Vein Center in West Des Moines, Iowa. But if the doctor detects this kind of thrombosis, you're sure to have some kind of treatment.

However your doctor decides to treat the problem, there are

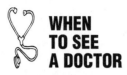

WHEN TO SEE A DOCTOR

Any type of phlebitis needs to be seen by a doctor to determine how serious it is. If you have been diagnosed with superficial phlebitis, call your doctor if you still have symptoms after 7 to 10 days or if the condition reoccurs. If you notice lumps, high fever, or overall pain and swelling in the limb, you may have developed deep vein phlebitis, and you'll need immediate medical attention, says Gabriel Goren, M.D., vascular surgeon and director of the Vein Disorders Center in Encino, California.

If you have deep vein thrombosis and are taking anticoagulant drugs, go to the hospital if you experience any unusual bleeding or signs of an internal hemorrhage, such as difficulty breathing, unexplained swelling, or chest, abdominal, or joint pain.

some ways to relieve the discomfort of superficial phlebitis and discourage blood clots from occurring.

Try This First

Heal it with heat. Apply moist heat to the affected area to soothe discomfort and speed healing. The heat especially improves circulation, which will help your body absorb the clot faster, says Dr. Olivencia. Cover the inflamed area with a towel that has been dipped in hot water and wrung out. Then cover the towel with a heating pad or hot-water bottle to maintain the temperature. Do this for 20 to 30 minutes at least twice a day.

Other Wise Ways

Rise to the occasion. Elevate the affected leg, which also will promote increased circulation and speed healing, says Dr. Olivencia.

Skip the aspirin. To relieve pain and inflammation, take ibuprofen instead of aspirin. It works better than aspirin in two ways. A more effective pain reliever, ibuprofen helps counteract the inflammatory reaction that generates pain and swelling in the vein, says Dr. Goren. Over-the-counter tablets contain 200 milligrams per pill, which is a relatively small dose. To control the pain and inflammation during an episode of phlebitis, you should take 400 milligrams, or two pills, three times a day after meals.

Put the squeeze on. Compression stockings help reduce the swelling and alleviate some of the discomfort caused by phlebitis, because they squeeze the veins and minimize the buildup of fluid in the leg. If you look on the package of compression stockings sold in pharmacies, you'll find that the compression is rated from light to extra-strong compression on a scale of one to four. Go with grade two, a moderate level of compression, to relieve superficial phlebitis symptoms, says Dr. Olivencia. "The stockings may be very uncomfortable if you have a clot behind the knee or if you have large legs. If the stockings are too uncomfortable, do not force yourself to wear them."

Increase your rate of return. To reduce your risk of developing phlebitis, keep your circulation moving whenever you are sitting

MANAGING YOUR MEDS

If you've been diagnosed with deep vein phlebitis, your doctor will prescribe an anticoagulant drug treatment, usually warfarin (Coumadin), to thin your blood and prevent additional clots from forming. The level of medication, however, must be carefully monitored. Severe internal and external bleeding can occur unless you have the proper dosage. This explains why most people who go on the medication need a short stay in the hospital while the doctor adjusts the level of medication. The adjustments depend on tests that show how fast your blood is clotting. The initial dosage for adults is generally administered for two to four days. It is then adjusted to a level required by the patient to maintain a proper blood-clotting time.

To avoid a potential drug interaction that could cause excessive internal bleeding, keep your doctor informed of all the medications you are taking, says Bernard Mehl, R.Ph., doctor of professional studies and director of the department of pharmacy for Mount Sinai Medical Center in New York City. Of the many types of drugs that can interact with anticoagulants and increase the risk of hemorrhage, there are three commonly used for people over 60, the prescription thyroid drug levothyroxine (Synthroid), nonsteroidal anti-inflammatory drugs (NSAIDs) such as ibuprofen, and aspirin. Some antibiotics such as erythromycin can also increase an anticoagulant's blood-thinning effect. And over-the-counter drugs such as cimetidine (Tagamet), used to treat heartburn and gastric ulcers, will decrease the activity of warfarin.

for more than a few hours, says Dr. Goren. Whether you're flying coast to coast or taking a long drive in the car, take a stretch break.

Once an hour, walk around for at least three to four minutes to return the blood in your legs back to the heart. While you're seated, flex the calf muscle every 10 minutes by moving your foot up and down.

Boost your B vitamins. Vascular diseases are more common in people with high levels of the amino acid homocysteine. Research has shown that the B vitamins folate, B_6, and B_{12} can reduce elevated homocysteine levels, says James Finkelstein, M.D., chief of medical service at the Veterans Administration Medical Center and professor of medicine at Howard, George Washington, and Georgetown Universities, all in Washington, D.C.

To maintain optimum health of your veins as well as your arteries, Dr. Finkelstein recommends taking supplements of 400 micrograms of folic acid (the synthethic form of folate) and 25 milligrams of B_6 daily. Because older people are at risk for vitamin B_{12} deficiency, they should also take 100 micrograms of B_{12} daily, he says. Folate-packed food sources include orange juice, spinach, asparagus, lentils, and navy beans. Bananas, lean chicken, potatoes, and watermelons are good sources of vitamin B_6. Vitamin B_{12} is found in animal products such as meat, milk, cheese, and eggs. But because people older than 50 years of age may not adequately absorb this vitamin from food, the National Research Council advises that they take foods fortified with vitamin B_{12}, such as ready-to-eat cereals, or use a supplement.

Note: If you've been diagnosed as not having the intrinsic factor, which aids in the absorption of B_{12}, you'll need to talk to your doctor about getting regular injections of B_{12}.

Improve the flow. Several studies indicate that vitamin E helps protect against clots, according to Joseph Pizzorno Jr., naturopathic physician and president of Bastyr University in Seattle. Vitamin E helps prevent platelets (components of the blood involved in clotting) from sticking to each other and to the walls of the blood vessels. To reduce platelet stickiness, Dr. Pizzorno recommends taking from 200 to 600 international units (IU) a day.

Note: If you are taking anticoagulants, you should not take vitamin E. Although vitamin E is generally sold in doses of 400 IU, one small study showed a possible risk of stroke in dosages higher than 200 IU. Consult with your doctor if you are at high risk for stroke.

PNEUMONIA

If you imagine having pneumonia, you probably see yourself coughing up a lung, barely able to breathe, and with a fever hot enough to cook an egg.

But as you get older, pneumonia may look a bit different if it takes hold of you. It doesn't manifest the way you think it would with the classic symptoms of fever, heavy sweating, coughing, sputum production, chest pain, and chills, says Henry Gong Jr., M.D., professor of medicine in the division of pulmonary and critical-care medicine and environmental health service at the University of Southern California School of Medicine in Downey.

Instead, pneumonia shows itself in ways you'd never expect and with symptoms that may seem completely unrelated. Some people seem suddenly confused or less aware of their surroundings or of people around them. Others exhibit weakness and fatigue. Rapid breathing, rapid pulse, or shortness of breath may also be signs of pneumonia. Others have symptoms like nausea and diarrhea, which we normally associate with intestinal problems. In fact, someone with pneumonia who has some or all of these symptoms may never utter a single cough.

If you notice these atypical symptoms in yourself or a loved one, you should go to a doctor. Although the advent of antibiotics knocked out pneumonia as the leading cause of death back in the 1940s, the disease is still dangerous, especially to people over age 65.

What causes pneumonia is still the same, no matter what age you are. It is an infection of the lungs caused by bacteria, viruses, or other organisms. Although the disease has more than 30 different causes, bacterial pneumonia is the most common. In this version, bacteria that's normally present in your throat when you're healthy starts multiplying in your lungs when your immunity is down. In viral pneumonia, a virus takes hold in your lungs and multiplies. A

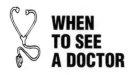

WHEN TO SEE A DOCTOR

The symptoms of pneumonia in older persons are often different from those experienced by younger persons, says Bruce Leff, M.D., assistant professor of medicine at the Johns Hopkins Bayview Medical Center Geriatric Center in Baltimore. Therefore, symptoms to watch for and contact a physician about right away include:

• Cough (especially if accompanied by colored phlegm)
• Fever
• Shortness of breath
• Chest pain
• Confusion

weakened immunity is also a common risk factor for contracting viral pneumonia.

In all kinds of pneumonia, the air sacs in your lungs fill with pus and liquid, which prevents oxygen from reaching your blood. Without enough oxygen in your bloodstream, your body's cells can't work correctly.

The well-traveled myth that a cold can turn into pneumonia simply isn't true. But it is so ingrained that Bruce Leff, M.D., assistant professor of medicine at the Johns Hopkins Bayview Medical Center Geriatric Center in Baltimore can't even convince his mother it's false.

People believe that a cold can directly lead to pneumonia because the one kind of illness sometimes precedes the other. But a cold just lowers your immune defenses, and when your defenses are down, you're more susceptible to another infection such as pneumonia. Both colds and pneumonia are more common during the winter months, says Dr. Leff.

Once you get pneumonia, you need to be under a doctor's care. Self-treatment can be dangerous, especially for older people, and it's important to remember that pneumonia can be deadly.

But rather than fight pneumonia just when it arrives, the better course of action is to prevent it. Pneumonia usually strikes when your defenses are already down due to another illness. So the best defense against pneumonia is to keep your immune system in top shape.

Try This First

Get shot. Ask your doctor for the pneumococcal vaccine, Dr. Leff says. No, this isn't a home remedy, but given the seriousness of pneumonia, you don't want to neglect this important form of prevention.

This vaccine, which protects you from certain strains of bacterial pneumonia, is recommended by the Centers for Disease Control (CDC) for everyone who is over the age of 65, chronically ill, or at risk for infection due to a weakened immune system.

Despite that recommendation, only about 28 percent of the over-65 population have ever received a pneumonia vaccine. A study by the CDC at a nursing home in Oklahoma observed that the vaccine probably could have prevented a pneumonia outbreak there that killed three people. If you're over 65, the CDC recommends that you get a booster shot if it's been over five years since your original vaccine.

Just one warning about getting a vaccine: Don't assume that because you got the injection, you can't get pneumonia. You can still catch a different strain of bacterial pneumonia, or you can catch viral pneumonia, which isn't affected by the vaccine, says Dr. Gong. So if you suspect that you have pneumonia, get to a doctor even if you have been vaccinated in the past.

Other Wise Ways

Take to the high Cs each winter. Deirdre O'Connor, naturopathic doctor in private practice in Mystic, Connecticut, tells all her older patients who seem vulnerable to upper respiratory problems to increase their vitamin C intakes during the winter months. She recommends a supplement of between 1,000 and 3,000 milligrams a day.

MANAGING YOUR MEDS

For the treatment of bacterial pneumonia, doctors will prescribe antibiotics. Some people are allergic to certain antibiotics, so talk to your doctor if you have had an allergic reaction before, says Bruce Leff, M.D., assistant professor of medicine at the Johns Hopkins Bayview Medical Center Geriatric Center in Baltimore. Also, check with your doctor before mixing antibiotics with anticoagulants such as warfarin (Coumadin). If you are given an antibiotic, be certain to take the full course of treatment.

This is in addition to making sure you fill your diet with foods high in vitamin C, such as broccoli, brussels sprouts, red peppers, sweet potatoes, and citrus fruits.

Vitamin C is necessary for a healthy immune system, Dr. O'Connor says. In studies, it has been shown to help older people who have severe respiratory infections, she says. Excess vitamin C may cause diarrhea in some people, so cut back on your dosage until you find a comfortable level.

Put some muscle in your immunity. Make sure your daily multivitamin has 15 milligrams of zinc in it, Dr. O'Connor says. In older people, this mineral isn't always absorbed properly from diet alone, so some people develop deficiencies. Immune cells are so dependent on zinc that they can't fight off infection unless they have this mineral. You'll find zinc in meats, poultry, eggs, dairy products, and oysters.

Whip up immunity soup. Start with a basic vegetable broth, then toss in red peppers, winter squash, carrots, garlic, onions, and any other colorful vegetables. Make this tasty meal frequently during the winter and especially when you are sick, suggests Dr. O'Connor. She calls it her carotene soup in honor of beta-carotene and other carotenoids that enhance the work of the immune system.

Carotenoids are especially prevalent in brightly colored vegetables such as carrots and squash. It's best to get carotenoids from foods, says Dr. O'Connor, because natural carotenoids are better absorbed and work better than synthetic supplements.

Make your eyes and mouth water. During the winter, Dr. O'Connor urges people to cook with lots of garlic and onions. These two related foods may have antiviral and antibiotic properties, she says, so they can help your immune system fight off both viral and bacterial pneumonia. Garlic and onions go with everything from mashed potatoes to meat or fish, and they're especially good in soups.

Favor foot motion. Take a brisk daily walk for half an hour a day. There's no guarantee, but daily walks may help keep pneumonia at bay. "Regular exercise keeps your immune system functioning very well," Dr. O'Connor says.

If you prefer other activities such as cycling or swimming, go ahead and enjoy them, she says. Any daily or regular exercise will keep your immune system strong. She also recommends trying different workouts like yoga.

POOR APPETITE

Experts agree that appetite can begin to malfunction as people age, though the exact reasons are not known. Many factors affect your yen for food. People who take various medications may have loss of appetite as a side effect. Ongoing health problems like upper-respiratory disease and diabetes can steal your appetite for food in some cases.

An age-related decline in your ability to taste and smell may also contribute to lowered appetite, says Susan Schiffman, Ph.D., professor of medical psychology at Duke University Medical School in Durham, North Carolina, because those senses trigger the first responses of the gastrointestinal system in preparation for digestion. "They set up the whole appetite response, so if you don't have taste and smell, you're not motivated."

"There's a whole complexity of changes going on," says Barbara Rolls, Ph.D., professor of nutrition at Pennsylvania State University in University Park. "For some people, it's a lack of ability to feed themselves, a lack of social interaction, poverty. For others, there are genuine changes in the mechanisms for making them hungry."

What happens to your weight when you lose your appetite? Some people will lose weight, but people also may gain weight if their eating is not regulated by a sense of hunger, says Susan Roberts, Ph.D., professor of nutrition and psychiatry and chief of the energy metabolism laboratory at Tufts University in Boston.

If your appetite has waned, there are actual strategies you can adopt to recapture your yearning for food. Here are some strategies that doctors recommend for recovering good digestion, appetite, and health.

435

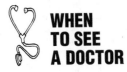

Try This First

Go ahead—be bitter. Some naturopathic doctors suggest eating bitter herbs to stimulate the production of gastric juices that provoke appetite response.

For a quick response, Thomas Kruzel, naturopathic physician in private practice in Portland, Oregon, recommends a formula of tinctures of the herbs burdock, Oregon grape, and gentian in equal parts.

The tinctures, diluted plant extracts, are available in health food stores. Mix the three tinctures and take about 20 drops of the mixture in some water 10 to 15 minutes before you eat, advises Dr. Kruzel.

Other Wise Ways

Toast your way to a better appetite. A glass of red wine with dinner may improve your appetite by aiding digestion. The tannins in the wine help the digestive tract to secrete digestive enzymes, according to Dr. Kruzel. In addition to helping jump-start the digestive process, it helps you to absorb more nutrients, which could be very important if you're eating less.

"Basically, beer and wine were initially used to help with digestion as well as being a part of rituals and religious ceremonies. A lot of the beer and the meads were peptic bitters, so they helped the person's gastrointestinal track to secrete enzymes," Dr. Kruzel says.

Try a vinegar cocktail. This alternative health remedy may not sound like the most appetizing cocktail, but a teaspoon of apple cider vinegar in a glass of water taken before a meal may help acidify your digestive system, which also aids in digestion. This is particularly important for older people, Dr. Kruzel says, because their stomach acidity naturally declines.

Eat when you're hungry. This requires a little detective work on your part, says Karen Chapman-Novakofski, R.D., Ph.D., professor

MANAGING YOUR MEDS

Some medications commonly used by older people have appetite loss as a side effect. Talk with your doctor about an alternative medication if your appetite seems to diminish from your drugs, says W. Steven Pray, Ph.D., R.Ph., professor of nonprescription drug products at Southwestern Oklahoma State University in Weatherford.

Some examples are:

- Prescription hypertension drugs such as spironolactone (Aldactone) and hydrochlorothiazide (HydroDIURIL)
- Prescription gold-salt compounds used for rheumatoid arthritis, such as auranofin (Ridaura) and gold-sodium thiomalate
- Prescription psychiatric drugs such as lithium (Lithonate) or fluoxetine (Prozac)
- Estrogens (Premarin)
- Some prescription heart medications such as nifedipine (Procardia), captopril (Capoten), losartan (Cozaar), propranolol (Inderal), and topical nitroglycerin patches

In addition to medications themselves, the way you take medicines can aggravate a poor appetite, says Karen Chapman-Novakofski, R.D., Ph.D., professor of nutrition with the College of Agriculture and College of Medicine at the University of Illinois in Urbana. If you take your medicine before your meal with a glass of water, you may be filling yourself up before you begin eating. "I usually tell people to talk to their pharmacists or doctors to see if those medicines could be taken after a meal so that they're not full by the time they start eating. That way, you're still taking your medication with food, as the prescription requires, but you're not spoiling your appetite."

of nutrition with the College of Agriculture and College of Medicine at the University of Illinois in Urbana. "You need to pay attention to when you are even the smallest bit hungry any time of the day," Dr. Chapman-Novakofski says. "And then you really need to capitalize on that. Have your main meal whenever you have a good appetite—even if it's 10:30 in the morning," she says.

Nibble like a bird all day. Some people may not be interested enough in food to eat the way we traditionally do—three large meals a day. Eating five or six smaller meals throughout the day may be more manageable and will give your body the energy you need, says Dr. Chapman-Novakofski.

Add some fiber to your diet. "Constipation will cause loss of appetite because you feel full," says Dr. Chapman-Novakofski. Adding a piece of fruit to each meal is a good way to increase fiber in your diet naturally.

If you add bran or other fibrous cereals, do it gradually and make sure that you drink enough water with it, she advises. Additional bran fiber takes some getting used to—and you might have to deal with gas at first. If you're getting your fiber with fruits and vegetables, you don't need to drink more fluids.

Ease off the caffeine. Dr. Chapman-Novakofski finds that retirees who are not very active can spend a lot of the day drinking coffee or tea. But, unfortunately, the caffeine in those beverages works as an appetite suppressant. She recommends switching to decaffeinated coffee or tea at mid-morning. Also, watch the volume you're drinking (two to three cups is a moderate amount), because this could make you feel full and eat less.

Keep 30 percent of your diet from fat. Older people are often very health conscious, says Dr. Rolls. They'll stuff their refrigerators and pack their pantries with low-fat foods.

But if your appetite is poor and you choose low-fat foods when you eat, you may not be consuming enough calories to keep up with your energy needs. This doesn't mean that you can go wild eating ice cream. But cutting down to nonfat or low-fat foods, particularly if you are older than 75, is inappropriate. "You should be getting 30 percent of your calories from fat," Dr. Rolls says.

Take a vitamin. If you fear that your poor appetite is not allowing you to consume all the nutrients you need, take a multivitamin every day, says Sherry Briskey, naturopathic physician and staff physician at Southwest Naturopathic Medical Center in Tempe, Arizona.

Thirst for hydration. Sometimes, people older than 60 forget to keep hydrated, because they usually aren't as active as they used to be and they don't sweat as much. Be sure that you drink six to eight glasses of fluids a day, Dr. Kruzel says. He recommends drinking a lot early in the day so if you have bladder-control problems you won't have to get up and go to the bathroom throughout the night. Good choices are filtered water and fresh fruit and vegetable juices. When replenishing fluids, you want to stay away from drinks that are diuretic or promote urination, such as coffee, beer, alcohol, and caffeine-containing sodas.

Get up off the couch. Exercise has the uncanny ability to help regulate appetite, says Dr. Chapman-Novakofski. "For people who are undereating, some kind of physical activity usually increases their appetites some." And it doesn't take much. A simple walk around your neighborhood will do.

Adjust your dentures. Make sure your dentures fit and are well-cleaned. Ill-fitting dentures can be painful, and that could cause you to lose your appetite. Poor denture and dental hygiene can leave unpleasant tastes in your mouth that also kill your appetite, says Dr. Roberts.

Eat breakfast for dinner. If you're too tired at the end of the day to prepare a meal, you may be tempted to go to bed without any supper. But skipping meals is bad because it sets up a calorie deficit. Try to nap in the afternoon to boost energy for the evening, or eat a bowl of fortified cereal with a glass of orange juice for dinner, Dr. Chapman-Novakofski advises. That breakfast is an easy meal with all the protein, carbohydrates, vitamins, and minerals you need. "Make sure you don't miss a meal completely, even if you eat something nonconventional," she says.

Make mealtime fun. Because depression and loneliness can be factors in loss of appetite, making mealtime an experience can prompt you to eat. Set the table with your good china. Add some flowers or candles. Do whatever it is that will make dining a special event for you. If eating in front of the TV set is a real treat, then do that, Dr. Chapman-Novakofski says. But make it a real meal, she advises—not just eating anything from a TV tray.

Try to eat with family and friends. People eat more in social groups than when they're alone, Dr. Rolls states.

Appeal to your other senses. Because the senses of taste and smell can decline as you age, visual presentations can become an important part of your culinary experience. Focus on colors, says chef Greg Tompkins of the National Baking Center in Minneapolis. Avoid a monochromatic plate. Help your green vegetables retain their color by steaming instead of boiling them. And be sure to include veggies such as carrots and sweet red peppers, which contain carotene and keep their strong colors no matter how they are cooked.

Try to arrange food on the plate so that it is asymmetrical and has some height to it. This design will cause your eye to move, creating visual stimulation and excitement about a dish.

Bring in the brine—first. An important thing to remember, says certified master chef Ronald De Santis, senior professor at the Culinary Institute of America in Hyde Park, New York, is not to begin your meal with a fatty appetizer that could fill you up and further dull your appetite. He recommends briny, vinegary foods like capers, or acidic foods like tomatoes that get saliva flowing. Save the fat for dessert.

POOR CONCENTRATION

More than 10,000 random thoughts and fleeting images zip though an average person's mind every day. They could include a snippet of a song, a momentary image of an old friend, or a fragment of a joke.

In most cases, these intruders are quickly banished from your mind so you can concentrate on the task at hand. But as you get older, it becomes harder to filter out these distractions and stick to a project, organize your thoughts, or follow the flow of a conversation, says Richard Restak, M.D., clinical professor of neurology at George Washington University School of Medicine and Health Sciences in Washington, D.C, and co-author of *The Longevity Strategy: How to Live to 100 Using the Brain-Body Connection*. Poor concentration also can affect your memory. So if you're doing the laundry, for instance, you may forget all about a boiling tea kettle in the kitchen until the smoke alarm goes off.

"It's just a natural part of aging," Dr. Restak says. "As you get older, it is simply going to take more effort to concentrate on complicated tasks like reading. It doesn't mean you can't do it, you just have to develop some new strategies." Here are a few ideas.

Try This First

Work in short bursts. Take a 5- to 10-minute rest every 30 minutes when you're working on a project. It will help you stay focused, Dr. Restak suggests. "As we get older, marathon work sessions become more difficult," he says. You'll simply need to take more frequent breaks in order to maintain good concentration.

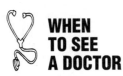

WHEN TO SEE A DOCTOR

Seek medical care if you or others around you notice a significant drop in your attention span or your ability to concentrate, says Richard Restak, M.D., clinical professor of neurology at George Washington University School of Medicine and Health Sciences in Washington, D.C., and co-author of *The Longevity Strategy*. If you find yourself losing track of the sub-plot in a novel or if you discover that filing your income tax suddenly takes you twice as long, don't simply assume that your mind is failing you. A number of correctable medical problems could be interfering with your ability to concentrate, including:

- Hearing loss
- Vision changes
- Poor circulation
- Thyroid diseases
- Severe depression

Other Wise Ways

Do first things first. Do one thing at a time. You're more likely to get distracted if you try to do several things at once, says Michael Chafetz, Ph.D., clinical psychologist in New Orleans and author of *Smart for Life*.

Keep your eye on the prize. Resist the temptation to get distracted. If you're paying bills, for instance, and need to go into another room to get some stamps, do that and immediately go back to your bill paying. If you do find yourself getting distracted while hunting down the stamps, pause, take a deep breath, and ask yourself, "What am I really here for?" Doing that will refocus your attention on what you really need to get done, Dr. Chafetz says. Otherwise, you may still be cleaning out your desk when the post office closes.

Zzzone out. Try to get at least six to eight hours of sleep daily, suggests Laura Slap-Shelton, Ph.D., clinical psychologist with a specialty in neuropsychology at Jeanes Hospital in Philadelphia. When you're tired, you'll have more trouble concentrating. Taking a brief nap in the middle of the day helps some people keep their minds focused on necessary chores and tasks.

Quiet your mind. Meditation is a simple and terrific way to boost your powers of concentration, Dr. Slap-Shelton says. "The mind is a noisy place, talking to itself and responding to all sorts of stimulation in the world around it," she says. "Meditation quiets the mind and can help filter out all the annoying distractions that make concentration difficult."

To try it, sit in a comfortable chair and begin to slowly breathe in for a count of four to eight seconds, allowing your diaphragm to expand fully, Dr. Slap-Shelton says. Hold your breath for several seconds, and then slowly breathe out as much air as you can. To see if you are breathing from your diaphragm, you can rest your hand on your stomach and feel it expand and contract as you practice your breathing. Whenever a distracting thought pops into your mind, just notice it and let it go, and keep your attention on your breathing. If you do this simple exercise twice a day, your ability to concentrate may improve, Dr. Slap-Shelton says.

Light a candle. Guided imagery can help focus your mind, says Elizabeth Ann Barrett, Ph.D., R.N., professor and coordinator of the Center for Nursing Research at Hunter College of the City College of New York in New York City. To try it, close your eyes and breathe out through your mouth and in through your nose. Breathe out long, slow exhalations and breathe in normally, but with shorter inhalations than exhalations. Notice that you are beginning to relax. Breathe in a feeling of confidence that can

MANAGING YOUR MEDS

Any medication that causes drowsiness can dampen concentration, says W. Steven Pray, Ph.D., R.Ph., professor of pharmaceutics at Southwestern Oklahoma State University in Weatherford. In particular, be wary of:

- Over-the-counter sleeping tablets that contain diphenhydramine (Nytol, Unisom)
- Over-the-counter antihistamines with diphenhydramine (Actifed, Benadryl)
- Antipsychotic medications such as risperidone (Risperdal) or haloperidol (Haldol)
- Tranquilizers like hydroxyzine (Atarax, Vistaril)
- Antidepressants such as imipramine (Tofranil)
- Antianxiety medications like diazepam (Valium), chlordiazepoxide (Librium), and other drugs known as benzodiazepines

improve your concentration, and breathe out the fear that you will be distracted.

Now imagine that you are lighting a candle. Focus on the flame and notice that any distracting thoughts cause the flame to flicker, Dr. Barrett says. Concentrate on seeing the flame burn brightly without flickering. Dismiss all distracting thoughts that create flickering. Each time you see a flicker, return to the steadiness of the flame. Notice how you can keep the flame burning brighter for a longer and longer time with fewer and fewer flickers. Keep watching the flame burning brightly. When you feel ready, open your eyes.

Do this exercise three times a day (morning, noon, and evening) for 21 days, Dr. Barrett suggests. After 21 days, the maximum effectiveness through one episode of repetition is over. Take a break to mark that one cycle is over. After seven days, begin again. Ideally, this 21-day cycle of guided imagery will become habit forming.

Clean out the attic. Store just a few bits of information in your head, Dr. Chafetz suggests. The more information you try to keep in your brain, the more distracting thoughts you'll have and the harder it will be to concentrate. So if you haven't done so before, start writing down phone numbers, birthdays, and other facts that you don't need every day.

Play mind games. Give your brain a good workout with chess, checkers, crossword puzzles, or board games like Scrabble at least twice a week, Dr. Chafetz says. These fun, mind-stretching activities can help keep your concentration in tip-top shape.

Poor Smell
and Taste

What do these things have in common?

- A loaf of homemade crusty bread just out of the oven
- A red Mister Lincoln rose, petals unfurling
- A walk in the woods after a spring rain shower
- Your grandchild's freshly bathed and powdered little body in your arms

If your answer is that they all still look and feel great but you can no longer smell them, then welcome to one of the most insidious parts of aging: a decline in the ability to smell and taste.

This change profoundly affects your relationship with food as well as many other sensory delights. When the senses of taste and smell are poor, food becomes less interesting. This often causes you to undereat, setting you up for energy and nutrition deficits. Or you might swing too far the other way, overeating in a misguided effort to find something—anything—that tastes good.

The sense of taste is limited to the perception of four basic taste qualities: sweet, sour, salty, and bitter. Smell is what we perceive with our noses. As you chew food, the vapors of the food will reach the olfactory (smell) receptors through the nasal cavity . The combined experience of taste, smell, texture, and temperature is called flavor.

When you lose the ability to taste food, it's really because your sense of smell is diminished. This is most often caused by a gradual increase in the obstruction of the nasal passages, as with sinus disease or by sudden viral infections such as a common cold or flu, says Miriam Linschoten, Ph.D., research associate at the University of Colorado's Rocky Mountain Taste and Smell Center in Denver.

Loss of taste and smell is more than just an impediment to gas-

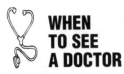

WHEN TO SEE A DOCTOR

tronomic pleasure. A loss of smell can mean that you don't know when something is burning on the stove.

Fortunately, there are some strategies that you can practice to help make eating a pleasurable, sensory experience again. Likewise, there are precautions you can take to ensure that you are safe in your own home.

Try This First

Trigger the trigeminal. The trigeminal nerve does not carry taste or smell information. Through its many branches throughout the nose, mouth, and face, it senses touch, warmth, cold, pain, tickle, and itch.

Take advantage of the trigeminal nerve to give you gustatory sensation by adding a little pepper, horseradish, mustard, or hot sauce to your foods.

"It means you take a mouthful of food and get some sensation from it—as opposed to nothing—and that's a positive thing," says Claire Murphy, Ph.D., professor of psychology at the Smell and Taste Clinic at the University of California, San Diego. "If you add hot peppers, then the food becomes appealing in its own right."

Menthol and mint flavors are also felt by the trigeminal nerve, so adding peppermint to cookies and ice cream and using mint in cooking are also good ideas.

Other Wise Ways

Add a little crunch. How your food feels in your mouth becomes more important when taste and smell diminish. Try to vary the textures of foods at meals. "You want one a little spongy, one a little crispy, one a little crunchy, and one a little chewy so that you can get more variety," says Susan Schiffman, Ph.D., professor of medical psychology at Duke University Medical School in Durham, North Carolina. Add croutons or crispy noodles to salads and soups. Sprinkle some chopped nuts over a main course. Toast bread even if you are eating it with dinner.

Give yourself an eyeful. "If you go into a French restaurant and things are served beautifully, that's so appealing," Dr. Murphy says. Contrast that dining experience with the sight of potatoes and pork or some other light-colored meat and a vegetable like turnips.

MANAGING YOUR MEDS

Many medicines can affect either the sense of smell or the sense of taste, causing what are called reversible taste perversions that can change the taste of your own saliva as well as the taste of the foods you eat.

Often, drugs affect certain parts of your tastebud palette. "You taste grapefruit and all of a sudden it tastes sweet," says Charles Lacy, Pharm.D., drug information specialist at Cedars-Sinai Medical Center in Los Angeles. This change in the way your tastebuds function leads to a perversion of what food used to taste like.

Some of the drugs commonly used by people older than 60 that can warp the senses of taste and smell are:

- Calcium channel blockers (Procardia, Vascor)
- Drugs used for Parkinson's disease (Levodopa, Dopar)
- Psychiatric drugs such as lithium (Lithane) and fluoxetine (Prozac)
- Adrenocorticoids used for nasal allergies and chronic bronchial asthma (Doxycycline)

Over-the-counter drugs such as pseudoephedrine (Sudafed) and aspirin also can affect your sense of taste and smell.

Anything with a high mineral content, including some vitamins, iron tablets, and zinc lozenges for the flu, can alter taste, leading to a metallic flavor in the mouth, Dr. Lacy says.

If your doctor changes your medication to one that impacts your sense of taste and smell less, it may be a while before you experience improvement because the effects of your previous medicine may linger.

Adding diversity to the color of the foods on your plate goes a long way toward making a meal look good. Chef Janos Wilder, who own Janos Restaurant in Tucson, Arizona, says reds, greens, and yellows actually make food more appealing. So instead of having a pale pork chop with mashed potatoes and turnips, try having it with bright red beets, dark green spinach, and multihued wild rice. And then sprinkle on some fresh green herbs such as rosemary and thyme. This not only adds color but also packs an aromatic punch.

Work in contrasts. "The easiest contrast in taste is sweet and sour," says Wilder. But don't limit yourself to contrasts in taste. Serving hot and cold items together, like a dollop of cold salsa on hot soup, Wilder suggests, is a contrast that adds some interest.

Cook in flavorful ways. When certified master chef Ronald De Santis, senior professor at the Culinary Institute of America in Hyde Park, New York, wants to add a flavor punch to food, he thinks about cooking methods. If you're cooking a food by poaching, boiling, or steaming, add herbs, spice seeds, and lemon zest to the water to infuse the food with additional flavor.

Roast and grill foods. These methods of preparation leave a nice browned, carmelized crust on foods that is appealing to the eye. That carmelization and some of the charred flavor found in grilled foods add a further flavor dimension.

Make food the focus. When you sit down to a meal, you want distractions kept to a minimum, says Richard Doty, Ph.D., director of the University of Pennsylvania Smell and Taste Center and professor at the University of Pennsylvania School of Medicine, both in Philadelphia. This means turning off the television and turning on the answering machine. Putting on a little music and lighting a candle makes a meal more of a sensory, leisurely event.

Take a while to thoroughly chew each bite. In addition to making your digestion easier, this little trick helps break down the cells of food and releases more flavor compounds, Dr. Schiffman says.

When serving older people in her own home, Dr. Schiffman likes to keep food covered as she serves it. She puts the plate of food right under the person's nose, then takes the cover off so the first smell is sudden and strong.

Switch-hit around your plate. Imagine walking into a kitchen where bread is being baked. The smell hits you at first, but wait a few minutes, and you won't notice it any longer. It's called adapting out. "That same thing happens when you eat three bites of food in a row," Dr. Schiffman notes. "The first bite is strong. The next bite is a little weaker. The third is weaker yet." To lessen this phenomenon, change from food to food around your plate as you eat.

Pucker up. The sense of smell is usually more compromised than the sense of taste, which detects sweet, sour, salty, and bitter. So eating foods that appeal to these taste groups can ensure that you have a sensory sensation. Because of the high-fat content in sweets and the risks of too much salt in the diet, it's better to stick with appealing to sour and bitter tastes. Doesn't sound appetizing? Beer, seltzer water, coffee, and brussels sprouts are examples of bitter foods that most people have learned to like. Lemons and lemon flavoring, pickles, pickled beets, and pickled eggs are sour foods that you might enjoy. Just know that sour, acidic foods like citrus fruits can eat away at teeth enamel, so it would be a good idea to brush your teeth after consuming them, says Daniel Kurtz, Ph.D., director of the smell and taste disorders clinic at the State University of New York in Syracuse.

Beware of leftovers. "I get quite a few people who lose their senses of smell for one reason or another and then get food poisoning," Dr. Linschoten warns. She suggests that people take freshness dates on foods seriously. Label and date your leftovers. If food has been around for a week or more, just throw it out rather than relying on your sense of smell to tell you if it's still good or not.

Think zinc. A zinc deficiency can affect taste and smell, so taking a zinc supplement may be a good idea, says Laurent Chaix, doctor of naturopathy and supervisor of the teaching clinic at the National College of Naturopathic Medicine in Portland, Oregon.

Also, people who are on dialysis tend to lose zinc, Dr. Kurtz says. Look for a zinc supplement or a multivitamin that provides the Daily Value of 15 milligrams, he suggests. You may also want to discuss with your doctor being tested for a zinc deficiency.

Make sure your dentures fit. Dentures can interfere with eating sensations by covering part of your soft palate and some of the tastebuds there. If your dentures don't fit well, they also could put pressure on and damage the nerves that convey taste information, Dr. Linschoten says. And if dentures aren't kept clean, they are a cause of bacterial growth that could coat your tongue and make the taste receptors harder to reach.

Be honest with yourself and family. If you think you may be having a sensory loss in the taste and smell department, let your family know, says Dr. Doty. You may be able to call on them to sniff out things in your home that you might be unaware of.

Not surprisingly, people who lose their senses of smell fear that others will detect their body odor. "People become insecure because they don't know whether they need a bath or whether they've put on too much perfume," Dr. Linschoten says.

Honesty is also important when you are cooking for others, because you won't be able to tell if a food is seasoned properly, according to Dr. Kurtz. Ask a friend or family member who will be dining with you to be a taste tester.

Invest in detectors. Smelling gas leaks and smoke from a fire becomes more difficult as the sense of smell declines. Buy smoke alarms and change their batteries twice every year. If you have gas appliances, you can use soapy water to check the gas pipes for leaks, says Dr. Linschoten. Every two months, put the soapy water on the gas pipes in your house. If there's a leak, the water mixture will bubble. But, of course, even that's not foolproof. If you can afford it, replace your gas appliances with electric, Dr. Doty advises.

In addition, it would pay to have a carbon monoxide detector ($30 to $50), Dr. Kurtz says. Carbon monoxide is a colorless, odorless gas that can't be detected even when you have a good sense of smell. But it's usually the by-product of a combustion process, and people take action such as identifying the cause or calling the fire department when they smell something burning. If you are unable to smell those combustion fumes, you are at a greater risk of suffering from carbon monoxide poisoning.

If you have a natural gas source in your home or office, it also makes sense to purchase a natural gas detector ($30 to $50) if your sense of smell is impaired.

PROSTATE PROBLEMS

For decades, a man's prostate is as meek as a lamb. But when it roars, watch out. A walnut-size gland that's wrapped around the urinary duct, the prostate has one job: to produce gobs of milky fluid that protects and insulates sperm when they are ejaculated from the penis. But as a man gets older, his mild-mannered prostate can gradually turn into the gland from hell, becoming vulnerable to infection and disease—including cancer—and often swelling to the point where it interferes with urination.

Virtually every man will have a prostate problem of some sort in his lifetime, doctors say. The three most common troublemakers are benign prostatic hyperplasia (BPH), a swelling of the gland; prostatitis, a bacterial infection; and prostate cancer, the most common malignancy among men over 50. But some doctors believe that men can reduce the possibility and impact of these conditions with a few dietary and lifestyle changes. Here's how.

Try This First

Seek herbal relief. Take 80 to 160 milligrams of saw palmetto standardized extract daily, says Thomas Kruzel, a doctor of naturopathy in private practice in Portland, Oregon. Several studies show that the seeds from this tree are effective in treating BPH. Consult with your doctor regularly when taking saw palmetto. In rare cases, people taking this herb have experienced stomach problems.

Other Wise Ways

Make whoopie. Tough medicine, we know, but regular ejaculation keeps your prostate from getting stagnant and inflamed, doctors say.

Go with the flow. Urinate when you feel the urge, doctors say. Don't wait, even if logic may tell you to train your bladder by

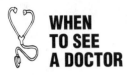

WHEN TO SEE A DOCTOR

holding out as long as you can. Urine from an overly filled bladder can back up into the prostate and irritate it.

Savor tomato sauce. As little as two servings a week of foods made with cooked tomato sauce, such as spaghetti, can help men halve their risk of developing aggressive prostate cancer, says Edward Giovannucci, M.D., assistant professor of medicine and nutrition at Harvard Medical School and Harvard School of Public Health. Tomato sauce contains an antioxidant called lycopene that fights off the cancer.

Drop the fat. A diet high in fatty foods seems to irritate the prostate and increase cancer risk, according to doctors.

The best meals for prostate health are low in fat and cholesterol and big on vegetables, whole grains, leafy greens, and fiber. Foods high in vitamins A, C, and E are particularly healthy for the prostate. Good sources of vitamin A include carrots, squash, and spinach. For vitamin C, load up on citrus fruits and juices, strawberries, and melons. Get your vitamin E from superfortified cereals, wheat germ, and almonds.

Stick with E. Preliminary indications are that this antioxidant helps protect against prostate disease, says Robert Cowles, M.D., a urologist in private practice in Atlanta. He recommends 1,000 international units a day. If you consider taking large amounts of vitamin E, check with your doctor first.

Snap up selenium. This mineral may help stave off prostate disease, Dr. Cowles says. It is still being studied in this regard. He recommends 100 micrograms a day.

RASHES

Lots of things cause rashes—plants, pets, jewelry, rubber, perfume, and fungi, to name a few. And if you've brushed up against poison ivy or developed athlete's foot after using the shower at the local swim club, you know where the rash came from.

Many times, however, a rash seems to appear out of nowhere. When the skin comes in contact with an allergic substance, the reaction is not immediate. A few days may pass before the rash takes hold—though once you have it, the rash can last a week or longer.

One way to figure out the cause is to look at the location. If the rash is caused by an internal trigger like food, medication, or virus, the rash will generally be more widespread and symmetrical. If something external like detergents or poison ivy caused the rash, it will be confined to areas of the skin that were exposed to the irritant, says Patricia Farris Walters, M.D., clinical assistant professor of dermatology at Tulane University School of Medicine in New Orleans.

Although the onset of allergies is less common in seniors, allergies may develop at any age. Plus, if you've recently retired and moved to a new location, you may find yourself exposed to a new allergy problem. And since people over 60 tend to have thinner skin, they can be more sensitive to rashes than ever before, and their skin can be damaged more easily, experts say. Most rashes need to be looked at by a dermatologist if they last longer than two to three days. But meanwhile, you'll want some methods to soothe the irritation, itching, and inflammation. Here they are.

Try This First

Cool with creams. An over-the-counter corticosteroid cream may provide relief from itching, burning, and irritation, says Thomas

453

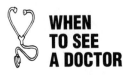

Fisher, M.D., dermatologist in private practice in Chicago. He says that application of 1-percent hydrocortisone applied thinly four times daily should provide some relief.

Or try an antibiotic ointment containing polymyxin bacitracin twice daily with hydrocortisone, Dr. Fisher recommends. Avoid over-the-counter ointments with neomycin, since it can cause allergic reactions.

Other Wise Ways

Cool it. If a rash starts oozing, Dr. Fisher recommends a cool compress with aluminum subacetate—Burrow's solution. You can make Burrow's solution from effervescent tablets that are sold in pharmacies as Domeboro.

To make a compress, soak a clean handkerchief or piece of gauze in Burrow's solution, then place the damp cloth on the affected area for 5 minutes. Repeat this process four times for a total 20-minute session. Do this 20-minute treatment three times daily. Follow each treatment with medicated cream.

Try a hot rinse. The itch of poison ivy can be turned off for extended periods by running hot water over the affected area, says Andrew T. Weil, M.D., director of the program in integrative medicine and clinical professor of internal medicine at the University of Arizona College of Medicine in Tucson. For 5 to 10 minutes, rinse the area with water that's as hot as you can stand without risk of burning yourself, he says. At first, the hot water will increase the itch, but after a few minutes, "the nervous circuits seem to get overloaded and the itching stops for a long time," he says.

Soak in soda. A half-cup of baking soda in a tub full of bathwater makes a rash-relieving soak. "You could also make a paste from a spoonful of baking soda mixed with a bit of water and dab that on your rash to soothe your skin," says Dr. Walters.

Soothe with salves. As an alternative to cortisone, Dr. Weil suggests calendula cream, made from the petals of a marigold-like flower that is prized for its healing effect on skin. Calendula cream is available in health food stores.

Cover with care. Ordinarily, you leave a rash uncovered, says Dr. Walters, but if it's wet, oozing, and blistering, you may want to cover it with a light gauze bandage to prevent an infection.

Take an antihistamine. To reduce swelling and itching, take a nonprescription antihistamine, like diphenhydramine (Benadryl), at bedtime, suggests Andrew P. Lazar, M.D., associate professor of clinical dermatology at Northwestern University Medical School in Chicago. Benadryl may make you drowsy, which can be an added benefit if the itch has been keeping you awake at night, he says. Before taking an antihistamine, however, be sure to check for any interaction with your prescription drugs, cautions Dr. Lazar. Some antihistamines can speed up your heart rate. And if you have an enlarged prostate, an antihistamine might impede urination.

MANAGING YOUR MEDS

If you are taking medication and develop a rash, call your doctor immediately, says Andrew P. Lazar, M.D., associate professor of clinical dermatology at Northwestern University Medical School in Chicago. Some medications, including antibiotics such as tetracycline (Sumycin), can cause an allergic reaction in the form of serious rashes. Your doctor may recommend that you stop taking the drug or switch to something else. Other drugs that can cause rashes are:

- All angiotensin-converting enzyme (ACE) inhibitors, such as captopril (Capoten), which are prescribed for high blood pressure
- All antidepressants, for example, monoamine oxidase (MAO) inhibitors such as tranylcypromine (Parnate)
- Over-the-counter and prescription nonsteroidal anti-inflammatory drugs such as ibuprofen (Advil)

Reading Problems

Since you're reading the words on this page, you have the vision power that it takes, and maybe you can zip along just as fast as you did when you were in your twenties or thirties. But many of us have to slow down. And after awhile, almost without noticing, reading becomes more of a problem.

It helps to accept the fact that your eyesight is less than it was—and, therefore, reading adjustments have to be made. "Your ability to focus deteriorates in a straight line from birth to death, but most people don't notice until their forties," says Joseph Kubacki, M.D., professor and chairman of the ophthalmology department and assistant dean for medical affairs at Temple University School of Medicine in Philadelphia.

You can do a number of things to make your reading environment as easy on your eyes as possible, whether you're reading for pleasure, using your computer, or searching for signs and labels. Here are some ideas.

Try This First

Get a bright light. Aging eyes need more light on the page, which means that the light needs to be brighter, says Pamela R. Oliver, O.D., director of the low-vision rehabilitative service at the Eye Institute at Nova Southeastern University and chairwoman of the low-vision subcommittee of the Florida Optometric Association in Fort Lauderdale, Florida.

The amount of light needed depends on the type of lightbulb as well as on the wattage of the bulb. If you've been using 60-watt bulbs, you might want to continue to use the same wattage but select a different kind of bulb, suggests Eleanor E. Faye, M.D., ophthalmologic consultant to Lighthouse International, a vision rehabilitation organization, and ophthalmologist in New York City. Instead of buying "soft white" or similar bulbs that are for general lighting, look for the bulbs that are "indoor floodlights." Such bulbs don't use more electricity but they provide double the illumination, explains Dr. Faye.

Other Wise Ways

Play with positioning. You'll get the most benefit from a bright light if it's positioned so it shines directly on your page. And the closer the light is to what you're reading, the easier it will be for you to see, says Dr. Oliver. Place your reading light over and behind your shoulder to eliminate shadows, she suggests. Then angle it so it shines directly onto your reading material.

Buy large print. The larger the print, the easier it is to read. In a large-print book, the type is this size rather than this size. You

MANAGING YOUR MEDS

Chances are, your reading problem is not related to any medications you're taking. The following medications, however, may cause blurred vision, which can make reading difficult. It is important to keep in mind that most vision changes are transient, says W. Steven Pray, Ph.D., R.Ph., professor of nonprescription drug products at Southwestern Oklahoma State University in Weatherford.

- Antiarthritis medications such as acetaminophen
- Anti-inflammatory medications such as ibuprofen
- Antidepressants such as amitriptyline (Elavil)
- Ophthalmic drugs used to dilate the pupil of the eye, such as pilocarpine (Isopto Carpine)
- Antibacterial treatment for the eye, such as ciprofloxacin (Cipro)
- Cortinsone-like drugs such as prednisone (Deltasone)
- Medicines that treat severe psoriasis, such as etretinate (Tegison)
- Antibiotics used to treat eye infections, such as norfloxacin (Chibroxin)
- Anticonvulsants such as phenytoin (Dilantin)

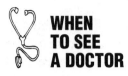

WHEN TO SEE A DOCTOR

Since a whole host of eye diseases could cause reading problems—from cataracts to macular degeneration to glaucoma—you should see an eye doctor any time you notice a change in vision. Also, try to get a checkup eye exam every one to two years.

can get large-print versions of many books, ranging from cookbooks, dictionaries, and the Bible to the latest romance novel. For large-print versions, contact the following organizations: American Bible Society, New York City; American Printing House for the Blind, Louisville, Kentucky; Doubleday Large-Print Home Library, Indianapolis; G. K. Hall and Company, Thorndike, Maine; and the National Association for the Visually Handicapped, New York City.

Get help from cutouts. If you need to read line by line to follow the text, you can make a simple focusing device, suggests Dr. Faye. Cut a thin rectangle in a piece of black construction paper or cardboard. The rectangle should be just as wide and tall as a single line of type. As you're reading, place this paper over the page, allowing just one line of text to show, moving it down line by line as you read.

Raise your computer font. Font refers to the type size. Every word-processing program has easy ways to make the font larger or smaller on the screen. If you use the computer frequently and would like larger-size type on the screen, check your manual or call the toll-free number listed in your manual to find out how to increase the font size. You'll have an easier time reading electronic mail or using a word processing program if you make the font size at least 13 or 14, says Dr. Faye.

Consider a screen change. See if you can change the colors on the computer screen. For easiest reading, choose a black background with yellow or white letters, advises Dr. Faye.

Wear tinted glasses. When trying to read food packages at grocery stores or when trying to read road signs, lightly tinted lenses can eliminate some of the irritating glare, suggests Dr. Faye. These glasses are especially helpful if you have cataracts or another eye condition that makes sign-reading difficult. For the grocery store, choose light amber- or yellow-tinted lenses. For the outdoors, you want polarized gray- or amber-tinted lenses, Dr. Faye says.

Use a big black pen. Whenever you write a note to yourself—a phone number, address, recipe—use a black marker that makes a thick line. Dr. Faye recommends Sharpies, which are available at most hardware or art supply stores.

Mark your medications. Do you have trouble reading the labels on medicine bottles? That can be risky because you can easily get your pills mixed up if you can't make out the small print on the labels. To avoid confusion, mark the bottles clearly with a black marker like a Sharpie, suggests Dr. Faye. For instance, put "BP" on blood pressure medication and "HR" on hormone replacement pills.

Restless Legs
Syndrome

Elizabeth Tunison struggles to sit still as she talks on the telephone in her Whittier, California, home.

"I'm massaging my right leg with my right hand right now. It helps relax my leg muscles a bit and keeps me still for a few moments," she says. "But I'm eventually going to have to get up and move. I can't help it. My legs just don't know how to stop."

Tunison, a retired college professor in her seventies, is one of the estimated 3 percent of Americans—many of them over 60—who have restless legs syndrome (RLS), a condition that causes odd sensations of creeping, crawling, or tingling in the legs. For many, walking provides the only relief. They don't have to walk far to rid themselves of the sensation. A stroll down the hallway or around the living room may be enough. But they often must do it over and over again. Because it usually worsens while lying down, people who have this syndrome seldom sleep well.

Restless legs syndrome typically starts at the onset of sleep, says Wayne Hening, M.D., Ph.D., research neurologist at the University of Medicine and Dentistry at Rutgers University in New Brunswick, New Jersey, and member of the Restless Legs Foundation's medical advisory board. In severe cases, it may be impossible to sleep. Even more unusual are instances where the movements are noticeable enough to wake a person. Typically, the "wiggles" will subside within minutes.

Doctors aren't certain what causes RLS, but it may have a genetic link since the condition tends to run in families, says Ralph Pascualy, M.D., medical director of the Sleep Disorders Center at Providence Medical Center in Seattle. Some researchers also suspect that RLS may be caused by low levels of dopamine, a neurotransmitter in the brain that helps regulate the body's nervous system. In fact, doctors have discovered that drugs like levodopa (Larodopa) and dopamine substitutes like pergolide mesylate (Permax), which are used to treat

Parkinson's disease (also linked to low dopamine levels), can relieve RLS. Pain medications and sedatives, and certain drugs for high blood pressure also can dampen the symptoms. In addition, these natural remedies can help you handcuff this sleep thief.

Try This First

Maintain a regular bedtime. Fatigue aggravates RLS, says Dr. Hening. Getting all of the shut-eye you can is important, particularly if you have a mild case of RLS that only flares up once or twice a month. Hit the sack at the same time each evening, he suggests. Even if you have to get up several times during the night to stretch your legs, a consistent bedtime should help you get an adequate amount of sleep. After all, adds Dr. Hening, a regular bedtime is known to generally promote better sleep, and clinical experience has shown that waiting for fatigue to set in before going to bed may actually worsen the condition.

Other Wise Ways

Splish and splash. Sitting in a warm bath or hot tub for 10 to 15 minutes just before bedtime sometimes helps relieve RLS, Dr. Hening

MANAGING YOUR MEDS

Any drug that reduces or blocks activity of the brain chemical dopamine, responsible for the transmission of nerve impulses, can worsen the symptoms of restless legs syndrome, says Wayne Hening, M.D., Ph.D., research neurologist at the University of Medicine and Dentistry at Rutgers University in New Brunswick, New Jersey, and member of the Restless Legs Foundation's medical advisory board. In particular, be wary of prescription neuroleptic tranquilizers including haloperidol (Haldol) and chlorpromazine (Thorazine). In addition, avoid:

- Alcohol
- Caffeine
- Prescription antinausea drugs containing metoclopramide (Reglan)
- Prescription tricyclic antidepressants such as amitriptylene (Elavil)

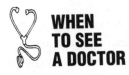

WHEN TO SEE A DOCTOR

See your doctor if:

• You have frequent "crawling" or other types of discomfort in your legs, occurring typically in the evening.

• You feel a overwhelming urge to move your legs or body to relieve the sensations.

• You find that the symptoms get worse in the late afternoon and keep you awake until the wee hours of the morning.

• You notice that the symptoms worsen when you sit or lie down.

says. If you have difficulty getting into a tub, stand in a shower and let the warm water gently pour over your back and legs.

Sleep in. If necessary, sleep in late, suggests Virginia N. Wilson, co-founder of the Restless Legs Syndrome Foundation and author of *Sleep Thief, Restless Legs Syndrome*, a guide to coping with RLS. Because RLS is usually worse at night, many people who have it don't get to sleep until 3:00 or 4:00 A.M. So avoid early-morning appointments because, odds are, you'll be groggy and irritable, she says. Wilson, for instance, usually sleeps until at least 10:00 A.M. and rarely schedules any activities before noon.

Zone out. Some people report that engaging in mentally absorbing games and activities like building jigsaw puzzles or solving logic problems stifles their attacks of RLS, Dr. Hening says. If you find an engaging hobby that requires intense concentration, it may help you control this condition, he says.

Find an aisle land. Ask for an aisle seat in the back of the theater when you attend a play or concert, Wilson suggests. If your legs begin to bother you, you will be able to stand up and walk around without blocking the view of other patrons.

Likewise, ask for an aisle seat when making airplane reservations. Try booking a flight that has one or two stops before your destination, so you can get off the plane and stretch your legs for a few minutes during each layover, Wilson says.

Try to schedule a morning flight, when discomfort is less likely, advises Dr. Hening. He also suggests asking your doctor if medication will help.

ROSACEA

In our youths, we may have loved seeing W. C. Fields perform his film antics. And certainly, his appearance was a big part of his act. His trademark bulbous nose made all his attempts at dignity, valour, and gallantry seem more buffoonish than even he could imagine.

But much as we coveted his wit and humor, few people longed for his nose. In fact, if Fields had been a star when color films began to appear, we might have been more distracted than amused by his sublime proboscis. Because along with the nose, he also sported a red rash and a bevy of broken blood vessels around his cheeks, nose, and chin.

Fields suffered from rosacea, a chronic acnelike condition that can turn your face beet red as blood vessels widen and engorge with blood. And today, long after the demise of the silent-film era, there are still about 13 million Americans who have to deal with the same condition.

Left untreated, rosacea tends to worsen over time and can spread to other parts of the face, including the eyes. With advanced cases, the nose may become red and swollen. On W. C. Fields, it was funny. But it's no laughing matter when it happens to you.

Unfortunately, rosacea cannot be cured and it rarely reverses itself. While the condition will get worse without medical treatment, patients who follow a treatment plan prescribed by a dermatologist can successfully control rosacea and even see marked improvement. These tips can also help.

Try This First

Fight flushing. Facial flushing, caused by the dilation of blood vessels, is the trigger mechanism for rosacea, says Mary P. Lupo, M.D., associate clinical professor of dermatology at Tulane Uni-

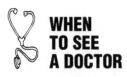

versity School of Medicine in New Orleans. So simply avoid anything that makes your face flush.

The top five flushing triggers are emotional stress, heat, humidity, spicy foods, and alcohol, Dr. Lupo says. Other triggers include activities that get you sweating, hot beverages, and sunlight. And certain foods, like chocolate, can bring it on.

But what bothers one person may not cause a problem in another. You need to pinpoint your personal flushing trip wires, according to the National Rosacea Society, then change your habits to avoid them.

Other Wise Ways

Apply a cold compress. When the flush hits, soak a washcloth in ice-cold water (or equal parts cold milk and ice water) and hold it on the affected area, recommends K. William Kitzmiller, M.D., dermatologist in private practice in Cincinnati. The cold will cause dilated blood vessels to constrict and will halt the inflammatory process, he explains. Apply for 10 minutes three times a day, as needed.

Reduce stress. Stress ranks high on the trigger list of many people with rosacea. What's the best way to reduce stress? Dr. Kitzmiller recommends the tried-and-true approach: regular healthy meals and snacks, reduced caffeine, regular exercise, and eight hours of sleep.

When you're feeling stressed, try deep-breathing exercises, he says. Inhale and count to 10, then exhale and count to 10. Repeat this exercise several times.

Cleanse with care. It is important not to use abrasives or astringents, says Dr. Lupo. She recommends extraordinarily gentle liquid cleansers, such as Cetaphil, that contain sodium lauryl sulfate. This ingredient cleans skin without any stimulation that might cause flushing. You can wash your face up to two or three times a day, but always use cool water, Dr. Lupo cautions.

Avoid products that contain alcohol or irritants. For a gentle wipe, you can combine one tablespoon of chilled witch hazel with one pint of chilled water, Dr. Lupo says.

Make for shade. "Stay out of the sun. Period," warns Dr. Lupo. "The sun will only set off a flare-up," she says, and no amount of sunscreen will prevent it. This is because sun exposure heats your skin, which dilates capillaries and leads to flushing, she says.

Of course, there are times when you have to cross the sun's path, and even in the shade you're exposed to indirect sunlight, Dr. Lupo

MANAGING YOUR MEDS

Certain drugs can cause facial flushing, resulting in rosacea flare-ups. Vasodilators, used in the treatment of cardiovascular and circulatory diseases, can worsen rosacea because they dilate blood vessels, says Mary P. Lupo, M.D., associate clinical professor of dermatology at Tulane University School of Medicine in New Orleans. Although you can ask your doctor to adjust the dosage, you should realize that you'll need to discuss the drawbacks and benefits of going off medication, says Dr. Lupo. If you have a circulatory problem, for instance, you may need the medication to maintain healthy blood flow to your limbs— even though you may not like what it does to the appearance of your nose or cheeks. So there's definitely a trade-off. "It's better to have rosacea than to lose your foot to poor circulation," says Dr. Lupo.

Also, long-term use of topical steroids, such as prescription-strength and over-the-counter hydrocortisone creams often used for rashes or itchy skin, has been found to aggravate rosacea or induce rosacea-like symptoms, says Dr. Lupo.

notes. She suggests using a sunscreen containing titanium dioxide, such as Neutrogena Sensitive Skin Sunblock. Unlike sunscreens made with other chemicals, titanium dioxide does not irritate rosacea-prone skin.

Drink with care. Alcohol dilates blood vessels, so it often induces flare-ups in people with rosacea. Monitor how your rosacea reacts to alcoholic beverages. If it aggravates your condition, reduce your intake or avoid alcohol entirely, advises Dr. Lupo.

Try chamomile. Chamomile is an herbal remedy that may soothe rosacea-ravaged skin, says Dr. Lupo. Steep a handful of pure chamomile or several chamomile tea bags in three cups of boiling water for 10 minutes, she says, then strain the liquid and put it in the refrigerator. When you need a cold compress treatment, dip a cotton cloth in the chamomile and apply it to the affected area until you feel relief.

SCARS

Like broken hearts and taxes, scars are an inevitable part of living. Some see them as unsightly marks on otherwise beautiful skin, while others view them as symbols of a life fully lived. Either way, they're with you for keeps, though they will tend to fade like the memories they represent.

A scar results when the skin repairs itself after being injured from an accident, illness, or surgery. Scarring is just a natural part of your body's healing process.

One of the little blessings of growing older is that when you get new scars, they're apt to be thinner and smaller than those that younger people get. Researchers says that young skin repairs itself rapidly and tends to overheal, producing thicker, larger, more unsightly scars.

In general, wounds on tighter skin produce more prominent scars. If you get nicked along your jawline, for instance, the scar may be easy to see. Scars on looser skin tend to be more difficult to make out.

The worst scars arise from wounds that penetrate below the surface layer of the skin and into the deeper layer called the dermis. Picking at a pimple or scratching at an itchy chicken pox lesion can lead to scarring of the dermis, which is why so many of these scars last a lifetime.

Depending on the severity of the wound, it usually takes a scar at least three months to dim. On the other hand, no scar fully disappears. The scar's color, or pigmentation, usually remains somewhat different from the surrounding tissue, though the difference in color can be hidden with makeup.

There are two ways to approach a scar. The first is to do all you can to minimize it in the wound-healing phase, and the second, to shrink it after it arises.

Try This First

Keep it clean. An infected wound is more likely to form a scar, says Frederic Haberman, M.D., assistant clinical professor of medicine (dermatology) at Albert Einstein College of Medicine in New York City and director of the Haberman Dermatology Institute in Ridgewood, New Jersey. Clean the wound thoroughly each day with soap and water and then apply some form of antibiotic ointment, recommends Dr. Haberman.

Other Wise Ways

Keep it moist. "A wound heals more effectively if it is kept moist, as opposed to keeping it exposed to the air and allowing it to dry," says Larry Millikan, M.D., chairman of the department of dermatology at Tulane University Medical College in New Orleans. "If the skin is moist, you're optimizing the environment for healing and for promoting healthy skin to grow over the wound. You can also cut the healing time in half."

Any of a variety of topical ointments, some of which contain mild antibiotics, are excellent for keeping the skin moist and promoting healing, Dr. Millikan says.

But if your medicine chest is out, apply petroleum jelly and even cooking fat, such as vegetable shortening, to the wound, says Dr. Haberman. Both will keep the wound moist and promote healing.

Keep it still. As much as possible, keep the injured skin immobilized because moving or rubbing increases the chances that the scar will become large and prominent, suggests Dr. Millikan. "The more you stretch or pull at tissue that's been injured, the more you interfere with the healing process, which increases the likelihood of a scar forming," he says. "The same goes for any friction you expose the wound to. Try to protect the cut from any type of trauma that would reinjure the wound."

Apply a moisturizer. Once a scar arises, you can still shrink the amount of scar tissue and its appearance by moisturizing the scar, says Dr. Haberman. "There are over-the-counter dressings that contain silicone or a silicone derivative that can be applied directly over the scar," he says. "These can be worn overnight and are effective at reducing the size of the scar. They literally can shrink the scar tissue."

Give it a good massage. After you have moisturized the scar, gently massage the tissue in circles, first clockwise, then counterclockwise, and then across, Dr. Haberman recommends. This will promote blood flow to the area and help to soften and break down the old scar tissue, promoting the growth of new and healthy tissue in its place.

Try Mederma. For decades, Europeans have used a product called Mederma, which is a combination of herbs that you apply directly over the scar. "We have seen improvements in patients with elevated scar tissue who have used this product," says Dr. Millikan. "It's a plant-based formula and you can get it over the counter. It promotes healing and reduces scar tissue." If your pharmacy doesn't keep Mederma in stock, ask your pharmacist to order it for you. Follow package directions for usage.

Reach for a multi. The antioxidants vitamins C and E and beta-carotene, and the mineral zinc all boost the immune system and promote healing, Dr. Haberman says. Use a multivitamin that contains 500 to 1,000 milligrams of vitamin C, 200 to 400 international units (IU) of vitamin E, and up to 2,000 IU of beta-carotene, Dr. Haberman recommends. As for zinc, take 15 milligrams, which is a safe and immune-boosting dose. Although vitamin E is generally sold in doses of 400 IU, one small study showed a possible risk of stroke in dosages higher than 200 IU. Consult with your doctor if you are at high risk for stroke.

Block those rays. Scars have very few pigmentation cells, says Dr. Millikan, which means they do not change color as much as normal skin does when exposed to the sun. This, of course, makes them more visible every time you get sunburned. Use a sunscreen with a sun protection factor of at least 15 to block sun and reduce the differences in color between your normal skin and scar tissue.

SCIATICA

If you've ever run a vacuum, cared for children, or tossed a few baseballs in the school yard, you've probably experienced a lower-back ache or two. Most people do.

But sometimes, lower-back pain isn't confined to the spine. It radiates, producing shooting pain or numbness into your buttocks and down your leg, below your knee, even into your foot and toes. When it does, you may be experiencing sciatica.

Sciatica is no respecter of circumstances, which is why its onset usually comes as a complete surprise. Maybe you've been weeding in the garden. As you rise to your feet, you suddenly feel as though someone has shot darts at your leg. Or perhaps you've been relaxing for an evening in your favorite reading chair with a cup of tea in one hand and a new novel in the other. But when you get up to refill that teacup, your lower-back pinches and your foot feels tingly. Either scenario portrays the beginnings of sciatica.

If you have sciatica, your symptoms are caused by irritation of the nerve that runs across your buttocks and into your thigh, calf, and foot, says John E. Thomassy, D.C., chiropractor in private practice in Virginia Beach, Virginia.

Sometimes, the rubbery disks between the back bones, or vertebrae, bulge and then press on a nerve root. This bulge may be referred to as a herniated, or slipped, disk. Poor posture, improper technique when lifting, and injuries may be contributing factors in this condition.

Over time, the disks experience more wear and tear. So by the time you reach retirement age, they're eager for some kid-glove treatment. As wear and tear catches up with you during your senior citizen years, the disks become compressed, vertebrae grow bony spurs, and nerve irritation becomes more likely, explains Dr. Thomassy.

The discomfort may be worse when you sit, and the pain in your leg or knee may be more severe than the one in your back, says Steven Mandel, M.D., clinical professor of neurology at Thomas Jefferson University Hospital in Philadelphia.

Forty percent of people will experience sciatica some time in their lives. For most, the pain will subside on its own, often within one month, says Dr. Mandel.

As a rule, anytime you have back pain for more than two to three days, you should see your doctor to rule out serious illness or injury, suggests Sheila Reid, therapy coordinator at the Spine Institute of New England in Williston, Vermont. But once your doctor rules out other things and positively identifies sciatica, here are some ways to find relief and help prevent future attacks.

Try This First

Get a chill. To help reduce pain and swelling, apply ice where you feel sciatica pain, Reid says. To protect your skin, place a towel between your back and the ice pack. Ice may be used for 15 to 20 minutes every hour. Or switch to the warmth of a heating pad, shower, or bath, she says. Heat relaxes muscles.

MANAGING YOUR MEDS

Although it's very rare, one drug may cause sciatica, says W. Steven Pray, Ph.D., R.Ph., professor of nonprescription drug products at Southwestern Oklahoma State University in Weatherford. Talk with your doctor or pharmacist if you experience sciatic pain while taking Zolpidem (Ambien), which is prescribed for insomnia.

To help with your sciatica pain, your doctor may recommend that you take acetaminophen, asprin, or nonsteroidal anti-inflammatory drugs (NSAIDs) such as ibuprofen. These types of medicine may interact with other drugs. Make sure to tell your doctor about any drugs that you are taking.

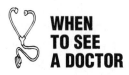

If you have shooting pains down your legs, don't just assume you have sciatica, says Steven Mandel, M.D., clinical professor of neurology at Thomas Jefferson University Hospital in Philadelphia. Any time back pain is accompanied by radiating, burning, or tingling, see your doctor. Several conditions can cause that kind of pain, including stroke, diabetes, and vitamin B$_{12}$ deficiency. It could even be caused by osteoarthritis, which afflicts more of us as we get older. Or you may have a fracture caused by osteoporosis (thinning bones). Since there are so many possible explanations, it's best to let a doctor determine what the problem is, says Dr. Mandel.

Other Wise Ways

Please sit up. Prolonged sitting may aggravate your discomfort because it reverses the normal curve in your back, Dr. Thomassy says. Sitting may compress disks and weaken lower-back ligaments and muscles. When you sit, maintain good posture. Don't slouch. Keep your knees level with your hips, your feet flat on the floor, and your back straight.

Get the angles right. If you are working at a desk or computer, adjust your chair so your elbows can be positioned at a 90-degree angle, with your forearms parallel to the floor, advises Dr. Thomassy. Tuck a small pillow behind your back to help you sit up straight and promote the normal curves in your spine.

Break things up. Take frequent breaks when you're working, Reid says. Get up and walk around every half-hour. If you're traveling in a car, avoid prolonged time behind the wheel or even in the passenger seat. Make frequent rest stops at least every hour or so.

Reach over the counter. Nonprescription pain relievers such as acetaminophen, ibuprofen, or naproxen may help relieve temporary discomfort, Dr. Mandel says. But be sure to ask your physician first. Even over-the-counter medicines can have side effects.

Step right down. Wear comfortable, low-heeled shoes, Dr. Thomassy urges. Heels that are higher than 1 to 1½ inches push your body weight forward and your spine out of alignment.

Get some Z. Try the Z position, suggests Augustus A. White III, M.D., professor of orthopaedics surgery at Harvard Medical

School, in the booklet "Back Care: How to Relieve and Prevent Pain from Low Back Problems."

Lie on your back on a rug or exercise cushion with your knees bent and your feet propped on a low table or chair. Your thighs should be nearly parallel to the floor. To get more comfortable, put a thin cushion under your buttocks and a pillow under your head. Then relax.

This relaxing position often provides quick relief, writes Dr. White.

Stretch it out. For sciatica pain, try this stretch from Dr. White. Stand with your feet apart and your hands on your buttocks. Push your hips forward and gently bend backward while looking up. Keep your knees straight. Hold for several seconds, relax, and repeat. You can do this several times a day, and it's especially helpful after sitting.

Lift safely. Even if your back feels better after an episode of back pain, you'll need to lift correctly to prevent a relapse. "Lifting is when most people are injured," Dr. Thomassy says. Whether you're lifting a laundry basket or toolbox, make sure your feet are square to the object, then crouch with your knees and hips bent and your back straight. Bring the object close to your body and when you rise, continue to keep your back straight. If you have to twist, bend forward, or reach out for an object, take the time to get into the proper position before you try lifting.If that's not possible, get help.

Sleep sideways. If you want to minimize or stave off back pain and sciatica, don't sleep on your stomach, Dr. Thomassy cautions. Instead, lie on your side, curl your legs, and slip a pillow between your knees. Or go belly-up with a pillow or rolled towel under your knees. If you like to sleep with a pillow under your head, don't strain your neck with a big one. Instead, use a smaller one that keeps your head and neck in line with your upper back.

Get around. Stay as active as you can while you're recovering from sciatica, even if you only walk around the house, Reid says.

After pain subsides, try gentle stretches and, later, mild aerobic exercise, Dr. Mandel suggests. Swimming and walking, for example, will help strengthen and condition your back and whole body. They may even make you less vulnerable to injury. "If people stretch and exercise," Dr. Mandel says, "they will reduce their chances of having back problems."

SHINGLES

If you had chicken pox as a child, you probably thought the virus that caused that itchy, blistering rash was gone for good. While it's true that you won't get chicken pox again, you may get its relative herpes zoster, or shingles.

The virus that causes both chicken pox and shingles hides in the nervous system of anyone who's had chicken pox, which is the majority of American adults. About 20 percent of us also will get shingles later in life. When that happens, the virus awakens with a vengeance, producing an oozing, blistering short-lived rash, and pain that can linger for months or years, long after the skin itself heals, says Karl R. Beutner, M.D., Ph.D., associate clinical professor and researcher in the department of dermatology at the University of California, San Francisco.

It is not known what causes the virus to reawaken. Stress, poor nutrition, and another illness may be triggers. "Attacks tend to occur during times of great stress," says Richard P. Huemer, M.D., holistic practitioner in Lancaster, California.

As the years roll by, your chances of shingles roll upward. Shingles is most common in people over 50, and about half of people over 80 will get the illness.

This condition is a trickster. The burning and stabbing pain often precedes the rash by one to three days, so many people don't realize the two are connected, Dr. Beutner says. Other early symptoms may include tingling, extreme sensitivity, or a dull ache on one side of the body, usually the trunk, buttock, or thigh. You may have fever, headache, or other flulike symptoms. If you have these symptoms, see a doctor right away. With a prompt diagnosis, you have the advantage of an opportunity for early treatment.

The rash occurs in the same area as the pain and quickly turns into pus-filled blisters that look much like the chicken pox you tried so hard to forget. The blisters themselves aren't painful, Dr. Beutner says. Although they may occasionally scar the skin, the blisters crust over and fade in about two to three weeks.

The pain, which emanates from nerve bundles, may not fade nearly as fast. In people over 60, symptoms may be more pronounced or prolonged. What's more, the pain can be severe enough to disrupt sleep and daily activities.

If you have symptoms of shingles, you need to see a doctor. But while you're at home, here are some additional ways you can keep discomfort at bay or even prevent shingles from paying you an unwelcome visit.

Try This First

Stay dry. You can't do a lot to get rid of the shingles rash; it must run its course. But you can help dry the oozing blisters, Dr. Beutner says. Apply calamine lotion or use Burrow's solution made from Domeboro tablets, both available in drugstores. As the wet solutions evaporate from your skin, they also steal moisture from the blisters.

Other Wise Ways

Say "aloe-ahhh." The thin milky liquid inside the leaves of the aloe vera plant may help soothe the blisters, Dr. Huemer says. If you have an aloe houseplant, cut a leaf and smooth the liquid over

MANAGING YOUR MEDS

Oral corticosteroids such as prednisone (Deltasone), taken for certain types of arthritis, allergies, and skin conditions, may weaken the immune system, causing shingles to appear, says W. Steven Pray, Ph.D., R.Ph., professor of nonprescription drug products at Southwestern Oklahoma State University in Weatherford. Using a nonprescription topical steroid such as hydrocortisone (Cortaid) on an area of skin affected by shingles could cause the lesions to spread further and last longer.

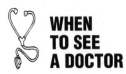

If you think you have shingles, you really need to see a doctor, says Karl R. Beutner, M.D., Ph.D., associate clinical professor and researcher in the department of dermatology at the University of California, San Francisco. Your doctor can determine if you have it by assessing the nature of your pain and the appearance of any rash. He can also give you an antiviral medicine that may reduce the length of your outbreak. The medicine is most potent if given early on, often before that telltale rash appears, Dr. Beutner says.

your skin. Or try an over-the-counter aloe lotion.

Get into a lather. Wash your hands regularly, Dr. Beutner says, especially if you have an oozing rash from shingles. The blisters contain varicella virus, so you could unknowingly infect someone with chicken pox. You also can cover the blisters with an antibiotic ointment, such as Polysporin, and wrap the area with gauze.

Pull the reins on pain. With your physician's okay, reach for acetaminophen or another mild over-the-counter pain reliever such as ibuprofen, Dr. Beutner says. Your doctor can prescribe stronger medicine for more serious discomfort.

Pack some heat. If your pain remains after the rash, you can smooth a capsaicin cream on the affected area three or four times a day, Dr. Beutner says. But be sure you have no more rash. Capsaicin cream is made from the extract of hot pepper. "On an open rash, it really hurts," he says. Capsaicin cream usually begins to work within two to four weeks, but it must be applied three or four times a day, every day. If the product is not used in this way, pain may recur in a few days or weeks. When you first apply capsaicin cream, you may feel a burning sensation on your skin, which should subside within a few weeks.

Take care of you. Because stress is a factor in developing shingles, relaxation is important. "Pace yourself," Dr. Beutner says. Stop and put your feet up or take an afternoon nap, especially if you don't feel well. "People should listen to their bodies and rest when they feel tired," he says.

Since the pain of shingles can interrupt your normal night's sleep, try to make up for lost rest at other times during the day, Dr. Beutner says. Getting plenty of rest will keep you healthier overall and may help you mend more quickly.

Eat to your health. "Probably the best prevention is a healthy lifestyle and immune system," Dr. Huemer says. Poor nutrition contributes to weakened immunity. The American Dietetic Association recommends eating at least five vegetables and fruits daily, along with an array of whole grains, dairy products, lean meats and fish, and small amounts of fat.

Look to lysine. Your diet also should include an amino acid called lysine, says Dr. Huemer. This amino acid, which prevents viruses from growing and spreading, may bring your bout with shingles to a quicker end. You can boost your lysine intake by drinking milk and eating potatoes and chicken. They are good sources of lysine, Dr. Huemer says.

It's hard to get enough lysine to prevent shingles outbreaks through diet alone. Luckily, lysine also is sold at stores. Take 500 to 1,000 milligrams three times a day during an outbreak, Dr. Huemer says. For prevention, use 1,000 milligrams a day.

Do Bs and more Bs. Vitamin B_{12} can boost your immune system and help you fight a shingles outbreak, Dr. Huemer says. A daily 500 microgram sublingual lozenge, which melts under your tongue, probably is worth trying, he says.

Bring in some big doses. For super-immunity during an outbreak, Dr. Huemer recommends a daily regimen of:

- 10,000 international units (IU) vitamin A
- 10,000 milligrams vitamin C
- 800 IU vitamin E
- 50 milligrams B complex
- 100 to 200 milligrams pantothenic acid
- 25,000 IU beta-carotene
- 200 micrograms selenium
- 60 milligrams coenzyme Q_{10}
- 25 milligrams zinc

Since most of these doses are way over the Daily Values for these nutrients, and supplements may cause problems at these high levels, these supplement levels should be monitored by a doctor. High doses of vitamin C, for example, can cause diarrhea in some people. Also, although vitamin E is generally sold in doses of 400 IU, one small study showed a possible risk of stroke in dosages higher than 200 IU. Consult with your doctor if you are at high risk for stroke.

See something completely different. When you're in pain, it's easy to wonder if it will ever go away, says Emmett Miller, M.D., mind-body specialist and author in Nevada City, California. That can make your perception of the pain worse, he says. Dr. Miller teaches patients to use visualization to see and feel their pain differently.

First, take a deep breath and relax as you slowly let it out. Close your eyes and allow an image that represents your pain to arise in your mind. Is it hot or cold? Is it moving? What color is it? Perhaps you see a twisting red-hot poker, Dr. Miller says.

Now, create a parallel image of something that would remove that object's harmful quality, and put it to use. You might picture a fire hose extinguishing the hot poker, or an Eskimo with a bucket of snow, Dr. Miller says. If you can learn to transform your mental image of pain, he says, you may feel less affected by it physically.

SLEEP INTERRUPTIONS

Ah, the beauty of great architecture. The Guggenheim, Versailles, the Great Pyramid of Cheops. Your nightly sleep. Yes, your nightly sleep. It has what sleep specialists like to call an architecture. But instead of a static architecture like that of a building, your sleep architecture is an active structure that refreshes your mind and body.

That is, it's refreshing if the next-door neighbor's Schnauzer, Pinkie, doesn't wake you up at 3:00 in the morning with a howl. Or if that late-night cocktail catches up with you, forcing a nocturnal visit to the bathroom. You see, in addition to being a thing of beauty, the architecture of your sleep can turn into a house of cards—particularly as you age.

"I've turned into such a light sleeper" is a common complaint of many older people. And it's quite true that older people catch less deep sleep, particularly the most restful and restorative kind, says Patricia Prinz, Ph.D., professor of behavioral nursing and adjunct professor of psychiatry and behavior sciences at the University of Washington in Seattle. As a result, you may find that you wake up a lot more easily than you used to. And once awake, you may find that it's devilishly hard to nod off again.

But why does this happen more to older people? Well, for one thing, the older you are, the more likely it is that you'll have some medical disorders, such as arthritis, restless legs, or heartburn. If you have pain or discomfort during the night, you're just more likely to wake up, says Dr. Prinz.

Of course, loud snoring or apnea could be your nocturnal wake-up call, so check the chapters about those conditions. And if you just can't fall asleep, that's an insomnia problem, which is also another chapter. But if you want to head off other disturbances that are short-changing your hours of rest, read on.

479

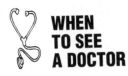

WHEN TO SEE A DOCTOR

If interruptions in your sleep leave you so fatigued that you have a hard time making it through the day, talk to your doctor.

Also, if you've been snoring and gasping in your sleep, consult a sleep specialist to see if you have sleep apnea. Sleep apnea is a condition where you stop breathing for brief periods, then wake yourself as you struggle to catch your breath. Waking with a headache or being tired during the day are tip-offs that you may have sleep apnea, says Patricia Prinz, Ph.D., professor of behavioral nursing and adjunct professor of psychiatry and behavior sciences at the University of Washington in Seattle. Sleep apnea can affect your blood pressure and heart health, which is all the more reason to see a doctor about it.

Try This First

Tire yourself out. Daily physical activity not only helps make you tired enough to sleep, but it can improve sleep itself, states Margaret Moline, Ph.D., director of the sleep-wake disorders center at the New York Presbyterian Hospital–Cornell Medical Center in White Plains, New York. People who are more physically fit generally have more deep sleep.

Get out and walk during the late afternoon, and you'll be less likely to wake up in the middle of the night, says Phyllis Zee, M.D., Ph.D., director of the sleep disorders center and associate professor of neurology at Northwestern University Medical School in Chicago.

Other Wise Ways

Sleep and rise at the same time. The regular pattern that helps prevent insomnia can also help ensure uninterrupted sleep. Put your body on a regular schedule, says Dr. Prinz.

Black out your room. You need to have a dark, quiet place to sleep, says Sonia Ancoli-Israel, Ph.D., director of the sleep disorders clinic at the Veteran's Affairs Health Care System in San Diego, professor of psychiatry at the University of California, San Diego, and author of *All I Want Is a Good Night's Sleep*. In darkness, our bodies secrete melatonin, which makes us sleepy, explains Dr. Ancoli-Israel. Be sure to cover the windows with dark blinds or drapes. To a light sleeper, the dawn's early light can be as wakeful as an alarm clock.

Quiet your restless legs. Older people may suffer from restless legs and periodic leg movements during sleep. These movements may be associated with vitamin deficiencies, anemia, thyroid disease, or peripheral nerve disorders. If you or your bed partner jerks a leg even a little, that can interrupt your sleep. When you have leg movements, get up and walk around, or massage your legs lightly to bring some relief, Dr. Zee says. For severe cases, doctors can prescribe medications to relieve restless legs.

Take some iron or folate. A lack of each of these nutrients can contribute to increased leg kicks in the night, says Peter Hauri, M.D., co-director of the Mayo Clinic Sleep Disorders Center in Rochester, Minnesota, and author of *No More Sleepless Nights*. Try an iron and folate supplement for two weeks and see if that one-two combination helps you sleep through the night. If it does, see your doctor to discuss your condition and long-term treatment.

Cut down on caffeine. Even if you are able to drowse off, too much caffeine can contribute to a light-sleep pattern. If you drink coffee, tea, or caffeinated sodas throughout the day, try to cut back to two servings before noon and none thereafter. If that doesn't work, you may have to avoid caffeine altogether, Dr. Hauri advises.

MANAGING YOUR MEDS

According to Peter Hauri, M.D., co-director of the Mayo Clinic Sleep Disorders Center in Rochester, Minnesota, and author of *No More Sleepless Nights*, anything that has a stimulating effect can disrupt sleep, including:

- Alcohol
- Nicotine
- Caffeine
- Bronchodilator drugs for asthma, bronchitis, and emphysema, such as albuterol (Proventil) or metaproterenol (Alupent)
- Some antidepressants, such as fluoxetine (Prozac) or venlafaxine (Effexor)
- Diuretics taken for heart conditions and other health problems, which increase your need to urinate at night

Make your nightcap nonalcoholic. Alcohol may initially sedate you, but after your body processes it, the alcohol can actually stimulate you enough to wake you up, Dr. Moline says. Try not to drink any alcohol in the evening.

Try pain relief. Chronic pain from conditions such as rheumatoid arthritis can disrupt sleep, so don't forget to ask your doctor for recommendations on which pain relievers to take before going to bed, advises Lauren Broch, Ph.D., director of education and training at the sleep-wake disorders center at New York Hospital–Cornell Medical Center in White Plains, New York. Or see other chapters in this book about relieving specific kinds of pain, and use some of those remedies for relief before you turn in.

Beat the heat. A cool room is more conducive to sleeping than a hot one. To stay cool, Suzanne Woodward, Ph.D., clinical director of sleep research and assistant professor of psychiatry at Wayne State University School of Medicine in Detroit, recommends that you wear cotton nightwear and sleep between cotton sheets and covers. It's also a good idea to take a cool bath or shower before bedtime—and keep some chipped ice or ice water near the bed to cool you down when you wake up. Even in winter, use a fan to keep the air circulating around your face and neck. Or stick your feet out of the blankets to help stay cooler.

Breathe deeply. Slow abdominal breathing is a relaxation technique that can help minimize a hot flash during the day, but it can also help a woman in the middle of the night if she is awakened by one. Men who are light sleepers are also helped by this technique, Dr. Woodward says. This type of breathing exercise increases your intake of oxygen and gives you something to focus on other than the fact that you are awake.

Concentrate on breathing regularly but a little more slowly, at a pace of 8 to 10 breaths a minute. When you breathe in, feel your abdomen rise, not your chest. To test if you are doing it correctly, place a hand on your chest and a hand on your stomach. It's the hand on your stomach that should be rising and falling, explains Dr. Woodward.

Hydrate early in the day. Seniors are no different than other age groups when it comes to needing eight, eight-ounce glasses of water a day. But because men often have prostate problems as they age, a drink of water too close to bedtime can mean that you have to get up repeatedly in the night. Try to drink more liquids early in the day, Dr. Zee advises. She recommends that you stop drinking two to three hours before bedtime and then urinate right before you go to bed.

Flummox reflux. The older you get, the more likely you are to be awakened by symptoms of heartburn or gastroesophogeal reflux. Eat a light dinner, and avoid caffeine, alcohol, smoking, and an after-dinner mint—all the things that can make reflux worse, advises Roger L. Gebhard, M.D., gastroenterologist at the Veterans Affairs Medical Center and professor of medicine in the division of gastroenterology at the University of Minnesota, both in Minneapolis. Or prop up the head of your bed to raise your head and chest a little higher than your stomach, he suggests. If you put the legs at the head of your bed on six-inch blocks, that may be enough to help hold off heartburn through the night.

SLOWED
REACTION TIME

Her slap shot doesn't zing off the stick anymore. She can't skate as fast as she once did. But Mickey Walker, a woman in her eighties, is still in the game. She believes that age is only a number and that seniors should think young and stay active. "We don't have to get old," she says.

"I've been playing hockey since the 1920s, and I'm still a good enough skater and stick handler to play recreational hockey every Monday night with people half my age and younger," says Walker, the oldest registered female hockey player in Canada. "I just love this game."

In a game that requires quick feet, quick thinking, and quick reactions, she is still swift enough to play—and win. "My reflexes are still real fast, and hockey has helped keep them that way," says Walker, who plays center for Mickey's Mares of Bala, Ontario. "I can take a deck of cards, put the edge of the cards over the edge of a table, tip them up, and catch them in mid-air. That's how fast my reflexes still are."

Okay, Mickey Walker is an extraordinary woman. But her nimbleness is well within the reach of all of us, says Charles Richman, Ph.D., professor of psychology and director of the martial arts program at Wake Forest University in Winston-Salem, North Carolina.

Granted, Mickey has maintained her physical and mental abilities through an inordinate amount of practice and exercise. "But I presume that anyone can do that. We all have the capability to slow down the processes that diminish reaction time as we age," Dr. Richman says.

In a sense, almost everything we do is a reaction. If you feel cold, you grab a blanket. If you see a pot boiling over, you instinctively reach for it. But as you age, your sensory organs—eyes, ears, nose, mouth, and skin—that help your brain stay in touch with the outside world all gradually wear down. Eyesight dims, hearing fades, smells and tastes become less distinct, and your sense of touch becomes less refined.

Meanwhile, the nerves that relay this sensory information to your brain and activate your muscles to get you moving become less efficient. As a result, it takes you longer to gather and process information about the world around you and then react to it, says Augustine DiGiovanna, Ph.D., author of *Human Aging: Biological Perspectives* and professor of biology at Salisbury State University in Maryland.

Even when we're in peak condition, reaction time slows about 6 percent every 10 years, starting at about age 30, Dr. Richman says. So by the time you get to age 80, even if you are in terrific health like Mickey Walker, you've lost about 30 percent of your ability to react quickly.

"As we get older, we become less competitive and stop doing the very things—like exercising and eating well—that would help us maintain good reaction time," Dr. Richman says. "We become grandmothers and grandfathers. The problem is that we assume our time is over. We sit back and allow whatever happens to happen. We shouldn't. We are still able to make things happen."

But even grandparents can have better than average reaction times for their ages, says Harry Jaffe, M.D., professor of internal medicine at Northwestern University Medical School in Chicago. Here are a few ways to keep your reflexes in tip-top condition.

Try This First

Keep your motor running. Swimming, walking, stretching, and other forms of exercise are probably the best ways to slash your reaction time, Dr. Jaffe says.

"The better conditioned you are, the better your muscles are going to work, and the better your reaction time will be, Dr. Jaffe says. "It's hard to ask a muscle to do something quickly if you've been sitting in a chair for 15 years."

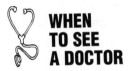

WHEN TO SEE A DOCTOR

Seek immediate medical care if you notice that one side of your body is reacting much more slowly than the other, says Harry Jaffe, M.D., professor of internal medicine at Northwestern University Medical School in Chicago. It may be a warning sign of a stroke.

In addition, consult your doctor if:

• You are suddenly more clumsy or accident-prone.

• You have a sudden onset of headaches that are unlike any that you've had in the past.

• You have sudden hearing loss in one ear, which might indicate wax that has plugged the canal, an infection, or a more serious condition.

He recommends doing a physical activity you enjoy—like ballroom dancing or gardening—for at least 20 minutes a day, three times a week.

Other Wise Ways

Visit the pyramid. Nerve and muscle cells work better and react faster if you eat a well-balanced diet, Dr. Jaffe says. The U.S. Department of Agriculture's Food Guide Pyramid recommends 6 to 11 servings of grains, rice, and pasta, 3 to 5 servings of vegetables, 2 to 4 servings of fruit, 2 to 3 servings of milk and other dairy products, and 2 to 3 servings of meat or fish daily.

See the sights, hear the crowd. Hearing and vision problems account for up to 80 percent of problems with reaction time, Dr. Jaffe says. So get your eyesight and hearing checked at least once a year after age 60.

Bridge the gap. Chess, jigsaw puzzles, and other challenging mind games not only keep your brain alert, they also may shave your reaction time, says Gisele Wolf-Klein, M.D., chief of geriatric medicine at Long Island Jewish Medical Center in New Hyde Park, New York.

"Even card games like bridge can help because you have to think quickly, you have to add quickly, and you have to move quickly to play," Dr. Wolf-Klein says.

Jack be nimble. Playing jacks, Ping-Pong, and other games involving hand-eye coordination can improve your reflexes, too, suggests Jim Buskirk, licensed physical therapist at Balance Centers of America in Chicago.

Play ball. Just playing paddleball for one to two minutes twice a day can help speed your reaction time, Buskirk says.

You also could cut out a variety of letters, small shapes, and colored pieces of paper and tape them to a ball. Then bounce the ball off a wall. As you bounce the ball, spot and call out one or more of the colors, shapes, or letters before you catch it, Buskirk suggests.

Earn a belt. Martial arts are a terrific way for seniors to improve their reflexes, Dr. Richman says. These ancient Eastern techniques build muscle strength, improve flexibility and concentration, and force you to react quickly.

"One of my tae kwon do instructors is 67 years old and his reaction time is great. It's not as good as some of the young football players in his class, but he certainly has better reflexes than most 40-year-olds," Dr. Richman says.

If you are over the age of 60, Dr. Richman recommends that you try tai chi, aikido, kung fu, or any other form of low-impact martial arts that focuses on developing fluid, dancelike movements. Check your phone directory to locate a martial arts school near you.

MANAGING YOUR MEDS

Avoid using sleeping pills, tranquilizers, and excessive amounts of alcohol. They can dangerously slow your reaction time in a crisis, says Gisele Wolf-Klein, M.D., chief of geriatric medicine at Long Island Jewish Medical Center in New Hyde Park, New York.

It's particularly vital for seniors to avoid these numbing influences. When your body is older, you don't metabolize drugs the way you did when you were younger, so they linger longer in your body, slowing down your reflexes. In fact, the effects of a drug like diazepam (Valium) can linger for up to three days after an older person takes it, Dr. Wolf-Klein says.

If you drink, limit yourself to one 12-ounce beer, one 4-ounce glass of wine, or a 1-ounce shot of liquor a day, she advises.

SLOW HEALING

If it seems as if your latest injury is taking a long time to heal, don't despair. With a few changes in diet and lifestyle, you can strengthen your healing forces and speed your recovery.

It's true, however, that your body's wounds are slower to heal when you're old than they were when you first bled in life's battles. "That's why it's so important for seniors to take good care of themselves, especially with their nutrition and activity levels," says Larry Millikan, M.D., chairman of the department of dermatology at Tulane University School of Medicine in New Orleans.

There are several reasons for this slowdown in healing. In women, hormones are a factor. Research has shown that women do not heal as rapidly after they pass through menopause and stop producing estrogen at their premenopausal levels. When women take estrogen replacement therapy (ERT) after menopause, they tend to heal at a faster rate—and that change can be attributed to the increase in estrogen. For men, the slowdown in healing is more often the result of chronically poor health and diabetes—and these are large factors for some women as well.

Once you have adequately cleaned and cared for your wound or injury, there are several things you can do to speed healing and recovery. If you're looking for a good place to begin boosting your wound-healing power, start with the dining room table.

Try This First

Heal with your meals. Even though you may not be as active or have as much appetite as you used to, your body still needs a regular supply of nutritious foods if it's going to be able to stay healthy and make speedy repairs. "All too often, seniors eat only one meal a day. Let's say it's dinner, but they've skipped breakfast and had a

488

candy bar for lunch. That's going to weaken their immune systems and slow down their healing," says Dr. Millikan. Try instead to eat three nutritious meals a day.

Other Wise Ways

Put in the protein. Your body requires about 45 grams of protein a day to repair damaged tissues. A three-ounce serving (about the size of a deck of cards) of fish, chicken or turkey, or cheese will provide about 21 grams of protein. A cup of milk will give you 8 grams of protein and a half-cup of beans will provide about 7 grams.

Boost immunity with antioxidants. Vitamins C and E as well as beta-carotene (a vitamin A precursor) are all antioxidants, which means they're particularly beneficial in boosting your immune system, helping to fight infection, and promoting more rapid healing, says Frederic Haberman, M.D., assistant clinical professor of medicine (dermatology) at Albert Einstein College of Medicine in New York City and director of the Haberman Dermatology Institute in Ridgewood, New Jersey.

"I tell people to take 500 to 1,000 milligrams of vitamin C, about 400 international units (IU) of E, and up to 2,000 IU of vitamin A after surgery," Dr. Haberman says. "They should also take about 70 micrograms of selenium." Although vitamin E is generally sold in doses of 400 IU, one small study showed a possible risk of stroke in dosages higher than 200 IU. Consult with your doctor if you are at high risk for stroke.

Be zealous about zinc. When it comes to wounds, the mineral zinc has strong healing power, according to Eleanor Young, R.D., Ph.D., a licensed dietician and professor in the department of medicine at the University of Texas Health Sciences Center in San Antonio.

Dr. Haberman recommends 15 milligrams of zinc per day. You can get it in supplement form, and it's also in foods like steamed oysters and most meat dishes.

Make multis part of a healthy diet. Take a multivitamin and mineral supplement, such as Centrum, says Dr. Millikan.

"The supplement provides the antioxidants and minerals they need to promote a stronger immune response," says Dr. Haberman.

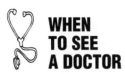

WHEN TO SEE A DOCTOR

Some injuries take longer to mend than others. But if a simple cut takes longer than a week to heal, or if the cut becomes red and swollen, see your doctor, says Larry Millikan, M.D., chairman of the department of dermatology at Tulane University School of Medical in New Orleans. Slow healing is often the sign of some other problem—a cold, an infection, or some more serious ailment, for example—that is interfering with your body's ability to heal quickly and properly. If your doctor can identify the real problem, there's a good chance he can correct that and speed your healing along.

Go for aloe. Buy an aloe plant to keep on the shelf as a houseplant, suggests Dr. Millikan. The next time you cut yourself, break off a leaf, split it lengthwise, and use the juice to speed healing. "Many of my patients firmly believe that this is a great help," he says. Research has shown that aloe can penetrate and numb tissue, prevent the growth of harmful bacteria, fungi, and virus, reduce swelling, and improve blood flow.

Walk your wounds off. People who exercise regularly tend to heal more rapidly and are more likely to have stronger immune systems. "The key is good blood circulation," says Dr. Millikan. As long as your tissues get enough blood, they're also getting adequate oxygen, nutrients, and immune cells—all the ingredients they need in order to heal. "On the other hand, people who have circulatory disorders tend to heal more slowly and can suffer from more infections," Dr. Millikan observes. One circulation problem that can slow healing is atherosclerosis, or hardening of the arteries, a condition that impedes blood flow. Another is diabetes—the inability to incorporate blood sugar, which leaves body cells deprived of nutrition and wounds more susceptible to infection.

For most seniors, the best exercise is walking, says Dr. Millikan. "You shouldn't adopt an exercise program, even walking, without first consulting your doctor to see how much exercise you can do safely. Once your doctor gives you the okay, walking is an ideal way to promote circulation and more rapid healing."

SMOKING ADDICTION

You've probably heard just about enough about the downside of smoking. You may have read somewhere that each puff contains 4,700 chemicals, including poisons like arsenic, formaldehyde, and ammonia, that raise your risk of cancer. Unless you're in a news-blackout zone, you realize that a single puff raises blood pressure, constricts blood vessels, and deprives the heart of oxygen. And you know that each puff sends a jolt of nicotine—the world's most addictive drug—surging into your brain.

But you probably didn't know that the average person who smokes a pack a day takes about 75,000 puffs a year. So if you're one of the 16 million Americans over age 60 who continue to smoke, you've taken at least 3 million puffs since you began lighting up in your teens. That's enough air to blow up about 300,000 balloons.

But even if you've been smoking for decades, it's not too late to quit and ensure that you'll have plenty of lung power to inflate your grandchildren's water wings well into your eighties and nineties, says Thomas Cooper, D.D.S., a nicotine-dependency researcher and professor emeritus at the University of Kentucky College of Dentistry in Lexington.

"It is a great feeling to be able to say I'm better off as a non-smoker," says Dr. Cooper, who smoked for 36 years before quitting in 1984. "There's nothing like knowing you have more stamina, you smell better, you breathe easier, and you like yourself better, all because you quit smoking. Once you get to that point, when you do see a cigarette, you can honestly say, 'No deal. I deserve better.'"

Admittedly, nicotine can have a pretty firm grip. "Nobody would get up at two in the morning and rummage around in a trash can for a toothbrush. But some people will do that in order to get a cigarette. It's that powerful of an addiction," says Mitchell Nides,

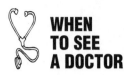

WHEN TO SEE A DOCTOR

Over-the-counter (OTC) nicotine gums or patches have helped many people over 60 quit smoking. If these products don't help you, see your doctor, advises John Slade, M.D., professor of clinical medicine at the University of Medicine and Dentistry of New Jersey Robert Wood Johnson Medical School in New Brunswick, New Jersey, and co-author of *The Cigarette Papers*. Your physician can review the problems that you have had with OTC products and offer tips or other support. It may also be appropriate to consider prescription drugs such as a nicotine nasal spray or an inhaler with nicotine, which can curb your urge to smoke. The doctor also may suggest a medicine like bupropion (Zyban), an antidepressant that has been shown to reduce nicotine cravings.

Ph.D., psychologist at the University of California, Los Angeles.

But you can beat it, Dr. Nides says. Even if you've tried to quit several times in the past, don't give up. Researchers have discovered powerful tools that soothe withdrawal symptoms and make it easier for you to become a nonsmoker.

Try This First

Set a quit date. You'll be more likely to stop smoking for good if you set a firm, unbreakable quit date, says Thomas Brandon, Ph.D., director of the Tobacco Research and Intervention Program at the H. Lee Moffitt Cancer Center and Research Institute in Tampa, Florida. Avoid picking stressful holidays like Christmas, and don't select a date that is months away. Odds are, your resolve will wilt by then. Instead, once you decide to quit, choose a day that falls within the next two weeks.

Other Wise Ways

Freeze 'em out. You'll have better luck quitting if you do it cold turkey, Dr. Brandon says. Gradually reducing the number of cigarettes you smoke only prolongs nicotine withdrawal and makes it easier for you to fall back into your old habits. If you quit cold turkey, you'll have no more than 7 to 10 days of withdrawal, but then the worst will be over—and chances are, you'll be a nonsmoker.

"We tell people that nicotine withdrawal is like the flu," Dr. Brandon says. "It's going to be a week when you're not going to be as productive, friendly, or charming as you usually are. You'd cut yourself some slack if you felt that way and had the flu. You need to make the same allowances when you are trying to quit smoking."

Throw away all of your tobacco products and anything associated with smoking, including ashtrays, lighters, and matches, Dr. Brandon says.

Get your dose without the smoke. Over-the-counter nicotine gums and patches can help you get through the first few weeks without smoking, says John Slade, M.D., professor of clinical medicine at the University of Medicine and Dentistry of New Jersey Robert Wood Johnson Medical School in New Brunswick, New Jersey, and co-author of *The Cigarette Papers*. These products release low doses of nicotine into your bloodstream and combat your cravings for a smoke.

If you are using over-the-counter nicotine gum, you should avoid chewing on a piece of it within 30 minutes of drinking any beverage, says Dr. Slade. Most beverages, including water, will change the acidity of your mouth and block the absorption of the nicotine in the gum.

Beverages have no effect on nicotine patches because the drug is absorbed directly through the skin into the bloodstream, Dr. Slade says.

De-stress for success. Gums and patches are only a short-term solution. To truly become a nonsmoker, you'll also need to make behavioral changes—such as learning stress reduction techniques—that will stop you from automatically reaching for a cigarette, says Dr. Slade.

Pen a note of certainty. Write a goodbye letter to your cigarettes or a love letter to your grandchildren, Dr. Nides suggests. Either one can solidify your determination to quit. Simply tell your grandchildren how much you care for them and that that's why you're quitting, he says.

As for cigarettes, "you could talk about how you once viewed cigarettes as true friends. But now, you realize that cigarettes aren't your friends, because they're killing you and making you look older and more wrinkled," Dr. Nides says.

Steer clear of smoke signals. Plan your day so you'll be less tempted to smoke, Dr. Nides suggests. If you know, for instance, that you get your worst urges to light up first thing in the morning and late in the afternoon, schedule smoke-free activities at those times. Try taking a dawn walk in a smoke-free shopping mall or having an early-bird dinner in a smoke-free restaurant.

Let your fingers do the walking. Keep your hands busy, particularly for the first three or four days after you quit, when the urges to light up will be strongest, Dr. Brandon suggests. Play with a pencil, doodle with a pen, squeeze a tennis ball, work on a jigsaw puzzle, or bake a cake (just resist the urge to eat all of it when you're done). Let your hands do anything except reach for a cigarette, Dr. Brandon urges.

Slice the space. During the two weeks before your quit date, gradually cut down the area of your home where you allow yourself to smoke, Dr. Nides says. Start by eliminating a room at a time, preferably the ones you use most often. When you're down to one room, begin chipping away at that area until you are down to a one-foot-by-one-foot space. Then quit completely.

"It will help decondition you from smoking in the places where you would have normally smoked," Dr. Nides says. "So when you do quit, you'll already have had the experience of sitting in the living room without smoking. It can make quitting a lot easier for some people."

Get an early start. Try to quit smoking on Monday or Tuesday of a busy week, Dr. Cooper suggests. "You don't want to quit smoking when you have a lot of time on your hands to think about it," he says.

Use the buddy system. If you're trying to quit, ask a nonsmoking friend or relative to provide encouragement and a sympathetic ear, says Fredrick J. Kviz, Ph.D., associate professor of public health at the University of Illinois at Chicago. In his studies, Dr. Kviz has found that people who recruit buddies to help them are twice as likely to remain smoke-free 12 months after quitting as those who don't.

Imagine that. Your imagination is a mighty weapon in your battle to quit. "Some people find that imagining life without cigarettes is a very effective way to quit," Dr. Nides says. "That's how former U.S. senator S. I. Hayakawa did it. Every day, he told himself he was a nonsmoker, and within a couple of months he quit."

Here's how to do it.

1. Take a couple of deep breaths and let them out slowly. Close your eyes for a few moments and imagine yourself not smoking in a situation where you normally would.

2. Imagine the vivid tastes and smells you can finally enjoy now that you don't smoke.

3. See yourself mingling with people who are smoking, but having no desire to join them, even when someone offers you a cigarette.

4. Now imagine yourself walking out into a bright, beautiful meadow filled with wild flowers. Take in an enormous breath of fresh air and let it fill your lungs.

5. As you slowly breathe out, say to yourself, "I choose not to smoke."

Begin doing this imagery for one minute five times a day at least two weeks before you quit, Dr. Nides suggests. Even if you smoke after doing it, the imagery will mentally prepare you for the day when you do become a nonsmoker. After you quit, do this imagery whenever a craving strikes.

It's a snap. Put a stiff rubber or elastic band around your wrist. Every time you feel an urge to smoke in the first two weeks after you quit, snap the band so that it gives you a sharp, uncomfortable slap. The snap can distract your attention from the urge to smoke just long enough that the craving will pass and you won't light up, Dr. Nides says.

Light up an apple instead. When blood sugar levels get low, smokers are used to reaching for cigarettes to perk them up, Dr. Nides says. Snacking on an apple twice a day for a couple of weeks after you quit will help boost your energy levels without lighting up, he says.

Knock off the booze. Alcohol dissolves your resolve and makes it easier for you to light up. Avoid alcohol for at least a month after you quit smoking, Dr. Cooper advises.

SNORING
AND SLEEP APNEA

If you snore, you're not alone. The National Sleep Foundation in Washington, D.C., estimates that 40 percent of adult Americans saw logs in their sleep.

But as people age, their sleep becomes lighter and more fragmented. Your spouse's snoring, which you may have been able to put up with 20 years ago, may be too disturbing now. And if you're the snorer, you may even be waking yourself up now.

What's more, the snoring may actually be a signal of a more serious problem. If the snoring occurs in loud gasping snorts that may ultimately cause you or your bedmate to stop breathing for brief periods of time, then there's a good chance that snore isn't just a snore—it's sleep apnea.

To avoid confusion, let's define the two right here: Snoring occurs as you inhale during your sleep and the soft tissues of your throat—the uvula and soft palate—vibrate against the back of your throat or tongue.

Sleep apnea, however, occurs when the muscles in the back of your throat relax during sleep. With this relaxation, breathing passages become narrower and may completely obstruct the passage for as long as 60 seconds. This causes a gasping type of snoring that can be serious if it isn't controlled, says Nancy Collop, M.D., pulmonary/critical-care doctor specializing in sleep medicine and associate professor at the Medical University of South Carolina in Charleston.

Apnea puts you at risk for high blood pressure. During apnea, when you obstruct the breathing passage, the levels of oxygen in your blood decrease. Your body treats this as a panic situation and starts pouring hormones into your bloodstream to wake you up or get you breathing again. An unfortunate side effect of this strategy is that the hormones cause your blood pressure to climb. When people with apnea are monitored all night long in sleep labs, researchers have found that their blood pressures go up at a time when blood pressure is normally at its lowest. In fact, that's one way researchers can tell if you have apnea.

"It's clear from research that in its severe form apnea produces high blood pressure and heart failure and depression and mental clouding," says Daniel Kripke, M.D., professor of psychiatry at the University of California, San Diego. For that reason, if you suspect that you have sleep apnea, it's important to see a sleep specialist to determine how serious the problem is.

If it turns out that you do have a less severe apnea or just a serious case of snoring, consider some of these tips to improve your slumber.

Try This First

Sleep on your side or stomach. Sleep on your back, and your tongue will relax back toward your throat, making it harder to breathe and easier to snore. Try sleeping on your side in a half-sitting position so that doesn't happen, suggests Dr. Kripke. It helps to have your head propped up with thicker pillows or more of them—but the main thing is to sleep on your side or stomach. Sometimes, a well-placed pillow can help you maintain these positions.

Because people move around in their sleep, you might be turning over on your back even if you start out in another position. Dr. Kripke says the easiest way to keep yourself from rolling onto your back is to sew a tennis ball into the back of your pajamas; you'll feel it when you roll onto it. "It's a very inexpensive way to train people not to sleep on their backs," he observes.

Other Wise Ways

Lose some weight. Excessive weight aggravates apnea and snoring. So give yourself an honest appraisal in the mirror: If you have more than one chin on the outside of your neck, Dr. Kripke says, you have fatty deposits on the inside that may be contributing to constricted airways. In fact, if your neck size is greater than 17

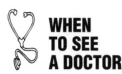

WHEN TO SEE A DOCTOR

Light snoring isn't a serious health problem, but see your doctor if you think you have apnea or if you are excessively sleepy in addition to snoring, says Peter Hauri, M.D., co-director of the Mayo Clinic Sleep Disorders Center in Rochester, Minnesota, and author of *No More Sleepless Nights*. When you have sleep apnea, you actually stop breathing, and this can cause your body to react in such a way that your blood pressure rises. That, in turn, can increase your risk of heart failure. If you do happen to have a severe case of apnea, a doctor can treat it, often with easy-to-use breathing devices.

inches, you're at greater risk for apnea. So change to a lower-fat diet and incorporate some exercise into your life to help trim off some of that fat.

Clear the airways. Any type of congestion, from colds to allergies, can aggravate a snoring problem. "The more resistance there is in your nose, the more you have to suck in to breathe," says Dr. Kripke. And that action can cause apnea. You can treat stuffy nose with a nonaddicting nasal spray that contains cromolyn sodium (Nasalcrom). Use this over-the-counter product before bedtime to help you breathe more easily.

Keep your nostrils spread. For some people, collapsing nostrils are a problem that can be helped with Breathe Right nasal strips. These strips, which are taped over the outside bridge of the nose to keep the nostrils from collapsing, are available at most pharmacies. There's a quick way to see if these strips might be helpful to you, Dr. Kripke says. Stand in front of a mirror, take deep breaths in through your nose, and observe whether the sides of your nostrils get sucked in as you breathe. If they do, then you can probably benefit from using the strip since it will help force your nostrils to stay open.

Don't do the dinner drinks. Alcohol has an initial sedating effect, and this can worsen snoring and apnea by increasing muscle relaxation, Dr. Kripke says. So you may want to avoid alcohol in the evening.

Snooze without sleeping pills. If you take sleeping pills, the medication might be contributing to apnea or making snoring worse,

Dr. Kripke says. The pills relax your muscles, including those around your tongue and throat.

Humidify the house. A lack of humidity can cause the membranes in your airways to dry out and swell, increasing the potential for one tissue to rub against another and vibrate, says Peter Hauri, M.D., co-director of the Mayo Clinic Sleep Disorders Center in Rochester, Minnesota, and author of *No More Sleepless Nights*. A humidifier in the bedroom can help you remain moist and may help you sleep more quietly.

Check for allergies. Allergies can cause swelling in the airway membranes, Dr. Collop says, leading to more friction, more snoring, and worse apnea. If you know you have allergies, take your medication regularly. If you suspect that allergies may be causing snoring, talk to your doctor about being tested for allergies.

Put down the cigarette. Besides all of the serious health consequences, smoking irritates the nose and throat, causing swelling that can make the vibrations of snoring more likely and make apnea worse, Dr. Hauri says. Kick the habit, and you'll snore less.

Get a good night's sleep. Most people, even seniors, need about eight hours of sleep a night. If you don't get enough, your body has a tendency to make up for a lack of rest by making your sleep deeper the next time you sleep, explains Dr. Collop. In deeper sleep, your muscles become more relaxed, setting the scene for increased snoring. So try to get your full night's rest. If you can't, try to take a nap during the day. You'll be better rested and less apt to snore.

MANAGING YOUR MEDS

The following types of drugs can all make snoring and sleep apnea worse, according to Daniel Kripke, M.D., professor of psychiatry at the University of California, San Diego. Talk to your doctor if you're taking:

- Sleeping pills (either prescription or over-the-counter) such as zolpidem (Ambien), flurazepam (Dalmane), temazepam (Restoril), or triazolam (Halcion)
- Sedatives such as diazepam (Valium) or lorazepam (Ativan)

STOMACHACHE

Medically speaking, there's no such thing as a stomachache. That's because what we think of as a stomachache could really be any of a number of abdomen-related pains—a dull ache, bloating, sharp cramps, acid pain, gas pain, or even pain related to diarrhea or constipation.

The possible causes are just as diverse: stress, dyspepsia (more commonly called indigestion), heartburn, gallstones, ulcers, lactose intolerance, or irritable bowel syndrome. You might be overeating or not eating enough. You might have eaten food that was ill-prepared, spoiled, or that simply didn't agree with you.

This much is certain: As you age, your digestive system may become more particular about what it can and can't handle, says Martin Brotman, M.D., gastroenterologist at the California Pacific Medical Center in San Francisco. And when your system has to deal with something it doesn't like, it will probably let you know about it—often in the form of a stomachache. But if you're armed with that knowledge, you can soothe or prevent most stomachaches, no matter what's causing them, with some simple strategies.

Try This First

Go through the process of elimination. Since your digestive processes get more finicky every year, that increases the likelihood that a certain food, beverage, or medication can cause a stomachache. "Try eliminating different things, such as aspirin, to see if you feel better," says Dr. Brotman.

Even chewing gum should come under suspicion. Some people get abdominal cramps and diarrhea when they chew sugar-free gum that's made with the sweetener sorbitol. Dairy foods and beverages such as ice cream and milk are other common offenders that can make you feel more gassy and bloated, as are many high-sugar or high-fat foods. If you suspect that a food is causing the problem, take it out of your diet for a few days. If the stomachache disappears, you've found your culprit, says Dr. Brotman.

Other Wise Ways

Give your belly a break. You can help your stomach recover from a bellyache by going on just liquids for the rest of the day, says Dr. Brotman. Stick to clear liquids, such as chicken broth, flat ginger ale, and water, and avoid carbonated or caffeinated beverages.

Loosen up. If you have a bloated, sore belly, make yourself more comfortable by wearing loose clothing. Loosen your belt. If you're wearing a tight shirt or pants, change into trousers, sweats, or pajama bottoms that have a bigger waistband, until your stomach settles down.

Warm your tummy. Turn a heating pad on low and place it on your abdomen until the pain subsides, says Dr. Brotman. "Warmth on the abdomen offers some comfort. If the pain continues for several hours and is new to you, notify your doctor."

Take time out. Soothe a sore stomach with rest. Put up your feet. Relax. "Close your eyes," suggests Roger L. Gebhard, M.D., gas-

MANAGING YOUR MEDS

Tummy troubles are a side effect of many prescription drugs. If you experience stomach problems after taking your medication, talk to your doctor about prescribing a substitute. Here are some common stomach offenders.

- Iron supplements taken to prevent or treat anemia, such as ferrous sulfate (Feosol)
- Caffeine in any form, whether as coffee, caffeinated beverages, or as a stimulant (Vivarin)
- Anti-inflammatory agents used for sprains, strains, toothache, or cold and flu aches, including over-the-counter products such as aspirin, ibuprofen, and naproxen (Aleve)

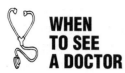

WHEN TO SEE A DOCTOR

If a stomachache is so severe that you're doubled over, or if it is accompanied by nausea and vomiting that lasts longer than one or two days or keeps coming back, let your doctor know, says Martin Brotman, M.D., gastroenterologist at the California Pacific Medical Center in San Francisco. And if the ache is accompanied by a change in bowel habits, such as the onset of constipation or pencil-thin stools, diarrhea that is persistent or getting increasingly worse and that is accompanied by fever, or blood in your stool, see your doctor.

troenterologist at the Veterans Affairs Medical Center and professor of medicine in the division of gastroenterology at the University of Minnesota, both in Minneapolis. "Find in your memory a place you've been to. A place of beauty, maybe a lake or a campground or a beach. Go back to that spot in your mind. Sit on a rock. Listen to the natural sounds. Breathe naturally."

Welcome a little BRAT into your home. When you are ready to eat a little something, try the BRAT diet—bananas, rice, applesauce, or toast. These foods are all easy for your stomach to digest. "Don't rush back into solid food by eating a steak dinner," says Dr. Brotman.

Call on chamomile. Chamomile tea is an age-old and, many believe, effective herbal remedy to ease a sore belly, says Mike Cantwell, M.D., clinician and coordinator for clinical research at the Institute for Health and Healing at the California Pacific Medical Center. Try two or three six-ounce cups a day, between meals. Chamomile decreases stomach activity and helps coat the stomach as well, says Dr. Cantwell. You can find the tea in most grocery stores. Follow the directions on tea-bag packages, or if you are using loose dried chamomile flowers, steep one teaspoon of chamomile in boiling water for 10 to 15 minutes. Very rarely, chamomile can cause an allergic reaction when ingested. People who are allergic to closely related plants such as ragweed, asters, and chrysanthemums should drink the tea with caution.

Stay regular. Constipation can certainly lead to stomach distress, so make sure that you're getting a healthy dose of fiber every day. Shoot for 25 grams of fiber each day, says Dr. Gebhard. Include apples, bran, cabbage, and raw vegetables in your diet—and drink eight, eight-ounce glasses of water a day to help keep you regular. "Peel the apple if the skin is hard for you to chew or digest," adds Dr. Gebhard.

Don't overfill with fiber. Believe it or not, stomach problems can also be caused by too much of a good thing—specifically, fiber. For some people, eating more fiber than they are accustomed to can cause gas and abdominal bloating, says Dr. Gebhard. It's best to introduce fiber into your diet slowly and a little at a time. Dr. Gebhard recommends starting with 10 to 15 grams a day, increasing by 5 grams each week to 25.

Work out stress. Tension and stress can cause plenty of stomach pain. To help relieve stress, put some regular exercise into your weekly routine. Try walking for half an hour three days a week, says Wanda Filer, M.D., family-practice physician in York, Pennsylvania. When you're active, you'll also find that your bowel movements become more regular, which is helpful if constipation is causing your abdominal distress.

Eat mindfully. "Mindful eating" is paying attention to the role of food in your daily life, says Amy Saltzman, M.D., internist for the Institute for Health and Healing at the California Pacific Medical Center.

"By bringing attention to when, what, where, and how you eat, you may improve not only your digestion but also the quality of your life," says Dr. Saltzman. "Try eating a mindful meal. Prepare the food with attention to what will be satisfying—and eat when you are hungry." When you sit down to eat, be sure to go slowly, Dr. Saltzman adds. Concentrate on eating, and taste each bite before you swallow.

STRESS

The images in the retirement-community ads certainly are alluring. A man fishing with his grandson. Golf seven days a week. A leisurely afternoon siesta. No worries, no problems, no stresses.

Dream on.

For many people who dream of such a stress-free nirvana, there may be a surprise waiting by the hammock. Stress doesn't retire. It can follow you like the flu. In fact, the retirement years often are among the most stressful in a person's life, says George T. Grossberg, M.D., director of geriatric psychiatry at St. Louis University School of Medicine. "Late life is a time of tremendous stress. You face numerous strains that you probably have never faced before, like the loss of loved ones, loneliness, disability, and unanticipated financial strain. And when you're 85, you're not going to bounce back from these stresses as quickly as a 25-year-old would," he says. "Consequently, the chances that stress will lead to chronic illness are much greater."

Researchers suspect that stress contributes to a multitude of physical and emotional disorders including high blood pressure, muscle spasms, chronic fatigue, insomnia, obesity, heart disease, digestive problems, anxiety, phobias, and depression. But it is particularly harmful after age 60, because the body can't physically adapt to the strain as well as it once did, explains Dr. Grossberg.

Under stress, for instance, an older person's blood pressure rises more rapidly and stays higher longer than a younger person's, because the older person's blood vessel walls may have lost some elasticity, increasing the risk of a heart attack or stroke, Dr. Grossberg warns.

Stress may take a greater toll as you get older because of a chemical imbalance—the body continues to crank out stress hormones at a steady pace, while the production of the hormones that counteract it declines dramatically as you age, according to Dr. Grossberg.

The result is like overinflating a balloon. You'll likely feel stretched—nearly to the limit. And that pressure can affect your mind, body, or spirit, says Frieda R. Butler, Ph.D., professor of gerontology at George Mason University in Fairfax, Virginia.

But it is never too late to learn how to deflate stress, Dr. Butler says. In fact, even if you've managed to corral stress in the past, you may have to develop new coping skills because the ones you used at 30 may not work as well at 70.

"As you get older, it takes longer to get yourself together after facing a stressful situation. So you'll have to adapt to maintain a healthy balance," she says. "Some of the old strategies may still work, but also you will have to take on new more effective ones."

Try This First

Take it in stride. "Exercise does more to relieve stress than a lot of other things combined," Dr. Butler says. "It helps get the blood circulating, improves mobility and muscle strength, and boosts morale. If you can move without pain, it changes your whole outlook on life. Exercise also has been shown to have a positive effect on mental abilities such as memory and in relieving anxiety."

Exercise also can improve your energy reserves so you'll feel more vigorous, says Robert E. Thayer, Ph.D., author of *The Origin of Everyday Moods* and professor of psychology at California State University, Long Beach. And the more energized you feel, the better you'll be able to cope with stress. If you feel slightly blue or worried, he recommends taking a brisk 10-minute walk at a pace as if you were late for an important appointment, but don't tense up as if you really were late.

Other Wise Ways

Stop peddling the news cycle. Computers, televisions, radios, and other forms of media offer staggering amounts of information instantaneously. But do you really need to know it all? Of course not,

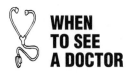

WHEN TO SEE A DOCTOR

People over 60 rarely admit that they feel stressed out, says George T. Grossberg, M.D., director of geriatric psychiatry at St. Louis University School of Medicine. Instead, they will complain about physical symptoms like heart palpitations or headaches. Ask your doctor to evaluate you for stress as soon as possible if:

• You have persistent insomnia.
• You have difficulty concentrating.
• You keep putting off important tasks.
• You have recently had stomachaches, headaches, and other vague aches and pains.
• You often feel dizzy or light-headed.
• You feel unusually irritable.

Dr. Butler says. In fact, letting go of news and information you don't need is one of the best stress busters for a person over 60.

"If you feel pressured to keep up with the world, then you may begin to feel stressed out. But who says you have to keep up with the latest music or styles anymore? Who says you have to read the newspaper or watch the evening news every day anymore? You don't. Only hold on to the information that is relevant for your new lifestyle. So if you golf, you may want to know who won the Senior Open, but not give a hoot about movies or politics. That's fine."

Get cozy. As you age, your natural ability to regulate body temperature declines, so you'll be more prone to stress in extreme cold or heat, according to Dr. Butler. Keep the temperatures in your house well within your comfort zone, and avoid venturing out on unusually frigid or sultry days, she suggests.

Inhale relief. Deep breathing is one of the simplest ways to keep stress under wraps, says Dr. Butler.

Practice it by doing the following:

1. Sit in a comfortable chair with your back straight.
2. Slowly breathe in and feel your lungs filling from the bottom to the top.
3. Focus your attention on your belly; let it expand as you breathe. It should feel as if your diaphragm, a muscular membrane separating your lungs from your abdomen, is being pulled down, as if it were attached to a string in your belly.

4. Slowly exhale, emptying your lungs from top to bottom.
5. Feel your diaphragm relax into its natural position. Then take another deep breath and repeat.

Do this exercise twice a day for five minutes, Dr. Butler suggests.

Anticipate power surges. Energy levels tend to be higher at certain times of the day than at others, Dr. Thayer says. Being aware of this cycle is very important because when you have low energy, you'll be more susceptible to stress. Every two to three

MANAGING YOUR MEDS

Caffeine, a prime ingredient in coffee, tea, cola drinks, and chocolate, is a stimulant that has a greater effect on the body after age 60, says George T. Grossberg, M.D., director of geriatric psychiatry at St. Louis University School of Medicine. Drink no more than one eight-ounce cup or glass a day to avoid feeling jittery and stressed out, he advises. Five ounces of dark, bittersweet chocolate has almost the same amount of caffeine as an eight-ounce cup of coffee. Milk chocolate has considerably less. Caffeine also is a major component of over-the-counter (OTC) stimulants such as No-Doz. Check with your doctor before using these drugs. Here are a few other common medications that can heighten feelings of stress or irritability.

- OTC sleep aids or cold and allergy medications such as diphenhydramine (Tylenol PM, Benadryl) and clemastine (Tavist)
- OTC decongestants, or antihistamines or antihistamine/decongestant combinations like pseudoephedrine (Sudafed), triprolidine and pseudoephedrine (Actifed), and clemastine and phenylpropanolamine (Tavist-D)
- Antihistamines found in some analgesics such as phenyltoloxamine (Percogesic)
- Antidepressants such as fluoxetine (Prozac), paroxetine (Paxil), and Zoloft (sertraline)
- Prescription and OTC asthma inhalants containing epinephrine (Primatene)

hours for three days, jot down on a notepad whether your energy levels feel high, moderately high, moderately low, or low. You should see patterns emerge that will help you make decisions, schedule appointments, and run errands at times when your energy levels are high and you are less apt to feel stressed, he says. So if you find yourself feeling drained around 2:00 P.M. each day, take a nap instead of balancing your checkbook or playing a chess game.

"This technique works particularly well for people over 60, who tend to not have the energy reserves that they once had," according to Dr. Thayer.

Head for the showers. Plunging into a steaming shower, bath, or hot tub is an excellent way to relieve stress, Dr. Thayer says. But don't stay in too long. Staying in warm hot-tub-like water for more than 10 minutes actually increases tension and can dampen your mood, he says.

SUNBURN

As good as sunlight feels, all the warnings about sun exposure definitely put a damper on the old-fashioned pleasure of basking in a beach chair. If you've heeded the warnings and shifted away from sun-worshipping habits, you probably rub on the sunscreen before you head for the beach. Interest in your own comfort as well as medical warnings may influence you to sun yourself at cooler times of the day. And if you can't remember the last time you had a truly uncomfortable searing from sunlight, you may feel like your skin is especially resistant to damaging rays.

But many people who have enjoyed the pleasures of sunning through their youth and middle age continue to bask when they're in their sixties and older. Often, older people get sunburned because they still follow the outmoded idea that a tan symbolizes attractiveness, youth, and fitness, says Jonathan Weiss, M.D., dermatologist and assistant clinical professor of dermatology at Emory University School of Medicine in Atlanta. Or they think that the damage is already done because of sunburns they had earlier in life. But the fact is, everytime you go out in the sun without proper protection, you're adding to any damage that the sun's ultraviolet (UV) rays may have already done to your skin, says Dr. Weiss.

That damage can go way beyond the red, painful skin you sport. In addition to the immediate discomfort, sunburn increases your chances of developing skin cancer, not to mention worsening wrinkles. Photoaging, the result of unprotected sun exposure, leads to tough, leathery skin that can make you look 15 to 20 years older than you are. Along with aging your skin, UV radiation can harm your vision, leaving you at greater risk for problems like macular degeneration and cataracts.

As a rule, the best treatment for sunburn, of course, is not to get it in the first place, says Dr. Weiss. But if you happen to find your

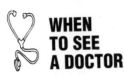

skin reddening after a few hours out in the sun, there's plenty you can do to soothe those burns—and to make sure that you don't get burned again.

Try This First

Preempt pain. When you know you've spent too much time in the sun, take aspirin or another nonsteroidal anti-inflammatory drug (NSAID) before you start feeling the burn, says Dr. Weiss. These over-the-counter medications offer two kinds of sunburn relief. They knock out pain and they reduce inflammation and swelling.

If taken soon enough, these drugs can help keep inflammation down and keep a sunburn from getting worse, says Dr. Weiss. He suggests taking the maximum dosage given by the package directions for 48 hours following the sunburn.

Other Wise Ways

Cool it. The best way to soothe sun-sizzled skin is to apply cool water as quickly as possible to prevent the sunburn from getting worse, says D'Anne Kleinsmith, M.D., staff dermatologist at William Beaumont Hospital in Royal Oak, Michigan. She recommends cold wet compresses and cool baths to bring down the heat of a sunburn. Do not apply ice, says Dr. Kleinsmith, because it could further injure the skin that's already been irritated by sunburn.

Just add milk. Whole-milk compresses are an excellent remedy for any kind of burn, says John F. Romano, M.D., clinical associate professor of dermatology at New York Hospital–Cornell Medical Center in New York City.

Dip gauze or a clean washcloth into milk, lay it on your sunburned skin, and leave the compress in place for 20 minutes or so, suggests Dr. Romano. Repeat every two to four hours, using milk that's room temperature or slightly cooler, but not ice-cold. Since milk leaves a residue that will soon have your skin smelling "sour," rinse yourself off with cool water afterward, he adds.

MANAGING YOUR MEDS

If the label of your prescription medication says, "Avoid the sun," don't overlook it, says Jonathan Weiss, M.D., dermatologist and assistant clinical professor of dermatology at Emory University School of Medicine in Atlanta. This warning label means that you'll sunburn more easily or become more sensitive to light as a side effect of taking the drug, says Dr. Weiss. Ignoring the "shun the sun" warning can give you more than a severe sunburn; it can affect how well the medicine does its job.

Among the drugs that commonly cause "photosensitivity" reactions are:

- Tricyclic antidepressants like amitriptyline (Elavil)
- Medications often prescribed as antihistamines, like promethazine (Phenergan)
- Tetracycline (Achromycin), used to treat infections and control acne
- Sulfa antibacterial drugs, such as the combination sulfamethoxazole and trimethoprim (Bactrim)
- Oral medicines for diabetes, such as glipizide (Glucotrol)
- Diuretics like hydrochlorothiazide (Esidrix)

If you're taking pills or liquid medications, your skin will resume its normal sun-sensitivity shortly after you stop taking the drug. But if you're using external salves or ointments on your skin, the photosensitive effects can continue after you stop applying it, so continue to maintain the precautions, says Dr. Weiss.

Alleviate with aloe. Aloe vera gel is probably the most soothing treatment you can apply to a sunburn, says Dr. Weiss. Apply it as needed to alleviate the pain and dryness of sunburned skin.

You can buy bottles of the pure gel in health food stores. Or try growing the plants around your house, and then just slice open a leaf and slather on the gel when needed.

Make yourself moisturized. Bland moisturizers (those without fragrances or irritating ingredients) such as Cetaphil cream or Eucerin cream can comfort sun-damaged skin, says Dr. Weiss. Smoothing on cream after a cool bath helps to lock moisture into parched skin, he says. Also, moisturizers with menthol or eucalyptus can add a cooling sensation.

Soothe with hydrocortisone ointment. An over-the-counter hydrocortisone ointment, either 0.5 percent or 1 percent, may help keep down inflammation and swelling, according to Dr. Weiss. Ointments are preferable to hydrocortisone creams since creams can contain preservatives that can sting irritated or blistered skin. Apply as directed on the label.

Flush your system. If your skin swells from a sunburn, that causes you to lose fluids from the rest of your body. To replace that fluid, you need to drink lots of water. Dr. Weiss suggests you drink at least eight, eight-ounce glasses of water a day until the sunburn no longer gives off heat.

Practice prevention. Your first line of defense should be a sunscreen. Get in the habit of putting it on every morning. Dr. Weiss recommends the use of products with a sun protection factor (SPF) of at least 15. Also, check the label to be sure that the lotion is designed to protect against both UVA (the deep-penetrating rays) and UVB (the sunburn-causing rays).

Dr. Weiss recommends looking for zinc oxide or titanium dioxide among the ingredients. These are inert, opaque compounds that block almost the entire spectrum of damaging rays, he says, without exposing you to the irritating effects of chemicals like paraaminobenzoic acid (PABA) found in many other sunscreens.

Apply sunscreen liberally—use about the amount that would fill a shot glass—per application for the average-size person. Apply evenly on all exposed skin, including your lips, nose, ears, neck, scalp (if hair is thinning), hands, feet, and eyelids, taking care not to get the product in your eyes, says Dr. Weiss. Be sure to put the sunscreen on 30 minutes before you go out, he adds. It takes about that long before it will protect you fully.

Know when your time is up. If you are careful to reapply sunscreen after getting wet, you can safely stay outside as long as the sunscreen promises. For instance, if you use an SPF 15 sunscreen, you can stay outside 15 times longer without burning than you could while not wearing sunscreen. If you would begin to burn after 8 minutes with no sunscreen, you can stay out for 120 minutes without burning by wearing SPF 15 sunscreen. But you can't "layer" sunscreen. Once your two hours is up, you can't reapply more sunscreen and stay out for another 120 minutes. Also, wearing an SPF 15 and an SPF 30 sunscreen does not make for SPF 45, says Dr. Weiss.

Cover up. Loose-fitting, long-sleeved shirts and pants or long skirts provide the greatest protection from the sun's rays. Tightly woven cloth is best, says Dr. Weiss. A simple rule of thumb is to hold the fabric up against the light: the closer the weave, the better the protection.

Don a hat and shades. Dressing for the sun should also always include a broad-brimmed hat and UV-protective sunglasses, says Dr. Weiss. He suggests a brim of about four inches all around and sunglasses that will block at least 99 percent of both UVA and UVB radiation.

Avoid peak exposure. Your chances of developing a sunburn are greatest between 10:00 A.M. and 3:00 P.M., when the sun's rays are strongest at all latitudes. The risk drops considerably before and after those times, says Dr. Weiss. It's also easier to burn more severely on a hot day because the heat increases the effects of ultraviolet radiation. In addition, you'll burn faster at high altitudes and in the mountains because there is less atmosphere to block ultraviolet rays, he adds.

Beware of clouds. People often discount the risk of getting sunburned on cloudy or overcast days. But you can't let your guard down even when the sun is in hiding, says Dr. Weiss. Up to 80 percent of ultraviolet rays can penetrate the clouds.

TELEVISION ADDICTION

Let's see what's on.

Click.

On channel 3, there's a rerun of *America's Funniest Home Videos*. Switch to channel 4—a movie called *Witch Academy*, in which the devil turns a sorority pledge into a monster. On *The Price Is Right*, a 20-year-old college student has just won a new car. On channel 8, there's an infomercial pitching a baldness cure. A few more stabs at the remote control, and suddenly there's a nude woman on a talk show—her private parts electronically camouflaged by the camera—angrily telling her husband, "I'm never going to wear clothes again, and I don't care how you feel about it."

Wow! Television certainly has come of age. From the primitive days of *I Love Lucy*, it has evolved into a 100-channel soap opera available 24 hours a day, seven days a week. Life—the good, the bad, and the ugly—is just a remote control click away, and all without ever leaving your home.

Is this retirement bliss?

Hardly.

For anyone with extra hours to fill, TV watching can actually become a health hazard. "Seniors can quickly become mentally and physically disabled if they watch too much television," says Kurt V. Gold, M.D., physical medicine and rehabilitation specialist who works with the Nebraska Spine Center in Omaha, Nebraska. Sound alarmist? As Dr. Gold sees it, there's a risk that "TV viewing replaces physical activity. And without regular physical activity, the heart weakens, bones become brittle, and muscles lose their tone and flexibility. So older people who watch a lot of television are really setting themselves up for falls, fractures, and other physical problems. In addition, TV viewing not only ages your body, it impairs your mind. Television simply isn't an activity that exercises your brain very much."

Yet many seniors spend a lot of time in front of the TV, according to a study conducted by the Americans' Use of Time project at the University of Maryland in College Park. An average senior devotes 26 hours a week or 56 days a year solely to the tube. No one intentionally spends one out of every seven years in front of a TV screen. Yet that's what you're doing if the daily shows consume 26 hours of every week.

"Once you start watching TV, it can be very engrossing," says Dr. Gold. But sitting around that much isn't good for anyone—especially older adults, he points out. "A senior who watches a lot of television will probably develop more aches and pains and will likely need more medications to get through the day."

If you're concerned about your viewing habits, here are some strategies to help pull the plug on TV dependency.

Try This First

Plan, don't scan. Get into the habit of plotting out your viewing schedule, says Matthew Lombard, Ph.D., associate professor of communication at Temple University in Philadelphia. Browse through a programming guide and mark no more than two shows a day that you want to watch. In addition, write down at least two tasks you want to do immediately after the programs end. Then stick to that schedule. Turn off the set as soon as each show ends, and dive into your chores, Dr. Lombard says. This will discourage you from channel surfing.

Other Wise Ways

Tune into reality. Get out of the house as much as possible, Dr. Gold advises. At least once a day, go for a walk, visit a museum, take a class, or do another activity that you enjoy. Odds are, when you do come home, you'll feel energized and ready to do anything except watch television.

Give it a rest. Make the television off-limits at least one night a week, Dr. Gold suggests. You'll be amazed at the mind-stretching things you can find to fill that time.

Get back to basics. Cancel your cable and limit your household to one television, recommends Dr. Lombard. The more channels and sets you have, the more tempted you'll be to watch.

Record while you play. If you own a VCR, record your favorite shows so you can get out and enjoy life, Dr. Lombard suggests. Taping will actually reduce your viewing time since you can fast-forward through commercials.

Taping will also help you weed out programs that aren't important to you. A good rule of thumb: If you don't watch a taped show within a week, perhaps you need to reassess why you're tuning in at all, Dr. Lombard says.

Place it out of sight, out of mind. Put your television in an awkward location. If it's in a room with no chairs, you'll have to make an effort to watch it, according to Dr. Gold.

Sound it out. Radio is a better companion because you don't have to be in the same room to enjoy it, and you'll be more apt to do other things while you listen, Dr. Gold says.

TINNITUS

I t's during the quiet moments that tinnitus is at its loudest.

People with tinnitus hear a noise in their heads that has been compared to everything from a tinkling bell to a jet turbine. In a more scientific description, Jack Vernon, Ph.D., professor emeritus of otolaryngology at Oregon Health Sciences University in Portland and a board member of the American Tinnitus Association, says the average tinnitus makes a 7,000 hertz tone. For comparison, the highest note on a grand piano makes a noise in only the 4,000 hertz range. With that in mind, you can see how tinnitus might monopolize your attention.

Because it is the real perception of a phantom sound, it can be difficult for the people around someone with tinnitus to understand what the person is going through, says Stephen Nagler, M.D., director of the Southeastern Comprehensive Tinnitus Clinic in Atlanta.

"Just because the sound exists only in your head doesn't mean you're crazy. The tinnitus sufferers have lost their silence. It's an incredible loss. It's incredibly real," Dr. Nagler says.

And it's surprisingly common. According to the American Tinnitus Association, almost 50 million Americans have tinnitus in some form and 12 million require medical help for it.

If you start getting it when you are older, it is particularly distressing because you may already have some hearing loss. Combine the constant, annoying ringing, buzzing, hissing, or thumping noises of tinnitus with an ever-present hearing problem, and it is a recipe for frustration.

The causes of tinnitus are varied and not completely understood. Trauma, exposure to loud noise, and toxic reaction to medicines can all cause ringing in the ear. It can be temporary or permanent. Whatever your personal experience with it, tinnitus is a sign of

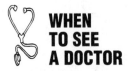

WHEN TO SEE A DOCTOR

If you experience a ringing in one ear accompanied by any bleeding or discharge from the ear, you need to see your doctor. Other symptoms that call for a doctor's attention are numbness of the face, balance disturbance, and headaches along with the ringing. These are all signs that you could have another more serious condition that could be anything from an ear infection to a tumor, says Jack Vernon, Ph.D., professor emeritus of otolaryngology at Oregon Health Sciences University in Portland and a board member of the American Tinnitus Association.

something gone awry in your auditory system, Dr. Vernon says, so be sure to see a doctor. Meanwhile, here are some remedies to help you cope.

Try This First

Mask the noise. Some people with tinnitus can mask the ringing. To determine if masking can help you, try this simple faucet test. Go to the kitchen sink and turn the water on full force. If the sound of that running water makes it impossible or very difficult for you to hear your tinnitus, then wearable tinnitus maskers will probably work for you, Dr. Vernon says.

You could purchase these maskers from some audiologists. Or you could simply create your own low-tech masker by tuning your radio to FM static (it's important to use FM since it's smoother than AM static). You can get a broad-band background noise that can distract you from your tinnitus.

Other Wise Ways

Let the band play on. Keep soft, gentle music playing. Classical music is a good bet, doctors say. Although it seldom masks the tinnitus, it can be soothing.

Listen to the sounds of nature. You may not be able to have a waterfall, an ocean wave, or a rain shower in your living room, but you can buy tapes of these natural noises. Play these noises softly to help cover up the tinnitus. They are unlikely to distract you from your daily activities. You are trying to avoid sounds that can attract attention, otherwise you will not be able to do something else, says Pawel Jastreboff, Ph.D., Sc.D., director of the University of Maryland Tinnitus and Hyperacusis Center in Baltimore.

Throw open a window. It's low-tech and simple. If you open your windows, the sounds of the outside world can help distract you from your tinnitus, Dr. Jastreboff says. The rustling of the wind, street noises, and birds chirping provide neutral background sounds that will distract you from your tinnitus but won't distract you from whatever task is at hand.

Try some ginkgo biloba. This herb may help circulation in the inner ear, says Michael Seidman, M.D., medical director of the tinnitus center at the Henry Ford Hospital in Detroit. He says some of his tinnitus patients swear by it for relief. If you take ginkgo biloba, Dr. Seidman advises that you purchase tablets with a 50-to-1 or 24-percent strength and take them three times a day. Allow three to six months for the herb to work. Natural remedies take a while to show their effectiveness, he says.

Add a niacin supplement. Niacin also improves circulation and may help relieve tinnitus symptoms. Begin by taking 50 milligrams twice a day. If you have no response after two weeks, you may increase the dosage by 50 milligrams a week, up to a maximum of 250

MANAGING YOUR MEDS

More than 70 medicines, prescription and over-the-counter, can cause ringing in the ears as a side effect. The most common are:

- Aspirin
- Narcotics such as morphine (Duramorph) and codeine
- Nonsteroidal anti-inflammatory drugs (NSAIDs) such as ibuprofen
- Antidepressants such as fluoxetine (Prozac) and amitriptyline (Elavil)

Some of the same drugs that can cause tinnitus symptoms are also used to relieve them, notes Michael Seidman, M.D., medical director of the tinnitus center at the Henry Ford Hospital in Detroit. Talk to your doctor about trying a different medication if you suspect that one you are taking is causing tinnitus or making it worse.

milligrams a day. Dr. Seidman warns that niacin may produce an uncomfortable pins-and-needles or flushing sensation, so you can try a "no-flush" niacin if you have these side effects from taking it.

Note: Doses of niacin above 35 milligrams per day should only be taken under your doctor's supervision.

Take a multivitamin. A deficiency in certain nutrients such as zinc or magnesium can cause or exacerbate tinnitus, so taking a general vitamin supplement every day might help, Dr. Seidman says.

Be smart about your schedule. Because tinnitus can be worse in the evenings when the noises of the day have quieted down, plan to use your noise generators at these times. Extremely high levels of noise, such as those made by chain saws, can trigger a bout of tinnitus or make the condition worse for a few hours, says Dr. Jastreboff. Wear earplugs for protection if you will be exposed to very loud sounds.

Be ready for an MRI. Seniors who may have to undergo magnetic resonance imaging (MRI) for other health reasons should wear earplugs during the scan. Dr. Vernon has had patients whose tinnitus was triggered by the loud noise an MRI machine makes.

Mind your menu. Caffeine and several other food items such as alcohol and the simple sugars found in candy bars can aggravate tinnitus, Dr. Seidman says. Try noncaffeinated beverages and more complex carbohydrates such as pretzels for snacks.

Dr. Nagler has also found that chocolate, spices, and red wine can temporarily aggravate tinnitus. He advises patients to make a prudent decision about whether to enjoy these foods or not. Though they don't do permanent damage, they can sometimes increase the risk of having a temporary problem.

Relax, there's hope. Experts agree that stress can aggravate tinnitus. Finding a good way to relax is an individual matter. For more information on tactics that might be helpful, see Stress on page 504.

Toenail Fungus

Toenail fungus sounds like such a nonthreatening condition. If you've had it for a long time, you probably put it in the nuisance category, along with things like dry skin, chapped lips, and age spots. Unattractive, maybe, but easy enough to ignore if you want to.

But after age 60, you need to take toenail fungus more seriously, says Neil Scheffler, D.P.M., podiatrist and president of health care and education for the Mid-Atlantic region of the American Association of Diabetes in Baltimore. As you age, your immune system is less able to fight off infection. When your nails get brittle—as happens when you have fungus—the sharp edges may puncture your skin, and germs can get in.

For people with diabetes, the risk soars. The danger of infection from a simple cut like that is much greater because of poor circulation. What started as a simple case of fungus can easily turn into an infection that can lead to gangrene if it's not treated, says Dr. Scheffler.

Technically called onychomycosis, toenail fungus is usually just that, a fungus. But yeasts and molds can trigger reactions that look similar, such as thickening and discolored nails. These things get passed around. Other people leave their footprints on the floors of health clubs, public swimming pools, or locker rooms, and if you step in the wrong place at the wrong time, you could pick up the fungus, yeast, or mold.

Despite its name, this fungal infection can also get on your fingernails. But the toes are the most common site. That's because toenails grow much more slowly than fingernails. A typical big toenail takes about 12 to 18 months to grow out, and that's about half the speed of a fingernail. So, once a toenail is infected, it's growing out at a very leisurely pace. Add to that an environment

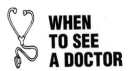

WHEN TO SEE A DOCTOR

Get nail fungus checked out by a doctor, especially if you have diabetes. "It's very important to take the medication that will help you get rid of it," says Alan J. Liftin, M.D., dermatologist in private practice in Livingston, New Jersey. Otherwise, you risk exposing yourself to potentially life-threatening infection. Your doctor may also prescribe an antifungal cream if the skin around your nails is also infected.

of sweaty, warm shoes, and you can count on toe fungus lingering quite awhile unless you do something about it.

Unfortunately, the only reliable way to rid yourself of toenail fungus is with an expensive prescription antifungal medication, says Alan J. Liftin, M.D., dermatologist in private practice in Livingston, New Jersey. Occasionally, fungus spontaneously makes a hasty exit from your nails. But don't bet your toes on it. After you go to the doctor, try the following home treatments to keep fungus from popping up again.

Try This First

Trim those nails. Short nails do not get damaged as easily as long nails, and damaged nails are welcome mats for fungus, says Dr. Liftin. Periodically, use a nail clipper to trim your toenails into a straight line. Then smooth the edges with a file. Make sure to sterilize the clippers after each use so you don't accidentally reinfect yourself with fungus.

Other Wise Ways

Treat your feet like your face. You may have been using alpha-hydroxy acids (AHAs) on your face for years to prevent wrinkles. Well, that same cream can do wonders for your feet. Smooth an AHA cream onto your feet before going to bed. This will buff the rough, scaly skin from your feet, and it's that rough, scaly stuff that picks up fungus more easily than smooth skin, according to Dr. Liftin. You should see a doctor if you have excessively scaly skin on your feet, because this could be a fungus, he adds.

Go up a shoe size. If your shoes are too small, they'll rub against your toenails, creating damage and making fungal infections pop up. Make sure you have at least a thumb's width between your longest toe and the end of the toe box, recommends Dr. Liftin.

Work on a hostile environment. Most cases of toenail fungus are really cases of athlete's foot gone haywire. This closely-related fungus thrives in sweaty socks and damp shoes. To keep your feet dry, change your shoes and socks as often as feasible, and wear open-toed sandals when you can, says Dr. Liftin. Also consider using an over-the-counter topical antifungal cream, powder, or lotion daily, he adds.

MANAGING YOUR MEDS

Your doctor will most likely prescribe itraconazole (Sporanox) or terbinafine (Lamisil) to treat your fungus. Antifungal drugs may interact with other medications, especially drugs commonly taken by people with diabetes, says Alan J. Liftin, M.D., dermatologist in private practice in Livingston, New Jersey. It is essential to tell your doctor which medications you are currently taking. Then your doctor can decide which brand of antifungal to prescribe. More than 70 prescription and over-the-counter drugs may cause adverse reactions. Here are a few.

- Acetaminophen
- Estrogens, such as estradiol (Estraderm)
- Antacids
- Antidepressents, such as fluoxetine (Prozac)
- The anticoagulant warfarin (Coumadin)
- Alcohol

TOOTHACHE

A toothache is usually an early sign of a cavity. But it also can be caused by inflammation of the gums, an abscess (an infection that develops in the tooth root or between the tooth and gum), a cracked tooth, or a dislodged filling. Each of these problems can cause different types of toothache, says Flora Parsa Stay, D.D.S., dentist in Oxnard, California, and author of *The Complete Book of Dental Remedies*. Your dentist will probably suspect that you have a cracked tooth, for instance, if you have pressure and pain while chewing. Severe pain accompanied by sensitivity to hot and cold could be a sign that a cavity has reached the nerve of the tooth.

The following remedies can help soothe your tooth pain while you're waiting for an appointment with your dentist.

Try This First

String it up. Sometimes, a toothache is caused by something as simple as trapped food between the teeth. These food particles actually irritate the gums, but the pain can radiate into the surrounding teeth, Dr. Stay says. So try rinsing your mouth with warm water to loosen any food particles. Then floss or use a water-irrigating device to clean between your teeth. But even if this technique relieves your pain, you should still consult a dentist to make sure other more complex dental problems aren't contributing to your toothache, she says.

Other Wise Ways

Gnaw a knot of cloves. Take a couple of cloves from a spice rack and place them between your aching tooth and your cheek—much like you'd use chewing tobacco. They can help soothe the pain, says

Richard D. Fischer, D.D.S., dentist in Annandale, Virginia, and past president of the International Academy of Oral Medicine and Toxicology. Let the hard seedlike cloves soak in your mouth's saliva for several minutes to soften them up. Then gently chew on them—like you would on a toothpick—so the soothing oils within the cloves are released into the area surrounding your aching tooth. Leave the cloves in place for about 30 minutes or until the pain subsides. Continue this treatment as needed until you can see a dentist, he suggests.

Lay on the ointment. If gnashing on cloves is unappetizing, then consider using an over-the-counter tooth-pain ointment such as Anbesol or Orajel, Dr. Fischer suggests. Be sure to follow the directions on the label.

Make some waves. Swishing warm salt water around in your mouth can help reduce gum swelling, disinfect abscesses, and relieve tooth pain. Mix a teaspoon of salt into an eight-ounce glass of warm water and use as needed for discomfort, Dr. Fischer says. Swish each mouthful for 10 to 30 seconds, focusing the salt water on the painful area as much as possible. Repeat until the glass is empty. Do this as needed thoroughout the day, he suggests.

If you have high blood pressure and are on a sodium-restricted diet, use epsom salt instead of table salt, he says. Epsom salts are made with magnesium and, unlike table salt, shouldn't adversely affect your blood pressure.

Pop a pain reliever. Simply taking a 325-milligram aspirin tablet every four to six hours can dampen a lot of tooth pain and gum inflammation, says Robert Henry, D.M.D., dentist in Lexington, Kentucky, and past president of the American Society for Geriatric Dentistry. If you can't tolerate aspirin, then try taking 200 milligrams of ibuprofen every four hours, Dr. Henry suggests. Ibuprofen is a potent anti-inflammatory that is gentler on the stomach than aspirin.

If you do use aspirin, never put it directly on the tooth or gums, Dr. Henry urges. Remember, aspirin is an acid. Keeping it in your mouth for more than a few seconds can cause a painful burn that will only complicate the treatment of your toothache.

Chill out. Wrap an ice pack in a towel and apply it to the outside of your mouth for 15 to 20 minutes every hour until your pain sub-

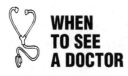

WHEN TO SEE A DOCTOR

Seek dental care for a toothache even if the pain diminishes or disappears completely, advises Richard D. Fischer, D.D.S., dentist in Annandale, Virginia, and past president of the International Academy of Oral Medicine and Toxicology. Although it may not still be provoking pain, an abscess or other underlying cause of your toothache could still be damaging your teeth and gums.

sides, Dr. Fischer suggests. The ice will reduce swelling and calm agitated nerve endings in your aching tooth.

Load up on minerals. Increasing your intake of calcium and magnesium can help soothe nerves and temporarily ease tooth pain, Dr. Fischer says. He suggests taking 500 milligrams of calcium and 200 to 300 milligrams of magnesium at the first sign of a toothache.

Note: People with heart or kidney problems should check with their doctors before taking supplemental magnesium.

Invite your teeth to tea. Herbal teas made with chamomile or echinacea often can quell mild toothache pain, Dr. Stay says.

To prepare a chamomile tea, add two tablespoons of dried chamomile flowers to two cups of boiling water and steep for 10 minutes. As for echinacea, add four tablespoons of the dried herb to eight cups of boiling water and steep for 10 minutes. After they have been strained, you can drink either of these teas as needed for pain, Dr. Stay says. You can also buy these teas premade in the tea section at your health food store. They may not be as strong as the do-it-yourself versions, but they're a little more convenient.

Note: Very rarely, chamomile can cause an allergic reaction when ingested. People allergic to closely related plants such as ragweed, asters, and chrysanthemums should drink the tea with caution. Don't use echinacea if you have autoimmune conditions such as lupus, tuberculosis, or multiple sclerosis. Don't use it if you're allergic to plants in the daisy family, such as chamomile and marigold.

Picture yourself pain-free. Your imagination is a powerful healer that can help you dampen tooth pain, Dr. Fischer says.

To try it, imagine swimming in ice-cold water or playing in the snow. Feel the chill of the water or snow penetrating your hands and feet so that they are almost numb. Now imagine that feeling of numbness enveloping your aching tooth, soothing it as if you were rubbing it with snow until all of the pain is gone, says Deena Margetis, certified clinical hypnotherapist specializing in dental care in Annandale, Virginia. Doing this imagery for one to two minutes as needed may relieve much of your pain, she says.

TOOTH STAINS

D azzling white teeth aren't just a modern obsession. As early as the fourteenth century, Europeans eagerly flocked to barber-surgeons for a crude form of enamel bleaching. These well-meaning quacks would file a patient's teeth with a coarse metal instrument. Then they dabbed each tooth with aqua fortis, a solution of highly corrosive nitric acid.

This procedure did whiten teeth, at least for a while. But the harsh acid so thoroughly destroyed tooth enamel that most people developed mouthfuls of painful cavities within a few years. Despite its obvious drawbacks, acid cleaning of teeth continued to be popular well into the 1700s, according to Charles Pánati in his book *Extraordinary Origins of Everyday Things*. Nearly 300 years later, dentistry has developed much safer and far less painful ways to satisfy the quest for brighter smiles.

"People in their fifties, sixties, and seventies want their teeth to look as good as their bodies," says Van B. Haywood, D.M.D., professor of dentistry at the Medical College of Georgia in Augusta. "This older generation is the first really healthy generation to come along. They jog, they swim, they run marathons. They're incredibly fit. But if you smile, and other people see yellow-brown teeth, that's a huge turnoff. I think if you're over age 50, tooth whitening will take about 10 years off your age."

As you age, teeth naturally begin to appear darker, says John E. Dodes, D.D.S., dentist in Woodhaven, New York, and co-author of *The Whole Tooth*. Over time, tiny potholes and cracks naturally form in your teeth. These microscopic crevasses are perfect magnets for hard-to-remove food, smoke, and drink stains. Meanwhile, the hard enamel covering your teeth naturally wears down from decades of chewing and brushing. The thinner the enamel gets, the more dentin, a yellowish inner layer of the tooth just be-

528

neath the enamel, shows through and makes your teeth appear stained.

Brushing and flossing daily, along with other good oral hygiene practices like professional cleanings every four to six months, should help minimize tooth stains. But if you are concerned about the appearance of your teeth, consult with your dentist, Dr. Haywood says. He will likely suggest several procedures that can brighten your smile, including prescription bleaching agents to remove most stains and resins that bond to your teeth to camouflage more difficult stains.

Once your teeth are stain-free, here are a few ways to keep them gleaming.

Try This First

Bank on baking soda. Toothpastes that are made with baking soda can help lighten tea, coffee, and other superficial stains on teeth, says Flora Parsa Stay, D.D.S., dentist in Oxnard, California, and author of *The Complete Book of Dental Remedies*. In fact, the brand you're currently using may come in a baking soda–fortified version.

"Don't expect a lot of whitening with these toothpastes, but they will help remove some mild stains," Dr. Stay says.

Other Wise Ways

Lighten up your brush stroke. Although it may seem logical that brushing hard would lead to cleaner teeth, that assumption isn't

MANAGING YOUR MEDS

Although it's rare, antibiotics like tetracycline (Panmycin) can stain the teeth of people over age 50, says Van B. Haywood, D.M.D., professor of dentistry at the Medical College of Georgia in Augusta. If you suspect that an antibiotic is causing tooth discoloration, check with your doctor or dentist.

WHEN TO SEE A DOCTOR

Tooth staining—particularly if it only appears on one tooth—could be an early warning sign of a cavity or abscess (an infection that develops in the tooth root or between the tooth and gum) and should be brought to your dentist's attention, says Van B. Haywood, D.M.D., professor of dentistry at the Medical College of Georgia in Augusta. And if tooth stains are bothering you and no home remedy seems to work, you may want to consult a dentist about some of the cosmetic treatments available to make teeth whiter.

correct, says Gretchen Gibson, D.D.S., director of the geriatric dentistry program at the Veterans Administration Medical Center in Dallas. In fact, up to 70 percent of seniors brush too hard, which can actually strip enamel off your teeth and make them appear darker, she says.

Ease back on the pressure whenever you put a toothbrush in your mouth, she says. Brush firmly but not forcefully, with a soft-bristle brush. Leave the vigorous scrubbing to your dental hygienist.

Reach for nature's toothbrush. Crunchy foods like apples, celery, and carrots act like little toothbrushes in the mouth, scrubbing away at stubborn stains, says Robert Henry, D.M.D., dentist in Lexington, Kentucky, and past president of the American Society for Geriatric Dentistry.

"Certainly, brushing your teeth is much more effective than eating an apple, but crunchy foods do have many of the same abrasive qualities of a toothbrush," Dr. Henry says. So make crunchy fruits and vegetables your first choice for between-meal snacks, he suggests.

Put out the fire. Need another good reason to quit smoking? Cigarettes literally bake tobacco stains into your teeth, says Dr. Dodes.

Make a fashion statement. To make your teeth appear whiter, select clothing colors that complement your complexion, Dr. Haywood says. In addition, the right makeup and lipstick can help a woman improve the look of her smile.

"In general, the color schemes that make your skin look the best will also help make your teeth look their best," he says. A wardrobe or beauty consultant at an upscale department store should be able to help you choose appropriate clothing and makeup, according to Dr. Haywood.

Don't nail it. Don't use your fingernail to remove tooth stains, Dr. Stay urges. "Believe it or not, the enamel on the outer surface of the tooth isn't as hard as a rock. So a fingernail can actually scratch the enamel," she says. Once it is scratched, debris can lodge in the enamel, worsening the appearance of the original stain and making the tooth more prone to cavities.

Sit on the bleachers. Avoid using over-the-counter (OTC) tooth bleach without talking to your dentist first, Dr. Haywood says. Even though these products are far less potent than prescription bleach, some are still so abrasive that they can dangerously erode tooth enamel and really make your teeth appear darker. OTC bleaching kits—particularly those containing a conditioning toothpaste, whitening gel, and polishing rinse—can increase gum irritation and tooth sensitivity. And since they just whiten your natural teeth, any discolored fillings you have will stand out like a Winnebago moored in a trailer park of Airstreams.

ULCERS

Ulcers were once seen as the scourge of stressed Type A executives and older people with weak constitutions. Now, revolutionary discoveries are changing the way doctors think about and treat painful ulcers. Unfortunately, the news hasn't made it to everyone who has ulcers.

Despite what many have thought for years, anyone at any age can get ulcers, and roughly 25 million Americans have them. The problem starts when a chronic sore develops either in the protective lining of the stomach or in the part of the intestine just below the stomach, which is called the duodenum. When your stomach's caustic acid seeps over this sore, you will know it by the burning pain you feel, says Martin Brotman, M.D., gastroenterologist at the California Pacific Medical Center in San Francisco. As you age, you can be at further risk for this problem, too. Taking too many painkillers like aspirin or ibuprofen can irritate your stomach lining and put you at greater risk. What's more, aging adults have a higher incidence of infection by a bacteria called *Helicobacter pylori (H. pylori)*, which is associated with virtually all duodenal ulcers. About 60 percent of Americans age 60 and over have *H. pylori.*

If you have burning abdominal pain—especially when your stomach is empty—or if you are awakened at night by this pain, see your doctor. He can determine what the problem is. If it is an ulcer, he will need to figure out where it is and what is causing it in order to treat it properly. He may, for example, order a blood test for the *H. pylori* bacteria. Whatever the cause, ulcers require prompt, supervised medical treatment to be healed properly, says Dr. Brotman. And while your ulcer is mending, use these tips to speed the healing process and to keep from irritating the sore spot in your stomach.

Try This First

Eat small. Although you might notice acid pain most when you have an empty stomach, the act of eating also signals the stomach to secrete acid to digest food. To keep that acid at manageable levels, try to eat smaller, more frequent meals rather than three big meals, says Roger L. Gebhard, M.D., gastroenterologist at the Veterans Affairs Medical Center and professor of medicine in the division of gastroenterology at the University of Minnesota, both in Minneapolis.

Other Wise Ways

Don't hold the onions. As a precautionary measure, add onions to your sandwiches, salads, and other meals. A study in the Netherlands found that the odorous sulfur compounds found in onions help fight the *H. pylori* bacteria, linked with ulcers and stomach cancer.

MANAGING YOUR MEDS

Ironically, agonizing ulcers not caused by *Helicobacter pylori* bacteria often develop from the use of common pain relievers. "The family of drugs known as nonsteroidal anti-inflammatory drugs (NSAIDs) interferes with the body's ability to maintain its protective lining in the stomach and intestine," says W. Steven Pray, Ph.D., R.Ph., professor of nonprescription drug products at Southwestern Oklahoma State University in Weatherford. NSAID-related ulcers occur more frequently among people over the age of 60, because they use these drugs more often than younger people do. If you need a pain reliever and you have an ulcer, are recovering from one, or simply want to avoid problems with ulcers, ask your doctor if acetaminophen would be suitable, says Dr. Pray. Popularly used over-the-counter and prescription NSAIDs include aspirin, ibuprofen, naproxen (Aleve), ketoprofen (Orudis KT), diclofenac (Voltaren), etodolac (Lodine), and oxaprozin (Daypro).

Any ulcer should be checked by a doctor. If you have stomach or abdominal pain that is eased by eating or if the pain wakes you up at night, call your doctor.

An untreated ulcer may bleed, leading to vomiting of blood or blood in your stools. If you are vomiting material that looks like coffee grounds or if your stools have turned black, get to a doctor as soon as possible, says Chesley Hines, M.D., a gastroenterologist at the Center for Digestive Diseases in New Orleans.

Perk up with pink. Over-the-counter stomach remedies like Pepto-Bismol can coat your stomach and provide temporary relief from acid, says Dr. Gebhard. Follow the instructions on the bottle when using any bismuth product such as this, as excessive use can be harmful, he says.

Be smoke-free. If you smoke, you have yet another reason to quit. Not only can smoking delay the healing of existing ulcers but also it may help cause them, says Melissa Palmer, M.D., gastroenterologist and liver specialist in private practice in New York City.

Can the citrus. Avoid high-acid citrus foods and juices; they may aggravate ulcer symptoms, says Marie L. Borum, M.D., assistant professor of medicine in the division of gastroenterology and nutrition at George Washington University Medical Center in Washington, D.C.

Abstain from alcohol. If you like a cocktail or a glass of wine with dinner, scratch it from your diet while your ulcer is mending, says Dr. Brotman. Alcohol stimulates acid production. What's more, alcohol can irritate your stomach lining.

Go easy on the milk. Dairy products, such as milk and yogurt, used to be recommended for those with ulcers. It is now known that they stimulate acid secretion, so it is probably not good to use them to soothe ulcer pain, says Dr. Gebhard.

For pain, take acetaminophen. If you have been taking aspirin or other over-the-counter anti-inflammatory medication for pain, switch to acetaminophen. Aspirin and other anti-inflammatories such as ibuprofen can increase your risk of ulcer and irritate your stomach lining, says Dr. Brotman.

Feel great with ginger. Ginger is considered an herbal remedy to help protect against ulcers. Take it in capsules, in root form, or as tea, says Mindy Green, director of education services at the Herb Research Foundation in Boulder, Colorado. You will find ginger in these forms at many drugstores and natural food stores. Fresh ginger is available in most grocery stores. To make tea from fresh ginger, cut a quarter-inch slice of a one-inch-round chunk of ginger, place it in a pot containing a cup of water, and simmer it for 10 to 15 minutes. While fresh ginger is safe when used as a spice, some forms of ginger aren't recommended for everyone. Ginger may increase bile secretion, so if you have gallstones, do not use therapeutic amounts of dried ginger or ginger powder without guidance from a health-care practitioner.

Choose vegetables for your vittles. Fiber and vitamin A from vegetables and fresh fruits may help protect against ulcers. Researchers at the Harvard School of Public Health studied the relationship of dietary factors and ulcer risk in nearly 50,000 men ages 40 to 75 years. Those with a higher consumption of fruits and vegetables were found to be less likely to develop ulcers than men who didn't add those foods to their fare. How fiber is of benefit in the reduction of ulcer risk is not yet understood, but the researchers believe that vitamin A may help protect the lining of the stomach and duodenum by increasing mucus production there.

UNDERWEIGHT

For many of us, the fun house at a carnival was a real treat. Especially the mirror that made a rather rotund person look tall and skinny. It was an instant, effortless, and ever-so-momentary diet.

Now, decades later, you may have noticed that you really are losing weight. If the undistorted image in the mirror tells you that you are beginning to look a bit gaunt—and you are not trying to lose weight—should you be concerned?

Perhaps, says Jan I. Maby, D.O., director of the Geriatric Medical Home Care program at Mount Sinai Medical Center in New York City.

Weight usually peaks in the early forties for men and in the fifties for women, says Dr. Maby. Then as a person creeps toward 60, the amount of muscle in the body naturally drops. By age 70, a typical woman has lost about 11 pounds of muscle, and an average man has lost about 26 pounds of it.

But a weight plunge may not stop there. Add in chewing difficulties, mobility problems, chronic intestinal upset, alcohol abuse, loneliness, and financial woes that hamper your ability to buy food, and you could be facing a major health problem, Dr. Maby says. In fact, involuntary weight loss or being severely underweight can touch off a host of related problems. As your body loses weight, your bones are also deprived, so bone loss, or osteoporosis, is accelerated. Other possible complications include liver problems, nutritional deficiencies, heart disease, slow wound healing, and arthritis. If you are severely underweight, the deprivation might impair your ability to think clearly, and it can contribute to dry, flaky skin and skin sores.

If you are 15 percent or more below your ideal weight or if you have lost 5 percent of your body weight in a month without really trying, see your doctor for an evaluation, Dr. Maby says. Once you have done that, here are a few tips that can help you regain your appetite.

Try This First

Beef up your diet. Although low-calorie, low-fat meals are great for younger people, they may not be all that terrific for seniors who are underweight, says David A. Lipschitz, M.D., Ph.D., chairman and professor of geriatrics at the University of Arkansas for Medical Sciences in Little Rock. In fact, for seniors who are underweight, the health risks of a low-calorie diet may exceed the perils of being a bit more lax in your eating habits, according to Dr. Lipschitz.

"The rules of good nutrition still apply here—you just need to consume more calories," says Marilyn Cerino, R.D., marketing director for Allegheny University Executive Health and Wellness Program in Philadelphia. "Carbohydrates are an excellent source of calories and can be combined with lean protein sources and limited amounts of unsaturated fats to help fill the void. Try mixing fat-free milk, fat-free milk powder, low-fat frozen yogurt, and bananas or strawberries in a blender for a high-protein, high-carbohydrate, low-fat drink. A bowl of cereal with fat-free milk and raisins can be a calorie booster as well," she says.

In conjunction with your doctor or dietitian, choose calorie-rich foods that are also loaded with nutrients, like red meats, pork, milk, and ice cream. Bagels, cornbread, and biscuits also can help you pack on some pounds. Also, consider eating regular portions of potatoes, avocados, nuts, eggs, peanut butter, kidney beans, puddings, custards, fruits such as peaches canned in syrup, and other foods high in calories, Cerino says.

"For a senior seeking to recover from a weight loss that is the result of an illness, you may want to relax the rigid rules of good nutrition during the initial recovery period and indulge in some of the foods that you normally limit to an occasional basis. Milk shakes, cheesecake, full-fat cheeses, and whole milk may appeal to a poor appetite. While they are not the recommended foods for everyday use, I would not deny them to someone who is attempting to recover a lost appetite. Oftentimes, you need to eat to get an appetite,

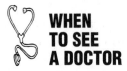

WHEN TO SEE A DOCTOR

See a doctor if you have any of the following symptoms or life circumstances.

• You notice that your clothing is becoming loose, and you can't explain why.

• You have an illness or condition that has changed the kind or amount of food you eat.

• You eat fewer than two meals a day.

• You have three or more drinks of beer, liquor, or wine almost daily.

• You have tooth or mouth problems that make it hard for you to eat.

• You don't always have enough money to buy the food you need.

• You aren't always physically able to shop, cook, or feed yourself.

and it is most important to at least get started—no matter what you initially choose. Of course, if there are medical conditions that require some dietary constraints, you must take those into consideration," Cerino says.

Other Wise Ways

Shoot for six. Frequent small feedings may help the depressed appetite, Cerino says. So instead of the traditional breakfast, lunch, and dinner, try eating six small meals a day, she says.

For instance, you might start your day with an omelet or poached eggs and a piece of toast, then have a midmorning snack like fruit. For lunch, you might have a bowl of soup with added pieces of chopped chicken or lean beef and rice, and a glass of low-fat or whole milk with some milk powder mixed in. In the afternoon, try having some rice pudding with a glass of juice. A good dinner might comprise a pork chop, a baked potato with butter and sour cream, squash or another vegetable, and milk as a beverage. Then finish off your day with an early evening snack like peanut butter crackers and milk, Cerino advises.

Use a timely reminder. Carry a small pocket alarm clock and set it to go off every three to four hours as a reminder to eat. Even if you only have a piece of bread or fruit, the alarm may help you establish regular eating times and tweak your appetite, Cerino says. If you wait for your brain to tell you to eat, you will lose even more weight, she adds.

Maximize each mouthful. Adding extra calories and nutrients to your favorite meals is actually quite easy, Cerino says. Here are some suggestions.

- Use milk in place of water in soups and sauces.
- Sprinkle milk powder into regular milk, casseroles, and meat loafs.
- Use pureed tofu in spaghetti sauce.
- Mix nuts, wheat germ, beans, cheeses, or cooked or chopped meat into pastas, casseroles, and side dishes.
- Top oatmeal and other hot cereals with melted margarine, pureed fruit, or vanilla ice cream.

Pack in the protein. Your appetite may diminish, as it often does after age 60, even if you are not ill. If that happens, increase the amount of protein in your diet to help your body retain lean muscle

MANAGING YOUR MEDS

When you see your doctor about your condition, be sure to take with you any medications—including over-the-counter preparations. It may help your physician pinpoint the cause of your weight-loss or underweight problems, says Jan I. Maby, D.O., director of the Geriatric Medical Home Care program at Mount Sinai Medical Center in New York City. Possible side effects of many medications include cramping, nausea, diarrhea, malabsorption, and anorexia. A doctor's close examination could help evaluate the cause of your weight loss.

Drugs that can contribute to unintentional weight loss include:

- Certain prescription antidepressants such as fluoxetine (Prozac) and other serotonin uptake inhibitors
- Over-the-counter decongestants that contain phenylpropanolamine or pseudoephedrine, such as NyQuil, Contac, and Dimetapp
- Nonsteroidal anti-inflammatory drugs (NSAIDs) including over-the-counter products like ibuprofen, naproxen (Aleve), or ketoprofen (Orudis KT), which can cause stomach upset and can indirectly lead to suppressed appetite and significant weight loss

and keep your heart and other muscles working efficiently, Dr. Maby says.

She recommends that all adults, unless otherwise directed by their doctors, have at least 1.2 grams of protein for every 2 pounds of body weight. Protein content is listed in grams on all packaged foods. If you weigh 110 pounds, for instance, you need about 66 grams a day of protein from animal products such as milk, cheese, yogurt, and other dairy products; meats like beef and pork tenderloin; and tuna fish. Other protein-rich foods include kidney beans and soy products like tofu and soy milk, Dr. Maby says.

Forget the rules. Who says that you must have bran flakes for breakfast? If you want leftover lasagna for breakfast, have it, Cerino says. Don't lock yourself into eating certain foods at certain times of the day. Let your cravings reign until you regain your appetite.

Tune in. One in every three older people lives alone, and loneliness can shrink your waistline, Cerino says. So try watching television or reading an interesting book or magazine while you are eating if there is no one to share your meal with, she says.

Have a before-dinner nip. In moderation, alcohol stimulates hunger, Cerino says. So if you drink, prime your digestive tract by having no more than two ounces of wine or four ounces of beer about 20 minutes before you are going to eat.

Don't forget the appetizers. Low-fat tortilla chips dipped in low-fat guacamole are a great way to get extra calories into your diet and tweak your appetite for other foods, Cerino says. Plus, low-fat tortilla chips are a good source of fiber.

Eat with your eyes. Pay attention to how a meal looks, because it really matters, especially after age 60 when senses of taste and smell begin to wane a bit, Cerino says. Use colorful plates, place mats, and napkins. "Make an effort to vary the colors and textures of the foods you eat."

Spice up your life. If you have noticed a change in your ability to smell, then spice up your foods. Increase the flavor, says Cerino. "A great deal of the food-flavor connection comes from the ability to smell. Use a heavy hand with the seasonings to compensate." Also, warm foods will taste better than cold foods since the flavors are transmitted better when foods are warm, she says.

Urinary Tract Infections

Y ou have a nearly uncontrollable urge to go. But once in the bathroom, you have very little success, just lots of burning and pain. And almost as soon as you go back to what you were doing before you were so rudely interrupted, that insistent impulse is back again. Sound familiar? It could be a urinary tract infection (UTI).

UTIs are a common malady, especially as you age, accounting for about eight million doctor visits a year. They are caused when bacteria enter the urethra, or urine tube. If the bacterial infection stays in the urethra, it is called urethritis. If the infection travels farther up the urinary tract into the bladder, as it often does, it is called cystitis (or, simply, a bladder infection). Unless treated promptly, a bladder infection can move to the kidneys, leading to a serious condition called pyelonephritis.

Women are especially prone to UTIs. In fact, one in every five women experiences a UTI during her life. The reason is partly structural. Since a woman's urethra is shorter than a man's, bacteria can travel up to her bladder quickly.

Even though men are less susceptible in general, their odds of getting UTIs increase as they get older. In men, however, the problems usually stem from some urinary obstruction—such as a kidney stone or an enlarged prostate—or from a medical procedure involving a catheter. In fact, any abnormality of the urinary tract that obstructs the flow of urine sets the stage for an infection.

People with diabetes also have a higher risk of UTIs because of changes in their immune systems. Any disorder that suppresses the immune system raises the risk of a urinary infection.

Not everyone with a UTI has symptoms. But if you do, you may have a frequent urge to urinate. Or you may experience a painful burning feeling in the area of your bladder or urethra during urination. It is not unusual to feel bad all over—tired, shaky, washed out—and to feel pain even when you are not urinating, says Dorothy M. Barbo, M.D., professor of obstetrics and gynecology and director of the Center for Women's Health at the University of New Mexico in Albuquerque.

If you suspect that you have a UTI, you should see a doctor as soon as possible. A prescription of antibiotics will help kill the infection, says Dr. Barbo. But there are also some actions you can take yourself to help ease your discomfort and minimize the problem. The first few tips are for both men and women, but the rest apply to women.

Try This First

Flush the system. Many doctors suggest that you drink plenty of water when you are in the throes of a UTI.

Eight to 10 glasses a day of any caffeine- or alcohol-free fluid will cleanse the bladder and wash bacteria out of the urinary tract, says Phillip Barksdale, M.D., urogynecologist at Woman's Hospital in Baton Rouge, Louisiana. "Drinking plenty of water flushes out the system, reducing the amount of irritating bacteria." To pace yourself, have an eight-ounce glass of water every hour throughout the day, he advises. Drink enough water so that your urine is light yellow. Yellow- or amber-colored urine is a sign that you aren't consuming enough fluid, he says.

Even more fluid is needed if you are in a hot environment or exercise strenuously, says Dr. Barbo.

Other Wise Ways

Ward it off with cranberries. Cranberry juice—a popular home remedy for UTIs—actually can prevent bacteria from sticking to cells that line the urinary tract. A study by Mark Monane, M.D., gerontologist and director of Merck-Medco Managed Care in Boston, found that women who downed a 10-ounce glass of cranberry juice every day for six months had fewer UTIs than those who drank other fluids.

Apart from clinical research, plenty of anecdotal evidence shows that cranberry juice helps, says Dr. Barbo. "I know it works for my patients," she says. The juice increases the acidic quality of urine, which, in turn, reduces bacteria levels.

Dr. Barbo recommends drinking four ounces of diluted cranberry juice two or three times a day. If you have diabetes, be sure to select low-calorie cranberry juice, which Dr. Barbo says is safer for diabetics.

Avoid irritants. Certain foods and beverages can magnify UTI discomfort. The worst of the offenders are coffee, alcohol, spicy foods, citrus, and chocolate. Avoid them until the infection clears up, says Dr. Barksdale.

MANAGING YOUR MEDS

While no medications are believed to make you more prone to urinary tract infections (UTIs), you may already be on medication that can help you avoid UTIs. Estrogen replacement therapy (ERT) reduces the risk of UTIs, says Dorothy M. Barbo, M.D., professor of obstetrics and gynecology and director of the Center for Women's Health at the University of New Mexico in Albuquerque.

The urethra is sensitive to estrogen, explains Dr. Barbo. Lack of estrogen can cause the tissues of the urethra to become dry, thinned out, and more prone to injury and infection, which puts women who are past menopause at increased risk for UTIs. Estrogen improves circulation in all of the tissues of the genital tract and makes them more resilient and less susceptible to infection. This UTI protection is an added benefit of estrogen replacement, she says.

Don't hold it. Even though it might be painful to urinate when you have a UTI, don't resist the urge, says Dr. Barbo. In general, you should try to empty your bladder completely every three to four hours. "It's a wise way to prevent bacterial infection and to hasten recovery if you already have one," she says. Urinating frequently helps to eliminate bacteria before they have a chance to multiply.

Have a seat after sex. Women should urinate after they have sexual intercourse, says Dr. Barbo. During sexual intercourse, bacteria may enter the urethra. By urinating, you help wash out the invaders right away.

Soothe with heat. To relieve the pain and cramping that are sometimes associated with a UTI, try a warm sitz bath, says Dr. Barksdale. Fill your bathtub with three to four inches of warm water and sit in the water for 10 to 15 minutes. When you are out of the tub, resting with a heating pad on your lower abdominal area can also help, he says.

Wear nonrestrictive clothing. Women should avoid clothes that constrict the genital area, says Dr. Barksdale, particularly control-top pantyhose and tight jeans. Clothes with tight crotches put pressure on the inflamed urethral opening, he says, and can force bacteria back up the urine tube. Skirts, loose pants, and knee-highs are far more comfortable and therapeutic when you have a UTI, he says.

Take off that bathing suit. Avoid wearing a wet bathing suit for long periods of time, adds Dr. Barksdale. "Bacteria love to grow in warm, moist areas," he says. "A wet swimsuit provides an ideal environment for bacteria that cause UTI, so you are asking for trouble."

Keep moving. Even though the discomfort of a UTI may make you want to take to your bed, doctors say it is best to stay active since mobility aids bladder function, says Dr. Barksdale. "Exercise is always beneficial for the bladder, and it helps to get your mind off your discomfort."

Clean with care. Keep infections at bay by cleaning the vaginal area with a front-to-back motion, says Dr. Barbo. Many women were taught to wipe from back to front after a bowel movement, which can spread bacteria from your anus to your urethral opening, she says. Proper wiping can prevent a significant number of UTIs, especially among women who get them recurrently.

Ditch douches and sprays. Give up feminine hygiene sprays and scented douches—both can irritate the urethra and vulva, says Dr. Barbo.

If you feel the need to douche, don't do so any more often than once a month. "Frequent douching can introduce infectious bacteria into the vagina and rinse out the normal 'friendly' noninfectious vaginal bacteria," says Dr. Barbo.

VARICOSE VEINS

The heart can pump blood to the toes in one beat, but it needs to pump a full five beats before the blood can make the return trip up your legs. The constant uphill battle against the force of gravity eventually takes its toll on our veins. By the time we reach the age of 60, about one in four of us has at least one bulging, blue-tinged ropy reason not to wear shorts in the summer.

Varicose veins is a condition of the superficial veins of the legs, where the standing pressure in the veins is greatest. These enlarged, twisted, and swollen veins usually appear just under the skin of the inner calves or on the backs of the legs, but they can also appear on the thighs. "Imagine that the blood in your veins is like a swimming pool. The farther you dive down, the more the pressure increases," says Gabriel Goren, M.D., vascular surgeon and director of the Vein Disorders Center in Encino, California. "The pressure in the veins is directly proportional to the height of the person." In other words, in tall people with varicose veins the appearance and symptoms can be more severe than in short people.

Doctors say that genetics and gender play the biggest role. If you are a woman and one of your parents had varicose veins, then you probably have them, too, especially if you have had multiple pregnancies.

Actually, the heart has an ally in the upward-pumping process. Every contraction of your calf muscles helps push blood back toward your heart. In fact, almost 90 percent of all venous blood leaves your legs through the deep veins by the contraction of your muscles. Doctors call it the calf muscle pump or peripheral heart.

As the blood ascends your veins, a series of valves prevent it from flowing back down. "They are like swinging doors going into a saloon, except they only open one way," says Kevin Welch, M.D., dermatologist with the Medical Center of Pensacola in Florida.

Varicose veins start when the circulation slows, usually because of the lack of muscular activity. The blood begins to pool and stretch the walls of the vein. The added pressure in the distended vein pushes on the valve, eventually forcing the "saloon doors" to open the wrong way. "Instead of the blood being held in little compartments, it flows backward," says Dr. Welch.

The damage doesn't stop at one valve. As we age, more valves fail, and more varicose veins develop, says Dr. Welch.

On the bright side, varicose veins are not dangerous, although they can cause an achy, tired feeling in the legs, says Dr. Goren. Often, the legs swell, too, and that swelling worsens throughout the day. Pain is more common during warm weather or after a period of prolonged standing.

You should see a doctor if your legs develop a brownish, purplish discoloration with itching or scaling, particularly around the ankles. Anything you can do to keep the circulation moving and relieve the pressure in your veins will help relieve your symptoms, says J. A. Olivencia, M.D., vascular surgeon and medical director of the Iowa Vein Center in West Des Moines, Iowa.

Try This First

Give them some support. Graduated compression stockings will give your circulation a boost and reduce the circumference of your veins. "Like a stretched-out sock, veins become stretched out from pooling blood, and they lose their ability to contract," says Dr. Welch. "Put compression stockings on before you get out of bed in the morning, and wear them all day."

The compression level of graduated stockings, which is measured in millimeters of mercury (mm Hg), is greatest at the ankles and decreases gradually up the lengths of the legs to promote blood flow toward the heart. Wear moderate compression stockings rated in the 15 to 20 mmHg range, or labeled grade one or two. They are available in drugstores.

Do not substitute ordinary support pantyhose for graduated compression stockings. "Support hose is a misnomer," says Dr. Welch. "Support hose provide uniform compression from foot to thigh. Since the upper part of the leg is so much larger, this creates

WHEN TO SEE A DOCTOR

If you have varicose veins, you are at higher risk of developing phlebitis, says Kevin Welch, M.D., dermatologist with the Medical Center of Pensacola in Florida. You should call your doctor if you notice any of the following signs of possible clot in the vein.

• A hard lump on the vein that doesn't disappear even after you elevate your leg
• Localized pain and swelling with redness
• A burning feeling in your leg

Even if you have had varicose veins for several years, you should contact the doctor if you develop new symptoms or if aching and fatigue of your legs suddenly get worse.

a binding atmosphere. The compression may actually be greater at the thigh or calf than at the ankle, which can force blood down the leg instead of toward the heart."

Other Wise Ways

Put gravity on your side. Elevate your legs above the level of your heart three or four times a day for 5 to 10 minutes, recommends Dr. Goren. Prop your feet up on some pillows or sit in a reclining chair with your feet up. Getting gravity on your side will help drain excess fluid from your legs and relieve your discomfort. "The gravitational drainage will reduce elevated venous pressure and will ease the discomfort," he explains.

Flex those muscles. Don't stand or sit in one place for more than a few minutes at a time. "The blood in your weakened veins will pool. The pressure will increase and fluid will accumulate in your ankles and calves," says Dr. Goren. To prevent blood from pooling in your veins when you are sitting, wiggle your toes and flex your feet and ankles several times every 10 minutes to work the leg muscles that help pump the blood back to the heart. If you are at work or traveling, get up and walk around at least once an hour for 3 to 4 minutes. If you have to stand in one place, get the calf pump moving by moving up and down on your tiptoes.

Take a walk. Walking reduces the pressure in your veins by one-third. "Staying active will set your calf muscle pump in motion. Blood will be pushed uphill toward your heart, and the pressure in your veins should drop," explains Dr. Goren.

The improved muscle tone that you develop as a result of regular walking will also improve circulation. "A weak muscle doesn't pump as well as a strong one," says Dr. Olivencia. "A walking program is the simplest and most effective way to make the calf muscle pump work more efficiently." Slowly work up to one hour of walking, three times a week.

Watch your weight. Excess weight, especially in the abdominal area, presses on the veins in the upper thighs and groin, causing them to weaken. Circulation slows, resulting in increased pressure in the veins. If you are more than 15 percent over your ideal body weight, chances are that the excess pounds are putting stress on your veins in one way or another, says Dr. Olivencia. "When people are overweight, they become less active. Their clothing may be tight and constrict blood flow." And that constriction will only make varicose veins worse.

Shower at night. Your morning shower may be a lifelong habit, but when you have varicose veins, the wake-up cascade of hot water is an invitation for discomfort early in the day. "At night, during sleep in the horizontal position, even bad veins can regain a more narrow shape," says Dr. Goren. "Heat in the early hours of the morning will immediately distend the veins." This will make them more prominent and more uncomfortable for you.

Stay out of the hot tub. People who have varicose veins should avoid soaking in a hot tub or whirlpool bath, no matter what time of day it is. The hot water just makes your veins swell, cautions Dr. Goren.

Avoid high heels. High heels increase the pressure in your veins and reduce the ability of your calf muscle to pump. "Wearing heels occasionally will not cause problems," says Dee Anna Glaser, M.D., associate professor of dermatology at St. Louis University School of Medicine. "If worn regularly, though, high heels alter your ability to contract your calf muscles." That, in turn, makes it harder to pump blood back up to your heart.

Don't toast your tootsies. Ah, the heat from a warm, cozy fire. Doesn't it feel good on a pair of cold feet on a cold winter night? That soothing feeling, however, is short-lived. Heat dilates the blood vessels and encourages additional fluid retention and discomfort in the veins, says Dr. Goren.

The same principal applies to any heat source at the floor level. Close heating registers or reposition furniture so that heat is not blowing on your feet while you are sitting down, says Dr. Olivencia.

Sleep it off. Elevate the foot of your bed on one or two bricks and put gravity to work while you sleep. "Tilting your bed this way will encourage fluid to drain out of your legs," says Dr. Welch. Check with your doctor first if you have a history of heart trouble, emphysema, or difficulty breathing at night.

INDEX

Underscored page references indicate sidebars. **Boldface** references indicate illustrations. Prescription drug names are denoted with the symbol Rx.